Psychoanalytic Trends in Theory and Practice

Psychoanalytic Trends in Theory and Practice

The Second Century of the Talking Cure

Edited by M. Hossein Etezady, Inga Blom, and Mary Davis

LEXINGTON BOOKS
Lanham • Boulder • New York • London

Published by Lexington Books
An imprint of The Rowman & Littlefield Publishing Group, Inc.
4501 Forbes Boulevard, Suite 200, Lanham, Maryland 20706
www.rowman.com

Unit A, Whitacre Mews, 26-34 Stannary Street, London SE11 4AB

British Library Cataloguing in Publication Information Available

Library of Congress Cataloging-in-Publication Data

Names: Etezady, M. Hossein, editor. | Blom, Inga, editor. | Davis, Mary, 1949- editor.
Title: Psychoanalytic trends in theory and practice : the second century of the talking cure / edited by M. Hossein Etezady, Inga Blom and Mary Davis.
Description: Lexington Books, [2018] | Includes bibliographical references and index.
Identifiers: LCCN 2018009887 (print) | LCCN 2018010599 (ebook) | ISBN 9781498577878 (Electronic) | ISBN 9781498577861 (cloth : alk. paper)
Subjects: : LCSH: Psychoanalysis. | Psychotherapy. | Psychiatry.
Classification: LCC RC504 (ebook) | LCC RC504 .P7964 2018 (print) | DDC 616.89/17--dc23
LC record available at https://lccn.loc.gov/2018009887

∞™ The paper used in this publication meets the minimum requirements of American National Standard for Information Sciences Permanence of Paper for Printed Library Materials, ANSI/NISO Z39.48-1992.

Printed in the United States of America

This book is dedicated to Anni Bergman, PhD, whose commitment to reevaluating theory and practice from an integrative and developmental perspective, and pioneering work with Margaret Mahler, has directly influenced many of the contributors in this volume. This book came about because members of the Margaret S. Mahler Foundation for Child Development wished to evaluate and update the implications of concepts and practices, and to make the ideas accessible to new audiences. Long before her collaboration with Margaret Mahler and the publication of *The Psychological Birth of the Human Infant*, and long after, Anni's home was a meeting place for people from near and far, a space where thoughts, feelings, and play fostered meaning making and community. Anni's life and work has been dedicated to strengthening vulnerability and promoting connections, and as a result we are all better clinicians and colleagues, friends and family members.

Table of Contents

Introduction 1
M. Hossein Etezady, Inga Blom, and Mary Davis

1 Emotional Development and Affects 7
Harold P. Blum

2 A Developmental Model to Enhance Understanding of Therapeutic Action 25
Alexandra M. Harrison

3 Observing Development from Infancy to Parenthood: Separation-Individuation, Attachment, and Intersubjectivity in the Clinical Encounter 43
Inga Blom

4 Gender Fluidity and Analytic Fluidity 71
Gabriel Ruiz

5 Severe Emotional Disturbances in Childhood 83
Theodore Fallon Jr.

6 Narcissism: How It Develops and How It Appears 103
Mary Davis and M. Hossein Etezady

7 A Developmental Perspective on Trauma: The Analysis of a Severely Traumatized Adolescent 127
Ann G. Smolen

8 Depression: A Psychoanalytic Perspective 149
Corinne Masur

9 The Dissociative Disorders 179
Richard P. Kluft

10 Psychoanalytic Aspects of Psychosomatics 201
Richard Cruz

11 Back to Freud's Beginning: Looking at Neuroscience through a Contemporary Psychoanalytic Lens 227
Susan P. Sherkow and Kate Lieberman

12 Culture, Socialization, and Creativity in Analytic Practice 251
Monisha Nayar-Akhtar

13 Psychological Testing for Psychoanalysis 269
Michael S. Garfinkle and Sara Lynn Richardson

Index 291

About the Editors 295

About the Contributors 297

Introduction

M. Hossein Etezady, Inga Blom, and Mary Davis

M. Hossein Etezady, MD:

It was still the heyday of psychoanalysis when I started my psychiatric residency in the 1960s. The major trend was a transition from id analysis to the novel notion of defense analysis in parallel with character analysis. In the 1970s, when I started analytic training, the structural theory was replacing, or rather supplementing, the contributions of instinct theory, and questioning the assumptions of the topographic model. This was soon followed by an elaboration of object relations, the vicissitudes of aggression and the dynamics of narcissism, borderline states, and developmental deficits. Infant research and new conceptual models of attachment, representation, internalization, the sense of self and identity flourished in the second half of the century, aided by great advances in information technology. And of course there were pioneering analytic researchers that emerged after the second World War. Teaching, training, research, and clinical practice evolved and were radically influenced by the new cultural and sociopolitical realities of the extra-clinical environment, as well as doctrinal challenges and schismatic divisions within institutions and among members of same schools of thought. Self-psychology, intersubjectivity, relational approaches to treatment, and prevention became better known and more influential.

For today's students of psychoanalysis and their teachers, a clearly articulated update of concepts in theory and practice, concerning these various trends and contexts, under divergent cultural conditions, is an invaluable and necessary resource. We are again—or perhaps always—at a crucial moment of diversification and opportunity, and we need clear, finely tuned, and practical applications of the vast array of knowledge and experience accumulated in the nearly one-and-a-quarter century of psychoanalysis.

Whether parochial and elite, or eclectic and practice-minded, the reader of this edited volume is provided with the essentials of various concepts and their development, as we strive toward increasing integration and a more holistic viewpoint of our ever-expanding field.

The contents of this book are intended to provide a discretely focused emphasis on theoretical, clinical, and technical aspects of phenomena most commonly encountered in clinical practice. Each chapter offers a comprehensive yet concise literature review, designed to orient the reader to how theory has evolved over time, with illustrative clinical material that brings theory to light, and demonstrates the contemporary relevance of psychoanalytic ideas and practice. As in a textbook, the chapters include the basics and highlight special features in a concise manner.

As an edited volume this book brings to the reader the individually unique perspective, style, and synthetic narrative of a group of psychoanalytic clinicians and practitioners involved in research, training, education, and intervention. The great majority of the authors are child analysts serving on the board of the Margaret Mahler Mother-Child Research Foundation. They are intimately familiar with Mahler's Separation-Individuation Theory and its integrative capacity for connecting various developmental lines and potentials into a coherent preoedipal construct that sets the stage for the unfolding of the Oedipal phase as well as the mature relationships and parental functions of adult life.

In the past one-and-a-quarter century much has evolved, been discovered and freshly generated. With each innovative move, new finding, or novel discovery, we have witnessed waves of declarations regarding the obsolescence of Freud's ideas and the final demise of psychoanalysis. The late Selma Kramer, who was the director of the child curriculum at the Philadelphia Psychoanalytic Society and Institute, for more than three decades opened the annual Mahler Symposium in Philadelphia each year with an enlightening statement that in conclusion bore witness to how "psychoanalysis is still alive and kicking." This edited volume aspires to echo this confirming assurance of Selma's firm assertion.

Inga Blom, PhD:

My formal introduction to psychoanalysis accompanied a developmental milestone—that of leaving the familiarity of home for the adventure of undergraduate life. For most lifelong learners, fall evokes the experience of new beginnings, the anticipation of new ideas, books, and partners in learning. For me, fall also brings nostalgia for the leaves outside the big, old windows of Victoria College at the University of Toronto, where, as a very eager first-year undergraduate, I enrolled in a course called Psychoanalysis and Literature. More than a new subject, I recall this experience as an awakening. With each of Freud's works encountered that year came a growing certainty that I was finally discovering a language, a lens, through which the world—people, relationships, behavior, events, family—made sense. I spent much of that year staring out of those big windows, fantasizing about the mysterious and unknown path to becoming an analyst, which for me at that time just meant someone with the capacity to psychoanalyze, in theory or practice. Four years later, I graduated from Trinity College's Psychoanalytic Thought Program, knowing only about my professional life that it had to be founded on psychoanalytic ideas, and that it had to involve bringing these ideas to people who needed them.

Long after the heyday of psychoanalysis, but not yet at the height of cognitive behavioralism, psychoanalytic ideas were readily available in academic circles, but I didn't know too many practicing analysts. So I traveled through London to New York to see how I could put those ideas to work. Nowadays, the path to becoming an analyst is somehow no less mysterious to me, despite two decades spent finding and following analytic work. I am perhaps a little less lofty in my conviction of the universal application of psychoanalysis, but my conviction that psychoanalytic ideas are essential to understanding almost everything about the human experience has only grown more certain. But I'm still not sure what this means for practicing psychoanalysis. Over the course of my clinical training, I sought experiences that would bring me to a diverse group of psychoanalytically oriented clinicians and supervisors working in as many different kinds of settings as it is possible to find in New York City, in offices, clinics, hospitals, and community centers. I was excited and encouraged to build skills and exposure to psychoanalytic thinking in action at every turn. But of course, it still didn't seem to be "actual psychoanalysis": that required an institute and a couch. During my postdoctoral fellowship in neuropsychology, I (finally!) started institute training, beyond dissertation defense, licensure, and postdoc hours, the real "end" goal of it all. And yet, the more time I devoted to institute work, the more disillusioned I became with my office-with-couch-vision. My institute classes were often comprised of clinicians who were encountering psychoanalysis for the first time, and, with a few notable exceptions, classes presented them and me with a narrowing of ideas, limited scope of readings, and a lot of rules governing acceptable ideas, progression and practice (my supervisors provided the opposite experience, making it that much more confusing). For a while, the possibility of psychoanalytic work seemed to shrink.

Leaving institute training and pursuing psychoanalytic learning through various research groups, study groups, and supervisors has restored my sense of the importance of bringing psychoanalytic ideas to as many people as possible, and making them as accessible as possible. My career at present continues those beliefs, through clinical work, supervision, and program development—not at an institute, but at a busy city hospital and practice that includes short-term and long-term psychotherapy, group therapy, and assessment. Now, as a practitioner, fall brings other beginnings, as treatments need to be reestablished after summer breaks, supervisees arrive eager for wisdom and challenges, and new patients initiate contact as the energy of summer recedes back into the realities of life. The need for comprehensive and accessible psychoanalytic writing for a range of practitioners is what makes this book seem so valuable and, as my co-editor mentioned, timely. I am excited and humbled to have had a part in bringing this volume together, and to be included among some of the most influential and innovative clinicians and researchers.

Mary Davis, MD:

My road to psychoanalysis was different from that of both Hossein and Inga. I began in medical school wanting to be a family doctor, not a psychiatrist; but I found that truly knowing my patients required spending more time with them than internists or family doctors could manage. When I began in psychiatry, I knew nothing about psychoanalysis. Again, I found that truly knowing my patients required spending time with them, listening, and exploring as they discovered themselves in my presence. When I discovered psychoanalysis, during my child psychiatric training, it opened the door to a world in which I could understand not only *what* people do, but at least some parts of *why* they do it; and in which I could help them to understand themselves and make their own lives less painful.

Hossein and I met when I moved to Pennsylvania and began to meet with the Vulnerable Child Study Group, a group of child analysts who meet monthly to discuss issues in analytic understanding and treatment of children. This study group was established nearly 50 years ago, and was chaired by Theodore Cohen from 1969 until 2009. Since 2009, Hossein and I have been co-chairs. Through it I have met many talented and dedicated clinicians who have greatly enhanced my own understanding of psychoanalysis and of vulnerable children; and the chapter in this book by Hossein and myself began as a summary of discussions in the group about normal narcissism and its development. I have been fortunate enough to be involved through the Vulnerable Child Study Group with a Discussion Group sponsored at the American Psychoanalytic Association annual meetings; with a series of books based on the presentations at the American Psychoanalytic Association meetings; and with other publications and presentations, culminating with the opportunity to be a part of this volume, which I believe will establish a new "ground" for ongoing learning and growth.

The chapters in this book each deal with a different piece of how we work to understand our patients. Affect regulation, depression, psychosomatic responses to emotional turmoil, dissociation, narcissism both normal and pathological, gender issues, attachment and intersubjectivity, neuroscience: each of the chapters tells us some of what we need to know to understand human nature, each traces how we learned what we know, and each identifies questions that still need to be answered. We hope our readers will take what is offered here and use it to continue the growth and progress in the field.

Because the focus is on theory as it relates to practice, each chapter is rich in clinical material. It is important to note that names and identifying material have been altered in all clinical descriptions in order to ensure confidentiality and protect the privacy of our patients.

Chapter One

Emotional Development and Affects

Harold P. Blum

DEVELOPMENT OF AFFECT THEORY

Multiple affect theories coexist with regard to development and clinical application, but agreement among the different theories has been limited. Knowledge of the development of affects has been enhanced by new findings derived from neuroscience as well as from psychological studies of mother/infant interaction from birth. Both avenues of inquiry have been enriched in recent decades by technological advances. Attachment paradigms and the corollary of separation/individuation have been developmental blueprints supplemented by the new findings which particularly expand the interrelated development of affects and personality. The lack of consensual definition of an affect within psychological and neurobiological perspectives as well as in clinical work may be related to the subjective and objective complexity of affects (Shapiro and Emde 1992; Blum 2005). In this chapter I distinguish between the neurobiological substrates of affect, innate affect dispositions, and the psychological feelings, i.e., emotions, which are very important and consciously experienced in all humans.

Affects have external and internal dimensions; externally they have a communication function through facial expression, eye contact, gesture, and posture. Internally affects influence the body with somatic effects on the autonomic nervous system, stress hormones, temperature regulation, etc. Emotions are positive or negative, i.e., experienced as pleasurable or unpleasurable/painful. Emotions can be both suppressed and probably repressed, kept outside of conscious awareness. The independence of affects in motivation, alongside rather than as drive derivatives, was at first theoretically obscure. Affects are motivational systems that may be activated by external stimuli such as grief in response to loss of a love object, as well as internal stimuli such as pain, dreams, or memories. During development, affects are linked to cognition and mental representation, so that affects are far less isolated than formerly conceptualized. Nor are affects localized in any discrete area of the brain, although affects such as fear have a focus in the amygdala.

Affect theory originated in the revolutionary 1872 publication of Charles Darwin's *The Expression of the Emotions in Man and Animals*. He proposed that human emotions are homologous to those of animals. Darwin also proposed that a basic group of emotions (e.g., anger, fear, surprise, sadness) is present across human cultures and across species. William James's inquiry "What Is an Emotion?" in 1884 assumed that emotions are reducible to body changes in response to an emotional stimulus. The James-Lange theory has been criticized and modified over time to encompass both the emotional feelings and the accompanying body changes, and Cannon in 1932 noted the fight-flight-freeze response to danger. In 1990, McLean proposed that primitive emotion arose from the old reptilian brain and was modified in the course of the evolution of the midbrain and later in the neocortex and cortex. The human neocortex links affect and cognition and exerts control over the earlier systems.

This basic architecture of the evolution of affects remains, but with additions and refinements. The facial configuration, somatic, and skin manifestations of affect are no longer regarded as necessarily isomorphic with feelings in humans and apes. Basic human affects have individual, familial, and cultural variations. Shame, humiliation, and guilt have innate determinants, but are not present in earliest extrauterine human life. Humans, apes, and perhaps other primates are capable of dissimulation, of hiding or falsifying their overt emotional expression. False smiles and feigned grief have long been noted. Nevertheless, in humans, persons of different cultures and societies can often correctly read facial expressions of fear or anger in a young child, as well as in an adult. This tends to confirm innate, stereotyped affect expression while allowing for the modification by socialization and relatively well-disguised individual dissimulation and disguise.

Two prominent classifications of discrete innate affect have been proposed, by Tompkins (1962–1963), and more recently by Panksepp and Biven (2012). Derived from his joint research Tompkins (1961–1962), Izard (and Tompkins) (1977) listed ten affects with salient aspects of their facial expression; emotion was a subjective internal feeling which included memory of a similar feeling:

1. Distress/anguish/replaced by sadness: cry for help; tears at six weeks; infants' corners of lips down; red face.
2. Interest, excitement: intense gaze; eyebrows down; learning is rewarded.

3. Joy, enjoyment: smile; lips widened, up and out.
4. Anger, rage: red face; muscle tension; scream.
5. Shame: eyes downcast and looking away; head falls.
6. Disgust: Tongue projects; lower lip protrudes; nausea.
7. Contempt.
8. Fear, terror: eyes wide open; eyebrows raised and drawn together; face pale; hair standing up.

The current classification of innate affect dispositions by Panksepp and Biven is applied to all mammals. These are:

1. seeking
2. care (nurturance)
3. play
4. lust
5. rage
6. fear/anxiety
7. panic-grief related to separation.

PSYCHOANALYTIC CONCEPTS OF AFFECT

In his preanalytic early considerations of affect, Freud recognized that the psychological as well as biological aspects of affect were all important. Before introducing psychoanalytic drive theory, Freud considered affects to be primary agents in motivation, intention, and attention. Affect was essential for adaptation, for personality development, and for the understanding and treatment of psychological disorder. Freud (1894, p. 66) referred to the mind functioning with "a quota of affect or sum of excitation which is capable of increase, diminution, displacement and discharge and which is spread over the memory traces of ideas. . . ." Affects were then recognized as crucial in pathogenesis, especially the affect of anxiety. Dammed up or strangulated or buried affects were consequent to psychic trauma. The relation of affect to psychosomatic phenomena, i.e., to somatization as well as to motor acts and behavior, was readily observed. An anxiety reaction might be manifest in somatic responses of tachycardia and sweating palms, as well as tendencies toward flight, fight, or freeze. In the so-called cathartic method of preanalytic psychotherapy, treatment was based upon retrieval of buried, repressed memories of the trauma or other experience and their affective component. The trauma was retrieved from repressed memory, recalled in detail, and expressed verbally with connected emotions. Expressing emotions in language and verbal discourse was therapeutically essential in differentiating past trauma from present-day life, and in modifying and regulating affect storms, such as anxiety and rage. Although the abreaction of affect was also thought of in terms of discharge, the conscious retrieval of buried affect remains vital to recovery and mastery of traumatic experience (Krystal 1988). The verbal report of trauma with retrieval of the buried affect was called the "cathartic method" because of the release of pent-up emotion which had been kept out of conscious awareness. The cathartic method still offers valid treatment in many situations of acute trauma (Blum 1991).

Consideration of the development of affects followed the formulation of the role of affect in psychopathology as well as in dreams and fantasy life. In the early development of psychoanalysis, instinctual drive derivatives supplanted affect theory, and affects were considered subordinate to or also a derivative of the drives. The psychoanalytic sequential oral, anal, and phallic-oedipal phases of development were then paramount in psychoanalytic thought and both subserved and overshadowed affect theory. Anxiety was first related to dammed-up libido, which could have detrimental effects on somatic and sexual function. In early psychoanalytic theory, the bonds of the infant-mother dyad were primarily thought to be related to the infant's oral gratification and feeding rather than broader aspects of nurturance. Pleasure and unpleasure were considered important, but largely derived from the infant's oral gratification and/or frustration.

Currently, however, instead of the single pleasure-unpleasure principle as first formulated by Freud, psychoanalytic theory and neurobiology differentiate two separate principles, pleasure and unpleasure. Pleasure is associated with mastery, working toward and achieving goals, as well as being consequent to drive discharge (Hendrick 1943; Shapiro and Emde 1992). (Psychoanalysts and their patients have found pleasure in achieving insight and improved mutually affectionate object relations.) There is a difference between infantile affect and the complex, affectively laden, adult life. Not only do affects become modified and modulated, but they blend and amalgamate; negative and positive affects regarding a particular issue may coexist.

Although affects have a neurobiological disposition, they develop in the context of the earliest object relationships. The interplay of maternal affective responses to the affective signals of their infants is crucial for normal development. While there is always unconscious conflict about pregnancy, there is also the potential for great pleasure in becoming pregnant and becoming a parent. Despite the discomforts of pregnancy it can be a time of pleasurable anticipation for expectant mothers. The joy of new motherhood and a consciously dearly desired baby may far outweigh difficult painful labor and the new burdens of care and nurturance of the newborn. Holding her newborn, responding to her/his cries, surveying the neonate's face to see who the baby resembles, fondling the baby's fingers and toes, are all part of a gestalt of maternal gratification. Along with pleasure in fulfillment of feminine developmental aspirations, the earliest parent-child relationship may be colored by internal conflict, ambivalence, and at times postpartum depression or paranoia. Neurobiological changes after delivery such as the release of oxytocin foster bonding and care. Panksepp and Biven's 2012 elucidation of the innate affective dispositions of care and play lend support to the rewarding aspects of dyadic bonds. Fetuses are already attuned to the sounds of their mothers, to rate and rhythm of their speech as well as heartbeat and respiration. An affective preverbal dialogue develops between mother and infant (Spitz 1965; Schore 1994). While infants smile at two to three months in response to other stimuli, responses to the mother (or other primary caregiver) are more readily elicited and more intense. In states of negative affect, the mother's response may be a unique source of comfort. The social smile is engaging for the caregiver, stimulating reciprocal smiling and promoting affectionate dyadic bonds. The baby's social smile probably has the adaptive function of social interaction and reward of parental care. Freud's 1909 hypothesis about the beguiling enigmatic smile of Leonardo da Vinci's Mona Lisa was that it represented the warm smile of his biological mother and wet nurse, and that Leonardo sought to recapture the embracing love of his lost first mother. Similarly, the peek-a-boo game of caregiver and infant represents a loss and refinding of the mother figure in the pleasurable context of a secure holding by the mother (Winnicott 1965). Mutual pleasure is expressed and enhanced in smiles and laughter, in dyadic giggling. Laughter is a human response supporting social interaction with probably homologous precursors in other primates.

Not only do affects influence and develop from the bonds between infants and caregivers, but affective communication is critical in the regulation of behavior. A blend of human emotions and thought influences the body and behavior. Maternal behavior and affect expression influence infant behaviors and somatization and vice versa (Mahler, Pine, and Bergman 1975). In social referencing a person in a situation of uncertainty seeks a signal from an authority figure, and social referencing in infancy has been the subject of extensive research. Infants engage in advance or withdrawal from a visual cliff depending on the mother's pleasure, displeasure, approval or disapproval. If the mother conveys anger or anxiety or a frown of disapproval, it will profoundly influence her infant's response. Confronted with the illusion of a cliff with a 30-centimeter drop, if the mother's face appeared apprehensive or frightened, no infant crossed, but with maternal approval 70 percent of the experimental infant group crossed over (Feinman 1992). The "still face" research further demonstrated the affective responses of two-month-old infants to the mother or caregiver. Exposed to a silent mother instructed to display an expressionless nonresponsive face, her infant, will quickly try to convert her to their familiar interaction. Failing to obtain mother's visual response the infant will likely turn away from her with a dazed, forlorn facial expression. The infant's attempt to recapture mother's interactive participation implies intentionally motivated goal-directed behavior (Tronick 2007). Most infants anxiously attempted to initiate interaction with the mother (or other primary caregiver) and modify her response. Infants scan and infer mothers' emotional states from the face, voice, eye contact, holding, and gesture, suggesting primordial dyadic affect regulation. An infant responds to a human face and interaction as to no inanimate object. A moment-to-moment reciprocal interaction has been repeatedly demonstrated in the mother-infant dyad with instant electronic registration, not available in the original visual cliff and still-face research (Beebe and Lachman 2002). Genetic predisposition and the sensitizing reciprocal responsiveness of the caregiver activate affect systems which will be the foundation of the human personality. The human infant is preadapted to be stimulus seeking from the maternal object; no longer is the infant regarded as having an initial autistic phase. There are stimulus thresholds and filters rather than the now antiquated concept of a stimulus barrier. Freud's 1923 dictum (p. 23), "the ego is first and foremost a body ego," took into account "perceptions which are received from without [external sense perception] and from within . . . what we call sensations and feelings" (Freud 1923, p. 19). The affect messages from within and without vitally contribute to the emergent self and identity. Affect regulation interacts with evolving perceptual, cognitive, somatic, and social ego functions. Social regulation of affect proceeds from familial affect styles of expression and inhibition even before self, object, and their boundaries are established. The feeling, emotional reaction to the external world specifically from and to the caregiver alters the developing brain and the mind in formation. Furthermore, affects are at the core of temperament, which also has genetic neurobiological determinants in response to psychic and external reality.

AFFECTS AND MENTAL REPRESENTATIONS

The mental representations of self and object are differentiated from each other, and normally then serve as internalized models of behavior. The integration of affectionate mental representations and of aggressive mental representations constitutes an essential achievement of normal development. Symbiotic longings may persist after differentiation of self and object, but a symbiotic developmental phase is no longer regarded as tenable. Affect is an intrinsic component of mental representations with enduring influence on object relations (Kernberg 2012).

During the first year of life, the social smile, affectomotor dialogue, positive mirroring by mother of her infant, and maternal holding and containing contribute to affect modulation. Play has a significant role in human development, and in other mammals as well (Panksepp and Biven 2012). Playful interactions such as peek-a-boo occur with the mother's empathic attunement. This shared enjoyable interaction invokes what Stern (1985) termed state sharing and state complementing. The dyadic partners learn to read each other's emotions, cues, and communication, replete with feedback loops. Nurturance broadly encompasses not only pleasurable oral gratification and nutrition but a tactile holding relationship and an affective responsive dyadic dialogue. The primary love object (caregiver) must also survive the infant's omnipotent angry assaults, retaining her love of her infant.

ROLE OF ANXIETY IN DEVELOPMENT

Freud (1926) distinguished signal anxiety as a positive transformation of traumatic or automatic anxiety into a cognitive signal of danger. He considered that in the course of development the affect of anxiety was desomatized, so that the bodily effects on heart rate and respiration are relatively extinguished. The emotional feeling of anxiety is diminished, becoming a thought-like signal of danger, facilitating mastery of trauma. This modification of potentially overwhelming anxiety was designated in the analytic literature as signal anxiety, a developmental achievement. In contemporary psychoanalysis all affects are considered as being capable of modification in development to a signal function. Signal anxiety facilitates discrimination of real external danger and realistic adaptation to reality. Signal anxiety develops gradually and is critical for regulation and modulation of affect. While the signal function of anxiety was rapidly incorporated into psychoanalytic theory, a more general appreciation of positive, pleasurable signal affects was integrated in analytic theory later.

Stranger anxiety, typically beginning at eight months, indicates the vital attachment to the mother and possibly a fear of her loss. When anxious, the infant seeks the comfort of the mother, the familiar, and the predictable. The caregiver's cues may modulate or intensify the infant's response. Stranger curiosity is also present as the infant explores the object world as well as the world of toys and inanimate objects. Stranger anxiety is variable among infants and has perhaps been overemphasized. The lack of stranger anxiety is not in itself indicative of a problem in the parent-infant relationship.

Separation anxiety, however, is an even more significant element in early development. The quality of this crucial affective bond between infant and caregiver, "attachment," had been studied by Bowlby (1980). Building upon his work, Ainsworth (1978) identified patterns of attachment which greatly amplified prior studies of separation anxiety. Ainsworth studied this bond by means of an original research design in which reunion of baby and mother after a brief separation was observed. This replicable experimental paradigm differed markedly from Bowlby's earlier studies of protracted separation trauma in a small number of infants. As anticipated, reunion with mother after physical separation was normally pleasurable for both partners, but reunion responses of distress were also observed after the brief separation in a minority of infants. It is important to distinguish physical separation from internal separateness. Psychological separation depends on ego boundaries, on the boundary between self and object representation. This variation in preferred and predominant affective responses was used to categorize the quality of the parent-baby relationship. One attachment pattern was labeled "secure" while anxious/insecure infants were classified as avoidant or ambivalent, and disorganized infants did not have a strategy for managing separations. These early affective responses were found to be related to later development. Secure attachment appears to be correlated with resilience and greater capacity to compensate for loss and to master trauma. Insecure attachment suggests strong ambivalent feelings, and the insecure infant may be predisposed to later narcissistic personality disorder, borderline personality disorder, and depression.

In subsequent research Main (2000) utilized the "Adult Attachment Interview" studying, in part, the mothers' attitudes toward their own mothers; various aspects of the interview were analyzed and both form and content were found to be related to the mothers' relationships with their infants. The converse of attachment is the infant's development of intrapsychic and emergent self and object representations. It is the capacity of the infant to mentally represent the mother that helps the infant tolerate and master the anxiety accompanying physical separation. A theory of different minds gradually evolves, beginning in the second year of life. Mentalization, the awareness of the independent thoughts and feelings of self and others, permits and promotes the toddler's self-regulation of affect, identifying with mother's affect regulation. Reflection upon thoughts and feelings becomes possible with diminished defensive distortion (Fonagy and Target 2003). Mahler, Pine, and Bergman (1975) described affective shifts associated with the phases of separation-differentiation. They described the infant's pleasurable exploration during the practicing phase of separation-individuation at approximately one year of age. Having achieved upright locomotion, the infant ventures outside the maternal orbit, often with intense affective expressions of delight, only to return for "emotional refueling." Mother remains emotionally available, monitoring her infant's exploration. Though "the world is his oyster" the infant pioneer should not go too soon, too far. Optimal distance and playful adventure are pleasurable, but can frequently become conflicted for infant and mother, particularly during the subsequent "rapprochement" phase. After this phase, at about 18–24 months of age the toddler becomes aware of the reality of his/her limitations and infantile omnipotence wanes. With greater awareness of being dependent on the caregiver, the elation of the earlier practicing phase becomes modulated and affective storms associated with struggles over submission vs. rebellion may appear (the terrible two's). Affective, cognitive, and social development proceed as language and symbolic thought develop. The capacity for fantasy develops, and verbal communication is added to the toddler's repertoire. Affects acquire cognitive components and are further differentiated in infancy and early childhood. According to contemporary neuroimaging studies, the brain constructs emotions from affective, cognitive, perceptual, and social determinants. In this theoretical frame emotions are not innate, fixed, discrete entities; they are not "hard-wired but are overdetermined, synthesized outside of conscious awareness. Emotions are processed nonconsciously prior to being consciously experienced (Damasio 2012). The ability to label and verbally express negative emotions with precision and specificity, more than a very general comment such as feeling "in the dumps," facilitates a more adaptive response.

All affects may be developmentally tuned to signal function internally, as well as in object relations throughout life. The empathic capacity to feel what others feel follows from maternal mirroring of the infant's affects, adding her own organizing influence in her affective feedback to her infant. This response to seeing and hearing her infant's behavior with inference of intent has a neurobiological substrate in the mirror neuron system (Kohut 1984; Gallese 2009). The mirror neuron system, the mother's mirroring of her infant, and the capacity for empathy and cognitive evaluation of motive and intent utilize multiple affect signals and systems. Currently, it is known that different affect systems have different neurobiological substrates. The wish to repeat pleasurable experience, the safety of secure attachment to the caregiver, play, exploration: all involve signal affects other than only anxiety or negative affect (LeDoux 1996). Conflict between mother's motives and her toddler's demands increases with potential compromise and the personality advancing toward self and object constancy in the rapprochement phase of separation-individuation.

During the rapprochement phase of separation-individuation, struggles of varying degree emerge between mother and infant, occurring as the infant both shadows the mother and darts away. Mothers may be confused by perplexing tendencies toward both clinging and autonomy. At their most intense these struggles are considered a "rapprochement crisis" and if extensive may be indicative of a disturbed caregiver-toddler relationship. Giving and sharing pleasure may alternate with tantrums and attempts to coerce and control mother. Ours, yours, and mine are attitudes associated with asserting personhood and also serve to quell fears of passive surrender to mother (Bergman 1997). Assertion of independence and autonomy are evident in the toddler's increasing desire to dress and feed himself/herself (Blum and Blum 1990). The two- to three-year-old begins to develop the capacity for conscious and unconscious fantasy and later for persisting fantasy. Pertinent to negative affect, repetitive play may also symbolically represent attempts to master fear of loss of the object and of the object's love. The caregiver's stable affection, empathy, and tolerance of the aggressive aspects of the bewildering ambivalence of the youngster during this period are of paramount importance for his/her feelings of safety and security. Love of the caregiver may be overshadowed by hostility. Mother may in fantasy become a persecutory object with projection and/or dissociation of rage and hate. The toddler may be afraid of his/her own aggression, fear of retaliation, and loss of mother's love and protection. A "good enough mother" (Winnicott 1965) does not regress into a childish battle over power and control nor submit to coercion. She does not lose her temper nor respond to her toddler with rage, retaliation, withdrawal, or depression; she tolerates assaults on her confidence and self-esteem. Mother verbalizes for the toddler affects that are within or just beyond the toddler's capacities. The ordinary devoted mother's own affect regulation influences her toddler's affect regulation, discrimination, and modulation.

Language development burgeons, concurrent with and contributing to the emergence of affect self regulation. Increasingly complex verbal expression, including growth of vocabulary and syntactic complexity as well as greater receptive language, facilitates more controlled affect expression. More precise recognition and expression of emotion fosters internal regulation and resilience. The child's growing capacity for verbalization and symbolic representation permits greater precision, comprehension, and control in affect communication. The verbal dyad can communicate at a greater distance, not dependent on visual and tactile contact. Through verbalization in conjunction with mother's language response, the infant begins to verbally formulate experience. Aspects of reality can be mentally considered, including the recent past. Future plans can begin to be understood, making it possible to anticipate a pleasurable experience which might follow an unpleasant but necessary precursor, permitting modulation of negative affect. For example, a youngster balking about donning heavy winter clothes can anticipate a rewarding consequence and master his/her desire to protest. Mother rewards the child's successful delay or diverted gratification and helps to attenuate the child's frustration, disappointment, and anger. Ideally infantile omnipotence is negotiated by the dyad, achieving sensible compromises. During this transition, tendencies for the infant to dissociate idealization and denigration of object and self recede, facilitating integration of love and hate. The "good enough" caregiver is internalized as a consistent, reliable, predictable love object and role model. The little child then gains better control of affect and impulse with increasing self-confidence and adaptive skills. Testing and knowledge of external reality occur in tandem with increasing complexity of language, affect, and cognition in the context of object relations and socialization. Identification with the mother and other caregivers' affects and functions modifies internal self and object representations with their associated affects.

In addition to genetics and neurobiology, gender and culture influence affect expression in concert with object relations and psychosexual development. In persons who are multilingual the affects of childhood are often more readily revived and reexperienced in the mother tongue. The joys and sorrows of childhood are likely to be more accurately reproduced in their original language, which may influence retelling in a subsequent different language (Amati-Mehler, Argentieri, and Canestri 1993).

In much of Western culture boys have not been expected to cry with grief, and girls have been expected to limit aggression while being allowed to cry with grief and sadness. Male parents can now enjoy nurturing and playing with babies without being regarded as effeminate. Girls' pleasurable participation in competitive sports is now encouraged without their being considered "butch" or a tomboy. Some cultures limit affect expression in the face or eyes; girls in social settings may favor smiles rather than frowns or an angry mood.

Spoken language expands rapidly during the second year of life. The infant acquires the mother tongue in the context of the mother-infant bond and affective, sensory-motor dialogue. Linguistic expression expands concurrent with nonverbal affect communication, both of increasing complexity. During rapprochement the toddler begins to combine words and then phrases. Face-to-face, eye-to-eye contact, gesture, and posture are significant modes of communication. Body language can be a thunderous silence or may emphasize or contradict what is spoken. Despite relative consistency in reading and reporting facial affect expression, there is no definitely isomorphic relationship between overt facial expression and underlying emotion as registered by electronic instrumentation. Nevertheless, the face is an important aspect of self and identity (Ekman and Rosenberg 1997). A massive cosmetic industry attests to the social, sexual, and narcissistic significance of the face. Plastic surgery of the face attempts to conceal the sad loss of youth and beauty. "Loss of face" referring to the affects of shame and humiliation implies the disapproving, disparaging looks of authorities within the social surround. It is not surprising that neuroscience has found a site in the brain with the specialization of facial recognition.

PSYCHOPATHOLOGY OF AFFECT

There are many neurobiological and psychological determinants of disturbed emotional expression and comprehension of language. Although etiology has not been definitely established, a traumatic background has been proposed for the majority of individuals with the syndrome of alexithymia. Alexithymia is characterized by great difficulty in recognizing, feeling, and verbally expressing emotion. Speech tends to be devoid of emotion, with diminished imagination, fantasy life, and reports of dreams. Affect signals from others are not well understood and therefore cannot be reconsolidated into verbal communication. Alexithymic and anhedonic persons may have severe impediments in processing positive as well as negative affects. High intensity affects are avoided and without treatment life is colorless with little pleasure or excitement. Treatment is very difficult, especially if there is an innate neurobiological predisposition. Regarding the effect of early life experience, some alexithymic individuals may have had actual harsh parental disapproval of pleasure-seeking activity and/or have internalized a cruel superego which forbids pleasures of the body, play, and social interaction. Positive joyful affects are disapproved and object relations tend to be sadomasochistic or enveloped in anxiety and depression (Taylor and Bagley 2013). High anxiety or terror may result in flight or fight, freezing, fainting, or personality regression and disorganization. Abused children and traumatized adults may be subject to impoverishment of affect or anxiety and panic disorders, as well as frightening flashbacks, nightmares, and pathogenic somatization. Trauma may also have sequelae of affect lability, instability, and/or restriction to one affect, such as anger or depression. Always on alert hypervigilant persons with posttraumatic stress disorder are prone to impetuous or inhibited behavior without awareness of underlying affect-laden motivations. The sound of a siren may lead to irrationally hiding behind a desk without overt fright. A depressed person may weep without being aware of feeling sad or hopeless. The greater the personality disorder, the greater the risk of concomitant affect disorder and vice versa. If preoedipal narcissistic disturbance is prominent, shame or humiliation may be more pronounced than guilt and feelings of remorse. Guilt with pressure toward seeking punishment and/or self-punishment will also be associated with fear of retaliation. Where a rather helpless person has been brainwashed in child abuse or in a prison camp or other setting, anger and hate may be turned against the self in extremes of self-injury and other masochistic phenomena or hopeless depression. Extremes of negative and positive affect are found in bipolar disorder (formerly manic-depression). The bipolar personality may paradoxically feel elated, and later depressed, yet unable to tolerate the spectrum of intense affects. The range of affect tends to be similarly restricted in hypochondria. In hypochondria aggression and anger are turned against the body self or projected on the body self. The body self is the hypochondriac's persecutor, tormenting the dissociated good self-object. Addiction to pain (Valenstein 1973) may be associated with clinging to negative affects. The emergence of externalized and internalized hate in the latter half of the second year of life contributes to polarized love-hate ambivalence, which if untamed and unintegrated will interfere with later object constancy and oedipal phase development. Pleasurable experience fosters positive affectionate affect, whereas excessive unpleasant or traumatic experiences foster hate and rage (Parens 1979).

When there is a small group it is remarkable how a contagious affect such as pity or anger may be communicated to all present. Contagious affect will favor social cohesion or antisocial antagonism. An appeal to others may be complicated by not feeling listened to or understood. Children who have difficulty identifying their own emotions and expressing affect may have further difficulty in differentiating or decentering their feelings from others. Early deficits in empathy may lead to misunderstanding or lack of feelings and emotional reciprocity in object relationships. Affects in this context are impoverished and to a degree ineffable, as occurs in alexithymia. In the milder forms of cyclothymia, psychogenic conflicts are outstanding, and affect regulation is mainly maintained and/or can be readily reestablished. Polarized forms of optimism and pessimism may be observed in some traumatized personalities. Some traumatized persons cannot stop talking about their experience, inviting either a sympathetic or irritated response or both. They may shift between a positive confident view of the future or a depressive, negative outlook.

Any discourse on affect invites consideration of visual art and music and their emotional evocation and communication of emotion. Among the arts, music particularly embraces emotions without well-defined cognition. Music may express and elaborate feelings with complexity and subtlety that may surpass other forms of communication. Music is the universal language of emotion: "If music be the food of love, play on, give me excess of it" (Shakespeare 1623). "Music has charms to soothe the savage breast" (Congreve 1697). Music may be joyous, charming, sad, mournful, reflective, etc. Experiencing a musical mood may influence a personal mood, although the mood may not endure for long afterwards. Beginning in infancy we listen to vocal music and the words, carried to higher levels of abstraction in later development. Music is usually a well-regulated, primarily affective communication, the more poignant and touching in its special capacity to elicit and activate intense controlled and delicate emotional reactions. The relatively inborn capacity for the creation of music is related to the substrate of language and to human passions; emotional expression contributes to understanding and feeling understood. Visual art may also have a powerful influence on affect, mood, and thought. Contemplating a painting or sculpture may engender an internal dialogue with the artist. Art can be exhilarating, depressing, thought provoking, etc.

The recognition, differentiation, and expression of emotions develop in the context of early object relations, by identification as well as instruction. Sometimes uneducated culturally deprived parents require education about the importance of talking to their infants and verbally responding to their children's emotions and questions. A group of these parents has been taught to help their infants and children recognize and express their feelings in linguistic communication (Parens 2014). Human emotion involves and is modified by social, cultural, and educational experience. Learning related to problem solving and adaptation to reality most readily occurs during low affect intensity. Reduction and moderation of peak negative affect states are dependent upon partially innate capacities for self-soothing. Interdependent with endowment, the capacity for self-soothing and self-regulation is consequent to identification with affect regulation provided by the caregiver (Mahler, Pine, and Bergman 1975). Modulation of disruptive peak affect states may also contribute to the attenuation of ego dysfunction and restoration of ego-organized self-control. Adolescents may seek peak affects as a defense against the eruption of repressed fantasy, but also in the service of defining identity. Though peak affect states may appear to be without cognitive appraisal, there is usually an underlying unconscious or conscious fantasy involving a meaningful object relationship (Kernberg 2012).

While adult affect constellations are usually on the surface of consciousness, character traits of poise, smugness, enthusiasm, and serenity have been psychoanalytically reconstructed to preverbal development (Rangell 1954; Arlow 1957; Greenson 1962). However, the transformation of preverbal affect constellations which have never before been symbolized into verbal communication that can be reliably connected to the preverbal phase has remained questionable. The influence of later developmental phases and life experience on the mind and brain may have permanently transformed affect states of early infancy. Countertransference based conjecture might facilitate reconstruction of preverbal affect (Beebe and Lachman 2002). Analytic insight into unconscious fantasy is mainly conveyed in verbal expression, which contributes to the further transformation of affect. Moreover, affect within the ego syntonic formation of character is persistent and resistant to change. Narcissistic individuals may react to any nonaffirmation of their grandiose identity as a narcissistic injury evoking humiliation and withdrawal and/or narcissistic rage. Characterological grandiosity may defend against diminished, fragile self-esteem; excessive humility may defend against humiliation or arrogant self-aggrandizement (Kohut 1984).

Character traits elicit emotional responses from others and may have a powerful influence on object relations. No longer limited to oversimplified oral, anal, or phallic character types, character conveys affect constellations. In circular effects, character influences the form as well as the affective/cognitive content of linguistic communication. The volume, pitch, pressure of speech, whispering or shouting, speaking softly or in stentorial tones, all have vital affect determinants. Character is an aspect of identity and there are internal affect signals related to both positive and negative aspects of the self-representation. Character change may occur over the life span, and affect disorders may be modified with improved affect regulation and expression

(Kissen 1995). In favorable development a superior integration of somatic, subjective, and expressive dimensions of affect is achieved. Integration and regulation of the different dimensions of affect codetermine whether the ego will control and master trauma or will succumb to regression and disorganization.

GROUP EXPRESSION AND REGULATION OF AFFECT

Within a family one family member may provoke another to express approval or anger at another that is otherwise suppressed. A mother may provoke a father to punish their child, evading her own guilty feelings toward her child, as well as averting the child's negative feelings toward her. Borderline characters generally include narcissistic traits, but are not necessarily narcissistic personalities and are more ego-impaired. Intrapsychic mental representations split between idealization and denigration are associated with affect lability, restriction to one affect, lack of affect, or inappropriate affect.

The regulation and expression of affects in society is heavily influenced by social and political forces. Within society, subgroups may have highly diverse affective/cognitive constellations. Affect regulation or dysregulation will be powerfully influenced by the composition of the group, the qualities of leadership, and the relationship of the group to the larger society. Splitting of representations between the idealized leader and members of the group and devalued or demonized groups of outsiders may be accompanied by diffuse uncontrolled affect storms. Leaders may arouse intense affects and may exploit or manipulate them for both malevolent or benevolent purposes. A leader's anger and hatred may incite mobs through identification to angry aggressive behavior toward those outside the group. Bitter experience has repeatedly confirmed how readily mature ideals and values may be relinquished in concert with loss of affect and impulse regulation. Fortunately civilization and culture have survived with object love and preservation of affectionate intergenerational bonds and sufficient mastery of traumatic anxiety and depression.

REFERENCES

Ainsworth, M., et al. (1978). *Patterns of Attachment: A Psychological Study of the Strange Situation.* Hillsdale, NJ: Erlbaum.

Amati-Mehler, J., Argentieri, S., and Canestri, J. (1993). *The Babel of the Unconscious: Mother Tongue and Foreign Languages in the Psychoanalytic Dimension.* Madison, CT: International Universities Press.

Arlow, J. (1957). On smugness. *International Journal of Psychoanalysis,* 58, 157–170.

Beebe, B. and Lachmann, F. (2002). *Infant Research and Adult Treatment: Co-constructing Interactions.* Hillsdale, NJ: Analytic Press.

Bergman, A. (1997). *Ours, Yours, and Mine.* Northvale, NJ: Jason Aronson.

Blum, H. (1991). Affect theory and the theory of technique. *Journal of the American Psychoanalytic Association*, 39, 265–289.
———. (2005). The language of affect. In *The Language of Emotion*. edited by S. Akhtar and H. Blum. New York: Jason Aronson.
Blum, H. and Blum, E. (1990). The development of autonomy and superego precursors. *International Journal of Psychoanalysis*, 71, 585–595.
Bowlby, J. (1980). *Attachment and Loss, Vol. 3*. New York: Basic Books.
Cannon, W. (1932). *The Wisdom of the Body*. New York: Norton.
Congreve, W. (1697). *The Mourning Bride: A Tragedy*. (reprint) 2011 Hamburg,Germany: Tredition Classics.
Damasio, A. (2012). *Self Comes to Mind. Constructing the Conscious Brain*. New York: Vintage.
Darwin, C. (1872). *The Expression of Emotions in Man and Animals*. Chicago: University of Chicago Press, 1965.
Ekman, P. and Rosenberg, E. (1997). *What the Face Reveals*. London: Oxford University Press.
Feinman, S. (1992). *Social Referencing and the Construction of Reality in Infancy*. New York: Plenum Press.
Fonagy, P. and Target, M. (2003). *Psychoanalytic Theories: Perspectives from Developmental Psychology*. New York: Routledge.
Freud, S. (1894). The neuro-psychosis of defence. In Strachey, J. (Ed.). (1971). *Standard Edition of the Complete Psychological Works of Sigmund Freud, Vol. III*. London: Hogarth Press and the Institute for Psycho-Analysis. (Original works published 1893–1895)
———. (1909). Leonardo da Vinci and a memory of his childhood. S.E., 11. In Strachey, J. (Ed.). (1971). *Standard Edition of the Complete Psychological Works of Sigmund Freud, Vol. III*. London: Hogarth Press and the Institute for Psycho-Analysis. (Original works published 1893–1895)
———. (1923). The ego and the id. In Strachey, J. (Ed.). (1971). *Standard Edition of the Complete Psychological Works of Sigmund Freud, Vol. XIX*. London: Hogarth Press and the Institute for Psycho-Analysis. (Original works published 1893–1895)
———. (1926). Inhibition, symptoms, and anxiety. In Strachey, J. (Ed.). (1971). *Standard Edition of the Complete Psychological Works of Sigmund Freud, Vol. XX*. London: Hogarth Press and the Institute for Psycho-Analysis. (Original works published 1893–1895)
Gallese, V. (2009). Mirror neurons, embodied simulation, and the neural basis of social identification. *Psychoanalytic Dialogue*, 19, 519–536.
Greenson, R. (1962). On enthusiasm. *Journal of the American Psychoanalytic Association*, 10, 3–21.
Hendrick, J. (1943). Discussion of "instinct to master." *Psychoanalytic Quarterly*, 12, 561–565.
Izard, C. (1977). *Human Emotions*. New York: Plenum.
James, W. (1884). What is an emotion? *Mind*, 4, 188–204.
Kernberg, O. (2012). *The Inseparable Nature of Love and Aggression*. Washington, DC: American Psychiatric Press.
Kissen, M. (1995). *Affect, Object, and Character Structure*. Madison, CT: International Universities Press.
Kohut, H. (1984). *How Does Analysis Cure?* Chicago: University of Chicago Press.
Krystal, H. (1988). *Integration and Self-Healing: Affects, Trauma, Alexithymia*. Hillsdale, NJ: Analytic Press.
Le Doux, J. (1996). *The Emotional Brain*. New York: Simon and Schuster.
McLean, P. D. (1990). *The Triune Brain in Evolution: Role in Paleocerebral Function*. NY: Springer.
Mahler, M., Pine, F., and Bergman, A. (1975). *The Psychological Birth of the Human Infant*. New York: Basic Books.
Main, M. (2000). The organized categories of infant, child, and adult attachment. *Journal of the American Psychoanalytic Association*, 48, 1055–1095.
Panksepp, J. and Biven, L. (2012). *The Archaeology of Mind*. New York: Norton.

Parens, H. (1979). *The Development of Aggression in Early Childhood.* New York: Jason Aronson.

———. (2014). The evolution of an early parenting program, its follow-up and implications. In R. Emde and M. Leuzinger-Bohleber (Eds.). (2014). *Early Parenting and Prevention of Disorder* (186–199). London: Karnac.

Rangell, L. (1954). The psychology of poise. *International Journal of Psychoanalysis*, 35, 313–332.

Shakespeare, W. (1623). *Twelfth Night*, Act I, Scene I, 1–3.

Schore, A. (1994). *Affect Regulation and the Origin of the Self.* Hillsdale, NJ: Erlbaum.

Shapiro, T. and Emde, R. (1992). *Affect: Psychoanalytic Perspectives.* Madison, CT: International Universities Press.

Spitz, R. (1965). *The First Year of Life.* New York: International Universities Press.

Stern, D. (1985). *The Interpersonal World of the Infant.* New York: Basic Books.

Taylor, G. and Bagby, R. (2013). Psychoanalysis and empirical research: the example of alexithymia. *Journal of the American Psychoanalytic Association*, 61, 99–133.

Tompkins, S. (1962–1963). *Affect, Imagery, Consciousness.* Vol. 1–2. New York: Springer.

Tronick, E. (2007). *The Neurobiological and Social-Emotional Development of Infants and Children.* New York: Norton.

Valenstein, A. (1973). On attachment to painful feelings and the negative therapeutic reaction. *Psychoanalytic Study of the Child*, 28, 305–392.

Winnicott, D. (1965). *The Maturational Process and the Facilitating Environment.* New York: International Universities Press.

Chapter Two

A Developmental Model to Enhance Understanding of Therapeutic Action

Alexandra M. Harrison

In this chapter, I propose that a developmental model framed by a first principle of open systems theory, the Dyadic Expansion of Consciousness Model (DECM), offers a useful perspective on therapeutic action (Tronick 2007). In particular, two features of the model, the "*match, mismatch, and repair*" process, and the proposition of *multiple simultaneous meaning-making*, help explain the observations gained when the data from *videotape observation* is added to the more subjective data of the analyst's recall of the session. I will describe how this conceptual model helps me understand the play therapy I do with children. Then I will give a clinical case as an illustration. I have written on this subject in previous publications (Harrison & Tronick 2007; Harrison & Tronick 2011; Harrison 2013). This chapter represents further developments in my thinking on the subject.

My major focus is a key feature of the DECM of developmental change—*match, mismatch, and repair*—from the point of view of understanding how change takes place in psychotherapy. *Match, mismatch, and repair* describes how two individuals exchange speech, gestures, and facial expression in order to make meaning together. This process occurs in typical interpersonal exchanges as well as in psychotherapy. The *match, mismatch, and repair* process has its roots in the infant-parent relationship, and it is also acting between the two members of the therapeutic dyad, as well as within the individual. *Match, mismatch, and repair* is a continually evolving activity that has the characteristic of sloppiness, or "hit or miss."

I propose that various perspectives on therapeutic change in different psychoanalytic theories can be included within DECM's overarching concepts about developmental and therapeutic change, in fact an economical view of therapeutic change is that of a continually evolving process of trying to find a match and repairing the mismatches along the way.

Another key feature of the DECM that I will discuss is the pivotal idea of *multiple simultaneous meaning-making*. According to this concept, the meanings emerging from the match, mismatch, and repair, hit or miss process, are being made simultaneously in many different domains or systems of the human organism—physical and nonsymbolic as well as verbal and symbolic.

The evolving communicative exchange of meanings by the two individuals in the therapeutic dyad represents an effort to make new, more complex and coherent—in other words, adaptive—meanings of the patient's life experience and sense of himself. As two people make meaning together, many partial or emerging meanings that are offered by one partner are rejected or not accepted by the other. These moments constitute a mismatch, but the mismatch can be very brief, as the two implicitly agree to one choice between them in a brief negotiating process that results in one cocreated shared meaning. These interesting moments can be as short as a mishearing of a verbal communication that is corrected or ignored, or as long as a real back and forth negotiation of partial meanings until one is ratified by the dyad. This negotiation process is important, because the negotiation or repair of mismatches is a competency that the infant begins to learn in the first caregiving relationships and continues to practice with the same and different partners throughout life.

The complexity of this apparently economical process is due in part to the *multiple domains of meaning-making* in which the activity simultaneously occurs. The meanings being communicated are not exclusively in the familiar form of symbolic acts or language, as has been noted by other psychoanalytic writers (Jacobs 1973; Pally 2001; Harrison & Tronick 2007; Harrison & Beebe 2017, in press). In addition, a match and mismatch may occur simultaneously in different domains of meaning-making, such as in language, play, facial expression, gesture, physiological arousal state, among others hidden from view. For example, a couple may create a matching pattern by coordinating vocal rhythms and repeating a familiar narrative, when one of them suddenly becomes physiologically "triggered" by an association to a past trauma in her life. In this case, the match in vocal rhythm may persist for a time until the new symbolic and affective meanings take hold and disrupt the match.

Even though psychoanalysts now generally agree that meaning between patient and analyst is a joint creation, psychoanalytic theory has not fully integrated this idea. Also, clinical reports in the literature for the most part portray "sense" being made of a therapeutic encounter in a linear manner—e.g., P says something, A responds, P and A both agree that they have progressed in their understanding. This is in part because of the kind of narrative data the analyst relies on to make sense of the ongoing clinical process. By contrast, the broader perspective of the DECM suggests that all the meanings—including many meanings escaping awareness—that analyst and patient make together are important and constitute "soundings" in the hit or miss effort to create something new and more adaptive than what there was before. A study of videotape data provides the opportunity to observe (1) the unconscious or nonconscious choice patient and analyst make about which to address among multiple simultaneous meanings; (2) the small mismatches that occur continuously in the therapeutic exchange; and (3) the patterns of repair that build the trust or sense of security in the relationship that allow for taking risks. The DECM explains that this ongoing process of reciprocal exchange can lead to an emergent property of a single dyadic state of consciousness that is more complex and coherent than the initial state of consciousness of either individual (Tronick 2001, 2007).

In a study of videotape data from an early therapeutic session with an eight-year-old boy, I will demonstrate these three activities. I will show that therapeutic process—when it is going well—consists of a continuous process of matches, mismatches, and repairs of mismatches, many if not most of which occur out of awareness of the analyst and patient. This perspective represents an elaboration of the "moving along" process described in the Boston Change Process Study Group's first paper (Stern et al. 1989). In fact, the "moving along" process between "moments of meeting," as I will demonstrate, is highly articulated, though also in constant evolution.

I will first briefly lay out more of the theoretical basis I use for the paper. Then I will describe the different types of data used in understanding therapeutic action in order to highlight the unique opportunities offered by videotape analysis in this study. After this I will present the clinical material and the sense I made of it. Finally, I will end with some concluding remarks.

THEORETICAL BASIS

Tronick's DECM model is framed by a first principle of open systems theory: The system must continually gain energy and information to maintain and grow its complexity and coherence (Tronick 2001; Harrison & Tronick 2007; Tronick 2007). When human beings are viewed as systems, this means that they must continuously grow in the meanings they make about their experience. Therapeutic process is an example of that growth. In psychotherapy, two (or more) people communicate with the intention of making some kind of meaning together. Each therapeutic partner then takes that cocreated meaning and integrates it into his individual repertoire of meanings. The hope is that the meaning the patient takes from the therapeutic engagement is more adaptive and flexible than that which he originally made of his life.

Critical to this model of therapeutic action is the notion of "multiple simultaneous meaning making," in which different systems—bodily organs, physiological systems, musculoskeletal system, states of consciousness, and symbols including language—operate at different levels in the individual simultaneously (Tronick 2007).

Therapeutic action takes place as therapist and patient draw on their individual repertoires of making-meaning in relationships. This repertoire begins to emerge in the infant-parent relationship. These efforts at cocreating meaning are sloppy at best, even in the best of therapies, and many mismatches occur. These mismatches provide choice points in the process, as the two interacting partners may proceed to repair the mismatch or proceed to make a meaning about discord, conflict, and stalemate. Each "repair" also constitutes a choice of meaning among many. Some choices are explicit but most are implicit, especially in the moment-to-moment time frame. Thus the continuing mismatch states are not bad but an essential part of the fabric of the therapeutic process. Not only do they result in a "choice" of meaning; they can also inform the therapist about important aspects of the transferential "landscape" (Granic & Patterson 2006).

As patient and analyst communicate with the intention of making sense of the patient's experience, engaging in an exchange of their individual "takes" of what is going on, they increase the energy of the dyadic system. When successful in cocreating new meanings that are more complex and coherent than those that existed before, they fulfill the first principle of open systems theory of gaining resources and, critically, they experience pleasure and connectedness. By contrast, when they do not succeed in this process, there is often a subjective sense of malaise, of being stuck, that indicates the system did not gain energy and therefore is losing energy, becoming more rigid instead of more flexible.

Data Sources for Study of Therapeutic Action

Studies of therapeutic process take advantage of different types of data. The most common source of data, which forms the basis for most psychoanalytic literature, is case reports constructed from the analyst's memory or from process notes. This source of data is particularly valuable when it includes an account of the analyst's subjective experience. The limitation of this source of data is that it is constrained by the analyst's memory and focus of attention, both of which are biased by the need to construct a verbal narrative in order to make sense of the ongoing interpersonal exchange and to convey it to others. In other words, data that is not presented in symbolic form is often neglected, as is the nonlinear nature of the therapeutic exchange. This source of data is also limited by unconscious choices both analyst and patient make about which of the multiple meanings the patient offers at the outset of a treatment to address. I will demonstrate examples of such choice processes in the clinical section.

Another source of data is videotape of the analytic session (Beebe & Harrison 2017, in press). Analysis of this data illuminates different areas of therapeutic process, such as gestures and facial expressions, vocal tone and the complex process of turn taking, for example vocal turns (Jaffe et al. 2001; Harrison 2013). It also demonstrates the multiple potential choices presented by the patient regarding meanings about himself that cause him distress. The choice of which meanings to address at the outset of a treatment is often made consciously by patient or analyst, but just as often unconscious choices are made. This unconscious or nonconscious choice-making process becomes an important aspect of the narrative of the treatment and also of the domain of meaning-making that is chosen, as I will demonstrate. As two individuals get to know each other they develop characteristic ways of repairing mismatches. Since these patterns of repair are drawn from each individual's repertoire of patterns of interpersonal exchange, they retain some of the particularity of the individuals. In addition, since they emerge from the interaction, the patterns of repair are unique to the relationship.

Videotaped play therapy sessions offer a unique advantage in studying mismatches and repairs for several reasons. Videotape allows the viewer to observe exchanges that take place in very small increments of time. Also, the interpersonal exchange can be observed multiple times, offering the opportunity to make new observations in subsequent viewings. Finally, play therapy videotapes include motor activity and nonverbal communication of affect and intention, as well as examples of symbolic meaning.

Vocal Rhythm Coordination

I have used the method of videotape analysis developed by Beebe to study mother-infant pairs (Jaffe et al. 2001; Harrison 2013). By analyzing the vocal stream of the two partners, Beebe and her colleagues have demonstrated that the qualities and characteristics of the interactions of rhythms of young infants and their mothers are consistent with aspects of negotiating intimacy and control in a relationship (Beebe & Lachmann 2013). According to this technique, the duration of the vocal turns taken by two people (for example, mother and infant) in conversation are measured as well as the pauses between their vocal turns. In this chapter I have included only one such analysis of a 40-second dialogue between my patient and me. I offer it as an example of a characteristic pattern that the child and I return to during the course of our work together.

CLINICAL CASE

"Mattie" was eight years old when his parents consulted me because of temper tantrums and difficulties getting along with his two-year-old younger sister and his mother. He presented as a handsome boy with a cheerful attitude and an eagerness to play with me. The first two sessions—the focus of this investigation—occurred a week apart and represented an evaluation that initiated a longer treatment. I did not videotape the first session for mechanical reasons, but I will discuss this session as I reconstruct it from my notes and then explore the following videotaped session in greater depth.

First Individual Session (Not Videotaped)

At the beginning of the first session Mattie engaged me with a direct gaze and an apprehensive expression and asked me why my floors creaked. I asked him if he had an idea, and he replied that maybe it was because it was an old house. I agreed and asked him what creaky floors made him think of. He hesitated. I then suggested that maybe he worried that the house might fall down. He nodded vigorously. I said, "That was a scary thought and I don't like to have scary thoughts, do you?" He continued to look apprehensive and said that no, he didn't either.

He chose to build with magnetiles (a toy consisting of geometric shapes of brightly colored plastic that contain magnetized strips so that the edges stick together). He built a tall tower that was very tippy. He then chose a magician puppet who he said was magic. I asked the magician, since he was magic, what wishes he had. Mattie responded that the magician wished there would be no creaky floors. I said this was a good wish because that meant children would not have to be so scared. He added a puppet of a rabbit and said that the rabbit was a queen and decided that the building would be a castle for the queen. The castle had several levels. In a somewhat enigmatic remark, Mattie said that it was "against the law" to "go beneath the queen."

Second Session (Videotaped)

Therapeutic Process

In the second session Mattie again chose the magnetiles and the magician and rabbit queen puppets. He informed me that the magician and the rabbit queen did not talk, although between the two of them they could speak magic language.

Mattie then proceeded to create a prism shaped structure of the magnetiles and made a dog puppet admire it. Then a small *mismatch* occurred. He made squeaking sounds for the dog and explained that he "lost his voice." He added abruptly, "Like my dad lost his shoes once at a track meet and had to leave his phone behind." I said, "Oh, my gosh. Why did he have to leave his phone behind?" Mattie hesitated, his gaze averted from me as he placed tiles in an ongoing construction; then he remarked without emotion, "He got it back."

Commentary

This is a common type of mismatch in conversation, especially with young children. When Mattie made his interesting but confusing remark about his dad losing his shoes and then his phone, I was confused and perceived a choice of first focusing on either the shoes or the phone—both of which had been lost. Identifying the more general meaning of loss was a third choice, and if I had been more astute I might have said something like, "Oh, my gosh! He lost *two* things!" but I was not. Yet, one benefit of not being so clever is that it offers your patient a bigger role to play in the repair. Allowing the patient to initiate the repair supports the therapeutic goal of new competency in making meanings. Mattie's response, "He got it back," brought coherence to the communication because—while it may have been defensive—it also succinctly refocused the emphasis on "loss." As we will see, this kind of terse reframing also became a characteristic way Mattie used to repair a mismatch created when I chose a meaning he did not like.

My response was to accept his correction and retreat in my questioning, respecting his defenses and giving the initiative back to him. I think the reason he did not "like" my question had to do with the fact that he was not prepared to go into that subject at this early time in our relationship. It was as if the association to his dad's track meet was made in an unguarded moment and he did not wish to expose himself further. Whatever fantasy lay behind his remark about his dad's track meet had to wait until later for elucidation.

Continuation of Therapeutic Process

Immediately, there followed a second small mismatch: Mattie took out the turtle puppet and turned it to face me as if in greeting (The puppet is unusual in that it has four floppy legs.) and I said hello, asking if I could shake his hand. I reached for his right hand, and less than a second later, as I made contact with the turtle's right "hand," Mattie offered his left hand. He then oriented him to me so that his right hand was easier to reach.

Commentary

Again, this is the kind of experience one frequently has in typical conversations, as well as in play sessions. One would usually pay no attention to it at all; as a matter of fact, without videotape it would probably go unnoticed.

There are many possible reasons for this tiny mismatch. A likely one is that Mattie was not yet secure in distinguishing right from left. Another is that he was not anticipating my request to shake hands and offered me the "hand" that was nearest. Both meanings are likely.

The fact that neither of us verbally acknowledged the mismatch is perhaps significant. According to the idea of multiple simultaneous meaning making, there are numerous possible meanings to the exchange. Perhaps I was protectively avoiding pointing out Mattie's error. Perhaps we were also allowing ourselves to behave a little sloppily, communicating that it was OK to make mistakes, a formulation consistent with an "introduction" (the dog puppet and me) and also with the beginning of Mattie and my relationship. We were experimenting with making repairs of mismatches. Confidence that we could repair a rupture between us is of course critical in building trust in a relationship. The physical adjustment without verbal accompaniment that each of us made to correct the original mismatch added to our repertoire as another method the two of us would use to repair mismatches.

Continuing Therapeutic Process

The dog and the turtle admired the construction, which was ongoing. Mattie commented, "We could make a little shade," to which I responded, "Good." And Mattie said, "And a little private area." I said, "Oh, a little private area, great." As he built, Mattie said that we might need more space for the queen, because "queens need to think a lot and they need to walk around." He then proceeded to make "a private area" plus an "area for walking around." Here is a sequence that particularly well illustrates a matching pattern. It is illustrated in Figures 1 and 2 below. I have chosen this sequence because of the coming together of the salient symbolic theme of "privacy" and the remarkable coordination of vocal turn rhythms.

The two figures together comprise 40 seconds of consecutive action in the videotape. Here is the context: After declaring that we should make shade for the queen and a little private area, Mattie proceeded to make more space for the queen, who needed to "think a lot and walk around." As Mattie continued to add rooms onto the building, he declared that he has just made "a private area!" This is the beginning of the clip and of Figure 1.

The figures demonstrate the vocal turns and pauses in this 40-second sequence.

Above the central horizontal axis are Mattie's turns, and below are mine (AMH). The axis is divided into seconds beginning with 0 and ending with 20 in Figure 1 and beginning with 20 and ending with 40 in Figure 2. During the time period represented in Figures 1 and 2, I was sitting quietly on the floor near Mattie, and Mattie was moving the two puppets in and out of the spaces he had created with the magnetiles. Mattie's activity is represented in a line above his vocal turns; his individual action turns are not articulated in these figures.

DETAILED DESCRIPTION OF FIGURES 1 AND 2

Figure 1

The clip began as Mattie took a vocal turn 2 seconds after I had previously spoken (my vocal turn and pause occurring before the time represented in Figure 1), creating a 2-second pause. He took a 2-second vocal turn. His hand was over his mouth, and the first part of his speech was muffled (perhaps reproducing in action the theme of "private" or "secret"); he then stated, "private area."

Using Mattie's pause and turn pattern, I waited 2 seconds before taking a 2-second vocal turn: "There are a lot of private areas there." After approximately ½ second, in which Mattie was placing the queen rabbit puppet in the structure, I made another 2-second remark, "I think these two guys (magician and queen) must . . ." (I paused). Mattie reinstated the 2-second pause before finishing my sentence in 1 second—"like private." It seems clear that I was implicitly requesting a response from Mattie. As he completed my sentence, there seemed to be an agreement between us about the importance of the theme of "privacy," both in the articulation of the symbolic/verbal meaning and in the synchrony we created in our turn taking pattern.

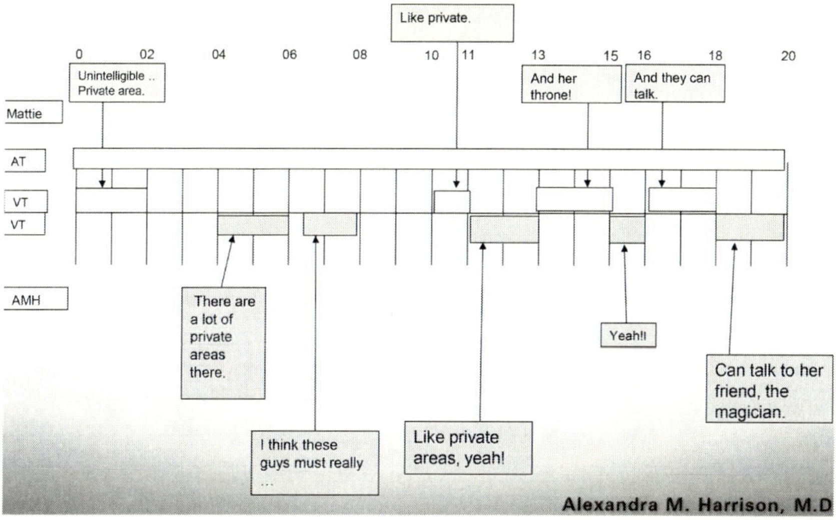

Figure 2.1.

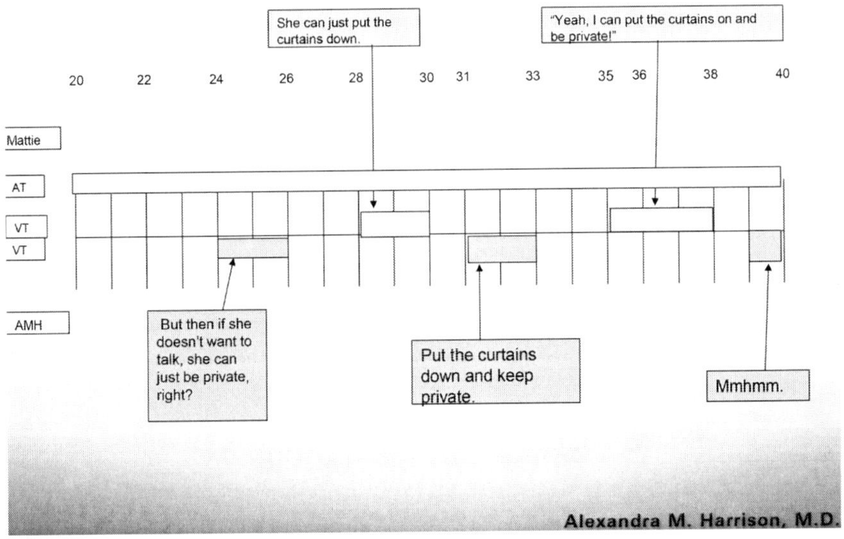

Figure 2.2.

As if to confirm an agreement about privacy, I came in immediately after Mattie "like private" with a 2-second vocal turn—"like private areas, yeah." With impressive attunement, Mattie followed this new pattern of tightly synchronized turn taking, taking a 2-second vocal turn, "and her throne." Next, I also spoke without leaving a pause, "Yeah!" Mattie again spoke immediately, taking another 2-second vocal turn—"And they can talk!" I again spoke without a pause, taking a 2-second vocal turn—"Can talk to her friend the magician." The 10-second sequence beginning with Mattie's "Like private" and ending with my "Can talk to her friend, the magician," comprises vocal turns of 1 second, 2 seconds, 2 seconds, 1 second, 2 seconds, and 2 seconds, with no pause between them. This unusual tightly synchronized pattern creates an emphasis on the meaning of "privacy" in the context of high mutual attunement.

Figure 2

Mattie moved the queen from room to room, bouncing the puppet slightly up and down, as if she were exploring her new space. Mattie's eyes were averted, and he had a soft expression of mild contentment on his face. After waiting 4 seconds, I took a 2-second vocal turn, "But then if she doesn't want to talk, she can just be private, right?" It is as if I wanted to allow Mattie privacy (waiting for 4 seconds) but I also wanted to maintain my connection with him and with the subject of privacy. Mattie waited for 2 seconds and responded with a 2-second vocal turn, "She can just put the curtains down." I waited for 1 second and then repeated his 2-second vocal turn duration, saying, "Put the curtains down and keep private." He waited 2 seconds and took a 3-second vocal turn, using a marked voice for the queen, "Yeah, I can put the curtains down and be private!" I waited 1 second before affirming his statement with a 1-second vocal turn, "Mmhm."

Commentary of Figures 1 and 2

Here is the sequence for the entire 40 seconds: Mattie—2-second (sec) pause (P), 2-sec vocal turn (VT); AMH—2-sec P, 2-sec VT, ½-sec internal pause, 1 ½-sec VT; Mattie—2-sec P, 1-sec VT; (Beginning of tightly synchronized exchange.) AMH—0 P, 2-sec VT; Mattie—0 P, 2-sec VT; AMH—0 P, 1-sec VT; Mattie—0 P, 2-sec VT; AMH—0 P, 2-sec VT (End of tightly synchronized exchange.) AMH—4-sec internal P, 2-sec VT; Mattie—2-sec P, 2-sec VT; AMH—1-sec P, 2-sec VT; Mattie—2-sec P, 3-sec VT; AMH—1-sec P, 1-sec VT.

In Figure 1, Mattie began with a regular rhythm of a 2-second pause followed by a 2-second vocal turn concerning the important theme of "private." I left a 2-second pause, following his lead, and also I followed his lead in terms of content, with my comment about private areas. I recognized that the theme of "private" suggested fantasies that Mattie might be anxious about exposing to me, and I did not want to intrude. I paused, and I saw that he was occupied with the action turns of introducing the queen to her new space. I wanted to maintain my connection with Mattie and support the development of the theme of privacy without intruding, so I took another vocal turn, saying that the guys (queen and magician) must really like. . . . Here, my pause indicated that I was hoping he would join me in a completion of this idea. Mattie did indeed complete my sentence, after a 2-second pause, saying, "like private." Mattie might have changed the subject after my "giving him the floor." The fact that he restated the same theme of "private" is significant to our meaning making and is an example of the back and forth, hit and miss—this time, "hit"—activity that constitutes the making of meaning together. So now we have cocreated an evolving meaning about privacy; privacy has to do with something you do in private and something you wish to keep private, at least at this point in a new relationship.

Convinced of the salience of this theme of "private" and eager to hold onto it, I came right in at second 11 with the unusual move of beginning immediately when Mattie completed his turn without leaving a pause. This pattern of turn taking is important, because it requires close attention and high synchronization (Jaffe et al. 2001). Here, I attribute the pattern to the importance of what Mattie was calling "private" and my recognition of it. This is a turn taking pattern I recognize in my work on previous cases

(Harrison 2013). It usually occurs when I want to "hold onto" a symbolic theme or an affect that I see as particularly important, to "keep it in the air," so that we can elaborate it.

My vocal turn at second 11 is followed by the now familiar 2-second duration. Mattie followed me, coming in right on the tail of my vocal turn, with another 2-second turn (second 13), the content of which expresses satisfaction with the queen's throne. I did the same at second 15, again not leaving a pause, affirming the positive feature of the queen's throne in a 1-second vocal turn. Mattie followed me again in the tight, no-pause pattern, taking a 2-second vocal turn at second 18, adding another positive feature of the queen's space—not only is she private, but she is not alone; she can talk to someone ("And they can talk."). I was imagining meanings related to the transference—maybe Mattie was communicating in the play his hope that he could entrust me (the magician) with some of his "private" thoughts and actions. I kept up the pause pattern of tight synchronization by not leaving a pause and by repeating his last speech with a slight variation, adding, "can talk to her friend, the magician."

Although I had ideas of my own about the symbolic meaning of "private" in the play, Mattie and I had not yet established between the two of us a coherent meaning for what the word "private" meant to him. Following Mattie's lead, I assumed that he was not yet ready to do this. However, with the rhythm of our voices we had communicated to each other that this ambiguous idea of "private" had salience and that we were "moving along" in a mutually agreed upon direction. This was an example of how the meanings we were making in different domains simultaneously were not synchronous. It was as if the synchronous vocal turn-taking rhythm was functioning as a carrier wave to hold the emerging but not yet established symbolic meaning in our awareness while we worked on it.

Figure 2 begins as I allowed a 4-second pause, while Mattie moved the queen puppet from room to room in a contented way as if taking possession of her new territory, or as if representing in play the exploration of his own or another's bodily spaces. When I said, "But then if she doesn't want to talk, she can just be private, right?" Mattie appeared to like my remark, because, taking up the familiar 2-second pause as well as the theme of "private," Mattie stated, "She can just put the curtains down!" I left a shorter pause, perhaps eager to affirm Mattie's initiative, repeating Mattie's remark again with a slight variation—"Put the curtains down and keep private." Mattie left the 2-second pause again, and this time declared in the celebratory voice of the queen, "Yeah! I can put the curtains down and be private!" I waited a respectful 1-second, before adding a 1-second affirmation.

The sequence diagrammed in Figures 1 and 2 demonstrate a match between us in terms of our implicit choice of symbolic content, but also in terms of the rhythm of our communication, and of Mattie's positive affect and my own. The vocal turn pattern is interesting in that Mattie and I demonstrated two turn-taking patterns—one the 1–2 second (primarily 2-second) pause and turn, and the other the tightly synchronized pattern of leaving no pause between the last speaker's and the next speaker's turns, what Beebe has referred to as representing high intensity and high attunement (Jaffe et al. 2001). It seems as if these two patterns represent two different types of "matches"—the tightly synchronized pattern indicating higher arousal and focused interest and the 2-second pattern a more relaxed, "moving along" pattern (Stern et al. 1989). The match in this 40-second sequence is similar to the "match" sequences of mother-infant play in terms of affect and intention, but it adds a match in the domain of symbolic meaning. Perhaps the highly synchronized pause pattern, which communicates salience, was a way we had of making a choice about what meaning we were going to work on together—something about "private" and the more relaxed pattern indicated the beginning of creating a process for doing that work.

Continuing Therapeutic Process

This match sequence was followed by the next mismatch event. Mattie tried on a kitty puppet but it fell off his hand. He cried out, "Ha! That hurt!" in a falsetto voice. I responded, "Hi, Kitty. You are so soft." It seemed clear that I did not hear Mattie's remark about the kitty being hurt. We made a repair initiated by Mattie, who proclaimed that the kitty's name was "Fuzzy," and I responded, "Fuzzy!" He said, "Mmhm," and I said, "That's a great name." The back and forth of our vocalizations, not illustrated in a figure, recruited the 2-second vocal turn, 2-second pause pattern.

Commentary

Although I missed the communication of the kitty being hurt, we made a repair in the domain of the nonverbal rhythm and the intention of getting back together "on the same page." We were experiencing the same positive affect, even though we missed an opportunity to address the negative affects associated with bodily injury. The missed choice of symbolic content regarding bodily injury is interesting; will we let it drop, or will it return as an option? If Mattie brought the theme back, it would have a more emphatic meaning than at its introduction, because in repeating the "hurt" theme, Mattie would be emphasizing its importance at this time in the treatment.

Continuing Therapeutic Process

There followed another comfortable, "matching" sequence, which seemed to allow for Mattie to risk a mismatch. This was a different kind of mismatch in that it was an internal one, a conflict within Mattie. Immediately after sitting back on his heels and admiring the work he had done, he moved to the couch and picked up the skunk puppet, saying, "Maybe, . . . if there's some room for the skunk." We retained our comfortable regularity in turn-taking rhythm as we entered risky content territory. I asked, "Yeah, where can the skunk go?" He had placed it between the kitty and turtle. Mattie remarked hesitantly, "But skunks . . ." He shrugged. Keeping up the same pattern, I finished his thought, "Mmm. They have bad smells, right?" He nodded and said, "But anyway let's make him a chair at the table." I agreed, "Let's make him a place at the table, OK." Mattie added, as he moved to place more tiles, "Everybody needs to eat." I agreed, saying, "I approve of that. Everybody needs to eat, skunks too." In that way, the carrier wave of our nonverbal rhythm supported Mattie's risk of introducing a theme of aggression—that we didn't pick up in the kitty falling (bodily injury often associated with aggression)—and allowed us to include its representation in the form of the smelly skunk into our play.

This led us to another step forward, as Mattie introduced other characters, first a hedgehog, who admired the tower and called it "magical," invoking the positive and even curative qualities of the magician. Mattie then took another risk in introducing a set of doll's house dolls. In a pretend voice, he cautioned the little boy doll not to "let anybody steal him," adding, "It's against the law!" an admonition Mattie had used in the first session to indicate the forbidden act of going beneath the queen. In the sloppiness of the process, I initiated a mismatch by suggesting a connection between the first session and the current play, asking whether it is against the law to be underneath the queen. He corrected me, explaining that it was against the law to *steal children*: "No, to be near here" . . . "stealing the children." "Oh, you mean somebody might steal the children?" Mattie nodded, "Mmhm." I said, "That's pretty scary." We have brought the theme of loss into the foreground again but with this frightening elaboration.

After a pause in which Mattie did not say anything, I asked again, "What did he say was against the law?" (I was trying to clear up the communication in the first session, which I was guessing has something to do with a combination of Mattie's sexual curiosity and his impulsivity). Mattie gave me a direct gaze and asked, "What did he say?" I responded, "Yes, he said something was against the law." Mattie answered, "It was just against the law because people can take people." I completed the repair, finally realizing that right now Mattie did not want to talk about whatever it was in the first session that was against the law. "Oh, people can take people, I see."

The final sequence of the session included Mattie shaking all the doll's house dolls out of the bag, including Fisher Price dolls that have holes in the bottom. He stuck these dolls on his fingers. I identified one boy doll as the one in the first meeting we had remarked to have a mad face. Mattie said, "He'd be like a T-Rex." Then Mattie replaced him with another doll. When I asked what happened to the boy, Mattie said, "He's still in the family," with his gaze averted.

Commentary

This last sequence of therapeutic process illustrates two interesting aspects of mismatch and repair. Both are becoming our characteristic ways of facilitating a repair—one that I frequently use, and one introduced by Mattie. My characteristic manner of initiating or facilitating a repair is to repeat the declaration of my patient with a slight variation, sometimes adding, "Yeah," or "I see." An example is how I tried to recover after my insistence on questioning the "against the law" theme—"Oh, people can take people, I see." Mattie's way of initiating a repair was perhaps more direct. When I pushed for including the boy doll (perhaps representing disavowed angry feelings) in the play, thinking that if the skunk got to stay for dinner, why shouldn't the angry boy get to play, Mattie's response was terse, "He's still in the family." This reminded me of when Mattie stated firmly and dispassionately, "He got it back," about his dad's phone. It is as if he were saying, "Get over it; we're not going in that direction right now." It is a pattern that he and I would use in the future.

We now had a set of symbolic themes only partially elaborated and without clear links to one another. The themes were "private," loss, bodily injury, and aggression. Of course, as a psychoanalyst I am familiar with the linking of aggression to fear of bodily injury and loss, and the theme of privacy suggested to me sexual fantasies, but I did not know for sure, and I knew I must wait for Mattie and me to put them together in our own way. We also were beginning to develop a set of ways of making choices about which symbolic meanings to elaborate and about repairing mismatches when we did not agree about those choices. As you can see by the description of the videotape material, the way these partial meanings were put together, the way Mattie and I made meaning together by negotiating choices about which symbolic content to address at what time, and the way we communicated this to each other through rhythmic turn-taking, facial expression, gesture, tone of voice, and other ways, articulated the "moving along" of the psychoanalytic process.

CONCLUDING REMARKS

Why call these mismatches instead of just saying that I am trying to clarify what a child is telling me about what is on his mind? It is because the notion of mismatches highlights a feature of the therapeutic process that is missing from more traditional conceptualizations. I have tried to demonstrate by videotape analysis that therapeutic process can be seen as made up of an infinite number of small bits of communication creating a continuous flow back and forth between two people as they try to make meaning together, and the bits and pieces of meaning that are communicated constitute small matches, mismatches, or repairs of mismatches in multiple simultaneous domains of meaning—affect, intention, physiological arousal state, motor activity, symbolic meaning, etc.—between the two partners. The creative process occurs primarily in the mismatches, as the two partners search for a way of fitting together the two sets of mismatched meanings. When they are able to "repair" a mismatch, the result is often a more complex and coherent meaning than either of the original meanings. On the other hand, in order to "move along," the new meaning may include an element of constraint (or "defense"), such as in the case of "he got it back" or "stealing people is against the law." In such cases, the moving along process is slowed a little in order to keep on going. Eventually, the constraint may be replaced with another less limiting meaning.

This calls to mind an explanation of aesthetic theory, such as in the writings of the art historian, Meyer Schapiro (1993). Schapiro described the observer's experience while viewing the tympanum sculpture of the pilgrimage church of Souillac (Schapiro 1993). Schapiro explains that the observer brings with him certain expectations (meanings) about the composition of the sculpture, expectations about symmetry originating in other familiar examples of similar sculptures. In viewing the sculpture, the viewer could then experience a dialogic exchange with the art—a conversation of sorts—in which he is confronted by certain dyssynchronies in the composition that disorganize his original expectations (meanings) and cause him to go through a process over time in which he—if he is successful—emerges with a realization of a symmetry at a greater—more inclusive and more complex—level of the sculpture's composition. Coherence can be gained, but only after an active disorganizing and reorganizing process between the viewer and the art, and only if greater complexity is allowed. This explanation of the aesthetic experience is also consistent with the conceptualization of development described in Tronick's DECM (2007).

The second feature of therapeutic process revealed by the concept of match, mismatch, and repair, is that therapeutic process is just one variant, although a specialized one, of the way two individuals try to make meaning together. This process begins in infancy in the infant-parent relationship and continues throughout life. The meaning-making process, according to nonlinear theory, is a necessary part of human life. We humans must continue to make meanings that are increasingly more complex and coherent, if we are to move forward in our development, if we are to continue to live our lives. When we make meaning with another human being we often gain access to greater resources than when we engage in the process alone. A psychoanalyst—skilled and experienced in making-meaning with many different indi-

viduals and at a profound level of emotional and symbolic signification—is a good partner in this process.

Where do we go from here in our study of therapeutic process? The DECM of therapeutic growth and development offers some suggestions. One direction would be in explorations of the various domains of meaning-making that are occurring simultaneously in human exchange. Experiments of physiological "biomarkers" such as galvanic skin response, heart rate, and cortisol measures provide a promising beginning in the study of these complex processes (Liu et al. 2016). More detailed analysis of videotapes of children and adults in psychotherapeutic sessions provides another method of investigation. Many other possibilities exist. Viewing therapeutic process from the perspective of DECM and principles of nonlinear systems theory allows us to recognize both disruption and continuity in patterns of meaning making in relationships from infancy to adulthood while also underscoring the cocreated feature of the meanings that result.

REFERENCES

Beebe, B. and Lachmann, F. (2013). *The Origins of Attachment: Infant Research and Adult Treatment.* New Jersey: The Analytic Press.

Granic, I. and Patterson, G. (2006). Toward a comprehensive model of antisocial development: A dynamic systems approach. *Psychological Review*, 113(1), 101–131.

Harrison, A. and Beebe, B. (in press). Rhythms of dialogue in infant research and child analysis: Implicit/explicit therapeutic action. *Psychoanalytic Psychology*.

Harrison, A. and Tronick, E. (2007). Now we have a playground: Emerging new ideas of therapeutic action. *Journal of the American Psychoanalytic Association,* 55(3), 853–874.

Harrison A. M., and Tronick E. (2011) "The noise monitor": a developmental perspective on verbal and nonverbal meaning-making in psychoanalysis. *Journal of the American Psychoanalytic Association*, 59(5): 961-82. PMID: 21980139

Harrison, A. (2013). The sandwich model: The "music and dance" of therapeutic action, *International Journal of Psychoanalysis,* 1746–8315.

Jacobs, T. (1973). Posture, gesture, and movement in the analyst: Cues to interpretation and countertransference. *Journal of the American Psychoanalytic Association*, 21, 77–92.

Jaffe, J., Beebe, B., Feldstein, S., Crown, C., and Jasnow, M. (2001). Rhythms of dialogue in infancy. *Monographs of the Society for Research in Child Development*, 66(2), Serial No. 264.

Liu, C., Snidman, N., Leonard, A., Meyer, J., and Tronick, E. (2016). Intra-individual stability and developmental change in hair cortisol among postpartum mothers and infants: Implications for understanding chronic stress. *Developmental Psychology*, 58 (4): 509–518, DOI 10:1002/dev.21394.

Pally, R. (2001). A primary role for nonverbal communication in psychoanalysis. *Psychoanalytic Inquiry*, 21(1), 71–93.

Schapiro, M. (1993). *Romanesque Art: Selected Papers, The Sculptures of Souillac* (102–121). New York: George Braziller Inc.

Stern, D., Sander, L., Nahum, J., Harrison, A., Lyons-Ruth, K., Morgan, A., Bruschweiler-Stern, N., and Tronick, E. (1998). Non-interpretive mechanisms in psychoanalytic therapy. *International Journal of Psycho-Analysis*, 79, 903–921.

Tronick, E. (2001). Emotional connections and dyadic consciousness in infant-mother and patient-therapist interactions, *Psychoanalytic Dialogues*, 11(2), 187–194.

———. (2007). *The Neurobehavioral and Social Emotional Development of Infants and Young Children*. New York: Norton.

Chapter Three

Observing Development from Infancy to Parenthood

Separation-Individuation, Attachment, and Intersubjectivity in the Clinical Encounter

Inga Blom

A woman sits nervously on the floor, legs crossed, head oriented downward, but often glancing at the room around her and the others in it. She speaks, rapidly then haltingly, her voice a bit shaky and uncertain and inflected with attempts to downplay her emotions. She is talking about her baby, the four-month-old who is moving about with some vigor on the colorful mat in front of her. The baby too looks at the face of his mother hovering above, and then to the scene beyond their space, his neck active in rotating his head and his arms and legs jolting outwards, sometimes in jerky bursts and sometimes in slow stretching movements.

The mother speaks about her wishes and fears, for herself and her baby, who seems both like a stranger and an extension of herself. Uneasy and uncertain about her decisions, she is hoping for the approval of the others in the room. At the same time, she is fiercely protective of ideas around what babies need and what babies do. She feels compelled to weigh in when others talk, yet is nervous about how people will respond to the things she says out loud.

A new mother, Serena, sits slightly separately from others in the group, quiet but watchful of others. She gazes longingly at the small baby in front of her, and hangs off the words of the other mother who is talking about painful thoughts, but remains quiet and skeptical of the scene in front of her. At times, she appears to disappear inside herself, her face stone still, even as her baby squeaks and rustles in front of her. At other moments, she is transfixed

by her baby, a smile hanging off her lips. These transformations seem independent of the scene in front of her. It is hard to know if her expressions connect to what is being said around her.

This description represents a composite of experiences working with new mothers and their babies, in private practice and clinic settings, in individual, dyadic, and group treatments, as well as reading hundreds of written observations and watching reels of film from the Master's Children's Center in New York City. It also represents experiences on the playground, in various mommy-and-me groups, and navigating the first years of motherhood as a therapist and a mother myself. My understanding of Serena and her experiences as a new mother is informed by the circumstances and theory of Margaret Mahler's research on normal child development, and many years studying Attachment Theory, with its gold-standard assessments and cross-cultural roots. This chapter will revisit the fundamentals of Margaret Mahler's Separation-Individuation Theory in the context of subsequent decades of research on infant development, nonverbal communication, attachment theory, and clinical work with mothers and babies. I will elaborate Separation-Individuation Theory at some length, given its disappearance from most reading lists and increasingly marginalized status outside psychoanalytic institutes. A discussion of two cases will demonstrate the utility of an integrative approach to understanding the dramatic, yet often invisible (or not consciously observable), dynamics at play during the birth of a mother and her baby.

As a clinician and researcher, Mahler came of age at a critical period when babies, and their caregivers (mothers), were capturing attention across a range of disciplines. Some of the groundbreaking work of the 1950s and 1960s was built on psychoanalytic principles put forth by Sigmund Freud, and the developmentally oriented observations of Rene Spitz and Jean Piaget, but while many of the pioneering baby-watchers paid homage to these works, each theorist's work and ideas developed in relative isolation from the others, for reasons to do with geography, discipline, and politics (national and psychoanalytic). It is wonderful to consider the ways in which integrating perspectives like Attachment Theory and Separation-Individuation Theory can enhance each other's scope and impact.

Mahler's desire to understand what happens in "normal development," which emerged after she spent years helping children and families in extreme circumstances, brought us into the everyday, mundane details of the life of a new mother and her new baby. This most pivotal and fundamental time and space had largely escaped scholarly attention until Mahler, and then Anna Freud, Winnicott, Bowlby, Ainsworth, and their students treated it as a starting point to understand development and its sequelae in their communities and around the world. Certainly psychoanalysts had privileged the inner life of babies, but much of what had been understood of the early mental life of babies came from retrospective theorizing from the couch, with little consid-

eration for the body of the baby and the mind of the mother (e.g., Freud, Klein) and certainly without much thought devoted to the social or cultural circumstances of the family. That is, unless there were problems in development, which were then seen as a reflection of poor mothering. In the decades that followed, an abundance of game-changing research, by Trevarthan, Meltzoff, Stern, Jaffe, Beebe, Bowlby, Ainsworth, and Fraiberg, for example, showed us the amazing nuance and power of the peripartum period, and completely changed the clinician and lay person's understanding of mothers and babies, as mothers and babies became the focus of intervention, and more recently prevention.

It is important to recognize how profoundly different the landscape was in the 1940s and 1950s, given the current preoccupation with pregnancy and parenthood that has seized much of the Western world. And interesting to note that it was the phenomenon of separations, big and small, that initially compelled both Mahler and Bowlby to focus on early childhood. In her early career as a pediatrician, Mahler was fascinated by dramatically different outcomes for sick children in two hospitals where she worked. In one, young children often died during hospitalization, and in the other they tended to go home: the main difference seemed to be rules around whether mothers and parents were allowed to be with their children in the hospital. This experience set in motion a lifelong pursuit of understanding what the early mother-child relationship does for development, the circumstances that lead to optimal, less optimal, and pathological development.

Separation-Individuation Theory emerged gradually from a research setting that would be unheard of today (Mahler, Pine, and Bergman 1975). The Masters Children's Center (MCC) was supported with funding from the National Institutes of Health for many years, and provided a treatment setting for disturbed children (where Mahler's Tripartite method was developed) as well as an observational research setting to understand the vicissitudes of normal development in as much detail as possible. It was one of only a few places that prioritized "a situation where the spontaneous day-to-day relationship of mother to child could be observed in a natural setting" (Mahler et al. 1975, p. 23) as the basis for investigating psychological and developmental phenomena. Babies and their mothers could attend daily, and were typically observed several times a week, often over the course of several years. Observations were supplemented by interviews with both parents, home visits, psychological testing, and developmental assessments. Participant and nonparticipant observers were assigned to each family, and daily observations were recorded and transcribed, and then discussed in regular meetings with Mahler and the entire staff. When technology allowed, babies and mothers were filmed. There were no instructions for time spent at the MCC, other than imposing separations when mothers were taken for regular interviews by research staff. The theory developed from there. Overall, almost forty babies and their mothers attended the MCC as part of the research into normal development.

Separation-Individuation Theory was developed by Margaret Mahler and a team of clinical researchers that included prominent clinicians such as Anni Bergman, Fred Pine, and John McDevitt. Other members of the team included individuals with backgrounds in child development. Pediatricians did regular developmental assessments and psychologists evaluated mothers and children. While Mahler always held an uneasy relationship with classical drive theory and ego psychology (Ainsworth 1969), Separation-Individuation Theory is also an early proponent of object-relations theory, focusing on the mother-infant pair as the basic, defining foundation of psychological development, and prioritizing the relationship as something that is internalized and that guides experiences of self and other. Like Bowlby, although certainly less so, Mahler also privileged the impact of biological processes as well as the temperamental characteristics of the baby, such that the unfolding of mental life is based on the quality of interactions between the infant and his caregivers, which are influenced by biology, environment, and family history. This further differentiates Separation-individuation Theory from other early psychoanalytic conceptualizations of early mental life, which minimize or reject the impact of situational and environmental factors. Separation-Individuation rests on the belief that all aspects of early development, including visual, tactile, and psychomotor skills, are integral to cognitive and emotional life. As a theory of early development, Separation-Individuation Theory uniquely sets the stage for making sense of experiences of self and other throughout childhood, adolescence, and beyond, and particularly during periods marked by identity changes and reorganization of roles.

Serena and the other mothers in the baby group, as well as the mothers at the MCC, show us that it is possible to think of new parenthood as a time when separation-individuation concerns reemerge as front-and-center dynamics in the birth of the parent, as they also unfold in the infant. Problems in infancy and early childhood contribute to problems in parenthood, as the "successful" parent must come to recognize the baby, in thoughts and behavior, as a separate being with his own experiences (Slade 2005). The new mother ideally achieved object-constancy through a loving and predictable early life, which sets the stage for her own transition to parenthood—ideally she has also engaged in a mutually satisfying partner relationship, in a reasonably good environment, that supports her and her baby, and any difficulties in her own separation-individuation process do not interfere with her ability to help her child achieve the milestones that define this process. Mahler and attachment theorists would agree that a mother's overall state of mind in regards to attachment is typically consistent over time, even in undesirable circumstances–but what can change, especially in the context of attachment insecurity and environmental instability, is her ability to delight in her child, to understand her child, and to sustain adequate attunement, i.e., her caregiving behavior. A mother's anxiety, depression, or past trauma can also get in the way (Mahler et al. 1975). Bowlby and Mahler also agree that predictability is critical for optimal development, and this is especially true in regards to a mother's predictable, flexible, and generally appreciative stance toward her infant. In the context of "good-enough" mother-child relationships, in which a mother is equipped to respond sensitively to her child's development much of the time, intrapsychic development proceeds smoothly along predictable lines, and eases later transitions, for example to parenthood. A number of studies have demonstrated the intergenerational transmission of early experiences (Fraiberg, Adelman, and Shapiro 1975; Steele & Steele 1998; van IJzenzoorn & Bakermans-Kranenberg 1997). Aspects of the separation-individuation process inform the process of entering motherhood, the emerging relationship between baby and mother, and the achievement of developmental milestones that belong to capacities that were identified later, such as the capacity for mentalization (Reflective Function).

The concepts fundamental to Separation-Individuation Theory will be elaborated next.

SEPARATION-INDIVIDUATION THEORY

Separation-individuation refers to two separate but overlapping developmental processes through which an infant gradually achieves a sense of self that is distinct and unique from others and the ability to function as an autonomous individual. Separation more specifically refers to an intrapsychic process of boundary formation, in which a baby establishes itself as separate from mother. Individuation is the formation of psychic boundaries that allow an individual the capacity to form thoughts, ideas, and experience independently from the reality of another person—or, more simply, self-representations that are distinct from object representations. Mahler repeatedly emphasized that "the biological birth of the human infant and the psychological birth of the individual are not coincident in time. The former is a dramatic, observable and well-circumscribed event; the latter a slowly unfolding intrapsychic process." (Mahler et al. 1975, p. 3).

Thus, development is a process, and while each child moves through early life via similar processes and trajectories across various modalities, there is a range of typical, normal behavior that occurs over a variable time frame (like A. Freud's developmental lines). Further, as the infant develops and changes, so must the mother adapt from a mother of an infant-in-arms to a mother of a toddler and so forth, and thus has her own parallel developmental process that might elicit a range of different capabilities, according to her circumstances and how they interact with experiences from her own childhood. Much of what unfolds occurs outside of awareness for both mother and infant.

Separation-Individuation Theory has been critiqued for Mahler's assertions regarding "the forerunners of the separation-individuation process," namely the symbiotic and normal autistic phases (e.g., Stern). In keeping with her time, Mahler stated that the neonate existed in a state of merger, an existence governed by physiological needs and defined solely by the mother's qualities and behavior (Mahler et al. 1975). The basic tenets of the "Normal Autistic" and "Symbiotic" phases of development are that physiological processes dominate over psychological ones, and that the baby experiences itself as in a state of undifferentiation from the mother.

These notions now read as quaint. We know a lot more about the first few months of life, and how action-packed they are. This includes how biologically wired human beings are for interactions, for a social existence that includes self-regulation, even in utero (e.g., Beebe 2014). Nowadays we might be more comfortable describing this period in terms of a state of mutual regulation, or overlapping coregulatory processes (e.g., Beebe, Lachmann, Feldstein, Crown, & Jasnow 2000). At three to four months of age, rather than emerging from a state of merger, infants have participated in achieving a nuanced emotional life; they can have a sense of themselves as understandable and knowable, and form expectations of others as available and similar-but-different. Likewise, they can also experience disturbed/distorted information processing and affective incongruence, inconsistent strategies vulnerable to alexithymia, dissociative disorders and behavioral issues. Mahler herself revised her stance based on subsequent research (e.g., Pine 1994; A. Bergman 2008), and focused on the intense intimacy that binds mother and infant at this time, perhaps like Winnicott's primary maternal preoccupation, which has been supported by subsequent research (Urdang 2016). Regardless of Mahler's errors, her appreciation for each baby's "drive," which includes basic or innate aggression as an organizing force in moving development forward, is valuable (Mahler 1971, 1981). Mahler's theories have been further critiqued by many of her advocates and detractors (e.g., Lyons-Ruth 1991; Gergely 2000; Beebe & Lachman 2002) as insufficiently acknowledging relational/intersubjective aspects of development and experience, and for appearing to normalize problematic behaviors or overvalue independence. I believe that it is possible to create a more collaborative space for many of these apparent differences, which could fill volumes of writing (e.g., Olesker & Steele, unpublished manuscript). For now, suffice it to highlight Mahler's focus on physiological development as influencing/influenced by the psychological, which was unusual for her time, and perhaps more importantly, the attention she paid to what was happening in the mind of the mothers, who figured prominently in recorded observations, and who were interviewed at regular intervals, even if she did not elaborate on this in her recorded theory. She was very much interested in how specific aspects of the relationship between the mother and her child set the stage for the development of the self and object constancy, and how they carried forward into adulthood.

SUBPHASES

There are four overlapping phases that make up separation-individuation, building on each other, so that adequate development in one is the foundation for adequate development in the next.

Differentiation and the Development of the Body Image

The differentiation subphase marks the beginning of psychological birth. Physiological development ushers in the primacy of sight and touch as growing capacities that organize the infant's experience, and as cornerstones of the development of a separate and consistent experience of self and other. The infant's whole body is involved in differentiating self-mother-not/mother in the world. This recalls Freud's position that the ego is "first and foremost a bodily ego" (e.g., Mahler & McDevitt 1982; Tyson 1992). The appearance of the infant's "hatched look" signals the arrival of differentiation around four to five months of age. Hatching is observed in the infant's increased alertness and orientation to the specific aspects of mother and the outside world, and discriminating responsiveness to stimuli. He now has a reservoir of "memories," of a caregiver who comes and goes, as well as pleasurable and unpleasurable experiences, small or big. Until now, the infant carries vague representations of significant caregivers when they are not immediately engaged in his care. By the end of this phase, the infant has achieved the precursors for object constancy, such as object permanence, a representation of mother that informs his experience even in her absence.

These developments are evident in the infant engaged in "customs inspection," whose hands wander painstakingly over the mother's face and objects that belong to her, who stretches to reach for things, and appears transfixed by his own fingers. Self and other touching builds the awareness of body boundaries. Cognition and emotion, beginning with distinguishing familiar from unfamiliar, and discrimination between various kinds and sources of stimulation and excitement, are increasingly unmistakable in the baby's behavior.

Similarly, preferential smiling refers to the infant's special smile that is reserved for mother, which ideally helps to sustain her focus and interest in her child's subtle behaviors and communications. The mother selectively responds to her child's cues. Together, they work out a system of predictable signals and responses. Peekaboo emerges now, and at first a passive observer, the infant becomes an active initiator of endless sequences of the game.

Also during this time mothers stake claim to an understanding of their children's experiences, needs, and intentions that is unavailable or unknowable to anyone else. Thus, the extent to which the mother can appropriately respond to her infant's increasingly individualized needs, as separate from her own, has a lasting impression on her infant's subsequent developmental tasks. The infant's development can be hastened, delayed, or complicated by his mother's particular ministrations, and separation and individuation can be affected differently. For example, a mother's distractibility or depression can hasten separation out of sync with individuation, compromising basic trust and the capacity for self-confidence.

As differentiation gives way to practicing, the infant has gained a sense of his own body as distinct from other bodies and objects, which he can direct toward specific aims and purposes. A specific bond with mother is evident in separation (and stranger) anxiety that occurs when mother moves beyond reach, and when the infant is confronted with unknown people. He has the tools to engage important others, like smiling and other gestures, and can associate objects with caregivers, especially mother.

Practicing

The hallmark of the practicing subphase is the infant's "love affair with the world." Around 10 or 11 months the infant becomes enamored with his own omnipotence and gleefully occupied with mastering his world, repeating sounds and motions that increase in complexity as new skills emerge. Early practicing is ushered in when, through a range of locomotor activities, the infant can move himself away from mother. The mother's emotional availability is ever paramount, but her physical proximity must be balanced against the need for exploration. Manuel Furer coined the term emotional refueling (Mahler et al. 1975) to refer to the normal infant's tendency to check in with mother, at first through touch, later through sight and offering objects.

Exuberance is characteristic of practicing, as the increasingly agile child is excited by his own abilities and his world. The infant's focus on mother, and things associated with her, spills over onto the world beyond. At this time, children are rather impervious to stumbles and pains. At times they are also oblivious to mother. Many caregivers during this time find themselves chasing after toddlers, who appear to have no sense of potential mishaps. Walking has enormous significance for development.

The extent to which a child is able to excitedly and confidently go out into the world depends, in part, on a foundation of basic safety provided by the mother, and the child's expectation of mother's availability. At this age, children develop the capacity for more complex representations of self, mother, and a hierarchy of other important caregivers. Stranger anxiety can intensify, and separations, even brief ones, can require careful navigation on the part of both mother and child. Mahler and her team often observed a state of low-keyedness, a subdued withdrawal from the environment that arises with the knowledge that mother is not at hand. This can signal that the child's internalized mother is available to him, even in her absence.

If a child experiences this phase with worry—that mother will be disapproving, will disappear, or be disappointed—this can have a damaging effect on his capacity to negotiate the environment and establish a sense of security. A mother who, on balance, communicates expectations, and confidence lays the foundation for self-esteem and the child's capacity for autonomy, separateness and competence throughout life. The capacity of the mother to sustain attunement and availability during this time will also more immediately influence the tremendous changes that Separation-Individuation Theory identifies in the second year of life.

Rapprochement

The central task of the rapprochement phase is for the toddler to master ways to manage conflicting experiences, emotions, and desires. Put differently, the rapprochement child is often caught with the dilemma of what he wishes to do and what his capabilities are, between a drive to independence and a desire for help from mother or others. Colloquially, this is known as the "terrible twos," although aspects of rapprochement can occur well before a child's second birthday, and intense struggles with autonomy and dependency are often easy to see in a three-year-old.

As the child actively experiences new things and new people, the exuberance of the practicing subphase gives way to painful knowledge of limitations, a wish to move further out into the world alongside knowledge of dependence. Misunderstandings and frustrations between mother and child are expected during this period; typically a mother is perplexed by her previously cheerful child's sudden neediness and demands for attention. Emotionally and cognitively the infant's representation of mother is also being renegotiated as he is able to sustain increasingly complex impressions over longer time periods, and positive and negative experiences of self and others are a source of confusion and conflict.

The ability of mother and child to recognize each other as distinct individuals with separate needs and desires, that are often complementary and often quite opposite, is an essential achievement. Toddlers must also contend with the unmistakable fact that their mother's attentions are needed and demanded elsewhere, and mothers must adjust to infants' abilities to master tasks on their own.

The mother's continued emotional availability from the infant's perspective is especially important during rapprochement. Availability is not the same as immediately meeting a child's needs and complying with demands. It is ideal for a mother to meet, understand, and solve her child's dilemmas with success in "midrange" as with so much else in early development. Mothers necessarily fail at times, or other things are more important than gratifying a child's needs, and an important task for the child is the capacity for frustration tolerance and delayed gratification.

The rapprochement crisis is the pinnacle of this time: the height of the toddler's new demands for managing frustration and integrating conflicting mental representations with adequate modeling by the mother. The way that the infant negotiates this has reverberations throughout life. Optimally, the child's anger, sadness, frustration, or disappointment does not compromise the representation of an otherwise loving and available mother. In less than optimal circumstances, the child's uncertainty regarding competence versus dependence, good versus bad other, separation and merger, persists and inhibits self-and object-constancy that would permit a flexible and satisfying engagement with the world.

On the Way to Object Constancy

Object constancy as Mahler defined it is very complex. It is both an achievement of early development and an ever-shifting goal that is never fully achieved: "the establishment of a sense of separateness from, and relation to, a world of reality, particularly with regard to the experiences of one's own body and to the principal representative of the world as the infant experiences it, the primary love object . . . is never finished." (Mahler et al. 1975, p. 3). By his second birthday, a child has more sophisticated strategies for existing as a separate individual in his own world, and for managing pleasure and anxiety on his own. From a different but parallel perspective, the child has achieved some capacity for autonomous affect regulation. Thus object constancy is also a measure of self-constancy.

The defining feature of object constancy is the achievement of an internalized representation of a fundamentally good and loving image (of the other) that provides the child a sense of safety and positive regard, just like his actual mother hopefully had. This representation is the basis of a lot of psychological functioning, including many cognitive capacities. The optimal relationship in infancy, and throughout life, is a balance of closeness and independence, and this develops out of a particular interactional history. The child who has internalized an available/predictable caregiver can engage in his environment with flexibility and find ways of meeting developmental needs across contexts. When the capacity for object constancy emerges from a sufficiently loving internalized representation of self and other, development should proceed relatively smoothly, and life's obstacles can be met with a degree of resilience. The internalized object representation of mother provides the infant with information about himself, as lovable or valuable or essential.

At this point, a fair amount of overlap with Attachment Theory and other contemporary perspectives on early childhood is hopefully obvious. For example, the concept of "emotional refueling" is a central feature of the concept of a "secure base" (Bretherton 1992). The mother's thoughts and feelings about herself-as-mother and her baby influence how her baby develops along motor, cognitive, interpersonal, intrapsychic domains. Other points of overlap have been described elsewhere in greater detail (Blom 2009; Blom & Bergman 2013). Overall, Mahler knew about Bowlby and others' work on the effect of brief and prolonged early separation on the developing child (Robertson & Robertson 1971; Bowlby 1973). She appreciated separation in basic terms, as an unavoidable and often frequent fact of life, in that separations accompany many interactions and daily activities (A. Bergman, personal communication, May 2008). Thinking about separation in that way, separation-individuation meets Attachment Theory at the point where the accumulated experiences of these separations, usually "minor" and momentary, although at times prolonged, but essentially unavoidable, define the quality and influence of the interaction between mother and child, and contribute to the infant's emerging understanding of both the self and mother as separate entities (Stern 1985). Separation-Individuation Theory emphasizes that both caregiver and child influence interactions and development, and also does not hold the mother responsible for everything that is both positive and/or negative in early experiences. Further, it emphasizes that the quality of the interaction between caregiver and child influences myriad aspects of social and relational development, including affect regulation, self-esteem, peer relationships, and psychopathology throughout life.

In line with evolutionarily based principles of Attachment Theory, and the microanalytic work of Beatrice Beebe, separation-individuation holds that the infant in his own right is highly participatory/influential in the development of the relationship with the primary caregiver in his own right. Because of the painstakingly nuanced research of people like Stern and Beebe in subsequent decades, we now also understand the specific ways in which togetherness and separation/separateness are predictably negotiated as early as four months of age (differentiation), and the strategies available to the baby to navigate his own emotional needs in the face of his mother's more-or-less predictable capacity for engagement. Like Mahler, Bowlby, and Winnicott in earlier decades, Beebe's research confirms that, even in the first few months of life, the optimal circumstance is one in which there is a midrange of coordination and in the modes of communication available to a mother and baby (vocal, touch, facial affect) (Beebe & Lachmann 2002).

Separation-Individuation Theory did not explicitly address the impact of what is in the mind of the mother on the experience of her child—of what becomes in the mind of the child. Mahler et al. (1975) certainly considered a mother's mental state as intricately wound up in the nuances, the day-to-day successes and failures, of psychological development. Regular interviews in which mothers and fathers were asked about their thoughts and experiences were central to how Separation-Individuation Theory developed. Mahler noted that a mother's wishes for her child can hasten or delay specific and nonspecific aspects of development. For example, a mother who relishes the closeness of a dependent lap baby may struggle with a determined toddler. Mothers can be more or less suited to their children, and more or less able to contend with specific developmental periods. Their data highlighted how adequate separation/separateness may be sacrificed while individuation proceeds. But they did not, could not have, offered specific ways of examining these potentialities in clinical situations (or other nonclinical ones). These considerations can be understood, nowadays, from the perspective of mentalization (Slade 2005) and the mother's ability to separate her own wishes, thoughts, needs, desires, from what her baby's might be. But at the time, as revolutionary and nuanced—and painstakingly data-bound—as these ideas were, they were limited by the extent to which they can be generalized. This may be one reason why separation-individuation has faded outside of psychoanalytic institutes.

As Mahler sought to capture development as it occurred in a nonclinical context, it bears emphasizing that normative developmental phenomena are not synonymous with ideal developmental phenomena. "Mahler's interest was less on the optimal circumstances for development of the self and more on the internal forces driving the toddler toward the realization of the separate self, even in circumstances of less than optimal availability of the mother" (Bergman & Harpaz-Rotem 2004, p. 561). Thus, Separation-Individuation Theory is a framework for understanding a wide range of phenomena in early childhood and beyond, that may be more or less adaptive or problematic. Much like the three main attachment organizations, Secure, Dismissing/Avoidant, and Anxious/Ambivalent, each represents an organized and adaptive system for managing attachment-related information and maximizing interpersonal experiences in a range of experiences (Main 2000).

SUBSEQUENT RESEARCH AND CURRENT RELEVANCE

There are a lot of avenues for considering the contemporary relevance of Separation-Individuation Theory and Mahler's legacy. Clinicians, mostly psychoanalytic, and often European, continue to use her concepts to guide conceptualization and technical considerations in work with children, adolescents, adults, and older adults. These include Blos's (1967) classic writings on separation-individuation in adolescence, Colarusso's (2002) writings pertaining to older adulthood, and Olesker's (e.g., 1998, 2011) ongoing exploration of the fluctuations and impact of early dynamics throughout development. These concepts have relevance in clinical work that has carried them forward, in spite of challenges in systematic evaluation and refinement of Separation-Individuation Theory—over the years, this has usually been on a case-by-case basis (e.g., Bergman & Fahey 2005; Kramer 1992; Olesker 1984; Tyson 1992). Nonetheless, Mahler's body of work remains one of the few systematic, comprehensive, and longitudinal evaluations of early development, examining what happens day-to-day, and how early experiences affect how we know ourselves, others, and resonate throughout life. In fact, this research is ongoing (e.g., Blom 2009).

Clinical researchers such as Beebe and Stern have worked tirelessly to examine and expose the minutiae of the baby's experience, and bring the life of the baby into the realm of adult treatment. Beebe and Lachmann (2002) conceptualized the long, intricate, and dramatic case of Burton, which was supported by Burton's own independent written account of his treatment with Beebe, largely in the language of Mahler and her peers, only to rewrite it and question the value of their original formulation. Nonetheless, it is not clear that Beebe and Lachmann's reconceptualization from a theoretical standpoint means that the actual work should have proceeded much differently (Olesker, personal communication, September 2015). Beebe embarked on this treatment firmly rooted in the perspective of Separation-Individuation Theory and related theories, and by all accounts the work was successful.

Bergman and Harpaz-Rotem (2004) write "the mother with the child creates a narrative about the child, about the mother, about their being together. This narrative is woven into the child's emerging representation of the self and the outside world. The mother takes on the new role of organizer into language of her child's affective life" (p. 564). They emphasize the role of separation-individuation in moving experience to the "level of representation," to use attachment terms (Main, Kaplan, & Cassidy 1985). Mahler "established a developmental framework for the first 3 years of life in which the developing drives, affects, object relations, cognitive and other ego functions could be understood and related" (Tyson 1996). While her work has receded from contemporary work on child development, it remains unique and uniquely relevant.

Aggression

Attachment theory and other contemporary research has helped elucidate the role of early experiences, and specifically the mother/child interaction, on emotional life (experienced emotions, expressed emotions, emotion regulation), but Mahler paid attention to important aspects of the role of affective experience in development in ways that other perspectives have neglected. Her work on understanding the role of aggression may be particularly worth reconsidering, given the immense difficulty that the appearance of aggressive urges and impulses can present to parents, especially those struggling with their role, and those who find their past intruding into the present. Mahler spoke about aggression, if permitted and tolerated, as something that moves development forward—it is an important driver of the separation-individuation process (Mahler 1981). Mahler also recognized the immense difficulties that can arise if the child's aggression is intolerable, threatening to the mother, or if the mother's aggression is not recognized, tolerated, or is too central a feature of the interactions, as will be seen in the case examples below. Certainly prior to Mahler aggression was recognized as important in the development and maintenance of psychopathology, and decades of research have clarified its role in attachment disorganization (Beebe, Lachmann, Markese, & Barhrick 2012), depression, personality pathology, anxiety, and a number of other psychiatric difficulties. It is less common to consider the positive, necessary role of aggression in early development and emotional life.

Aggression is thus an important consideration in conceptualizing and intervening in mother-child issues and treatments, where experienced or repressed aggression plays a central and pivotal role in most, if not all, cases. Aggression is a central concern in the cases discussed below, either as it is experienced as part of the self, emanating from others, in the form of intrusive thoughts, or concerns about living up to expectations and meeting disapproval. In addition to promoting understanding of normal displays of aggression in infants and young children, it is important to help adults identify and tolerate their aggression, to recognize it, and organize it in the therapeutic relationship in ways that may not have been done in early childhood, and to encourage the new mother to embrace aggression or aggressiveness as, if not desirable, then at least an expectable element in development and the mother-infant relationship.

The Body

In their recent paper, Fotopoulou and Tsakiris (2017) "ask" whether the self is primarily more bodily or social in origin, and bemoan the perceived neglect of the body in much of psychoanalytic theorizing in recent decades. While their highlighted philosophical debates are beyond the scope of this chapter, from a practical and clinical perspective this is certainly one area where Mahler's work can reclaim significance, and offer a bridge between foundational concepts of the past and the concepts of today. Fotopolou and Tsakiris's main goal is to place the body at the heart of mentalization, a concept that currently has the power to unify disparate psychological theories and practices. They emphasize the importance of homeostatic mechanisms on subjective experience, on the capacity to experience, and prioritize bodily states as the essential building blocks of mentalizing functions. Likewise, Mahler operated from Freud's premise that "the ego is first and foremost a bodily one." In Separation-Individuation Theory, the mother's body functions as a central and organizing presence for the baby, who should be allowed to explore it as an extension of his own body (customs inspection), and who should use it as a beacon of safety and familiarity when engaged in exploration (secure base). The mother's body and baby's body are inseparable for the purposes of the earliest in utero and postpartum experiences, and baby and mother experience increasing body boundaries through various biological and social processes. Just as separation-individuation occurs psychologically (at the level of representation) it should occur physically, so that the baby (via the mother's parallel experience) comes to know mine-not-mine and me-not-me. Relative comfort with, or concern over, physical closeness in all elements of baby care—feeding, dressing, bathing, sleeping—are central preoccupations for new mothers, often taken up in polarizing ways in popular culture—for example, around cosleeping, breastfeeding, baby-wearing. When this is disturbed or complicated, clinically significant problems arise.

Mahler's initial theorizing on the state of "merger" between mother and baby places the body of the baby and the mother at the center of the self and other. The separation-individuation process starts with a baby-mother whose physiological states are intertwined and interdependent—not merged but not separate, as the baby, in the process of differentiation, comes to increasingly recognize the not-me and his own body boundaries. The body is central in Mahler's work.

This is important for clinical work. There are many ways in which our patients experience their bodies as theirs/not theirs. For example, a patient experiences moments of depersonalization and derealization whenever she is reminded of her physical resemblance to her abusive mother. How new mothers experience the physicality of pregnancy and new motherhood, the sudden separation of the new baby from their internal bodily experiences and the ways they can feel more or less separate, after the baby is born are all important elements of the mother's and baby's interpersonal and intersubjective experience.

I will turn to two examples to illustrate elements of the separation-individuation process and its reverberations in adulthood, while integrating an attachment perspective to understand the experiences and presentations of two different women.

CASES

By most criteria, Sara and Serena come from disparate backgrounds, economic circumstances, and sociocultural eras. They are united by intelligence, curiosity for complexity and learning, and determination to achieve a stable and enjoyable family life. Furthermore, their experiences and capacity for meaningful and fulfilling relationships, with spouses, friends, and their children, have been imperiled by problems in the separation-individuation process, likely starting with differentiation, so that they each embody aspects of a dismissing attachment style. Important relationships are reduced to transactions or occasions to revisit their own childhoods, and their inner life and experiences in the world are bound to their early relationships with their mothers in a way that reflects a lack of successful individuation, and poor object constancy. Under times of distress, there are moments of poor body boundaries—experiences when their own and their mother's bodies are intertwined.

Explicitly, Sara and Serena value relationships and desire to give their children experiences of acceptance and closeness that they never experienced themselves. But these (conscious) intentions are derailed by ways of relating and communicating that are defined by anxiety, depression, anger, merging, and preoccupation with their own mothers. Smolen (2017) writes, "the infant brain is shaped by its early experience in the world of relationships. Children who are afraid of their caregivers, or cannot rely on them, cannot learn to trust. They often have grave difficulties in loving and accepting love. These children learn to protect themselves by avoiding or resisting others" (p. 211). In Sara's case, data from the MCC and follow-up testing, interviews, and therapy sessions in adulthood show how Sara's mother's difficulty tolerating aggression while actively promoting it, her detached emphasis on Sara's motor achievement at the expense of physical/emotional closeness, and Sara's lack of pleasurable engagement with her mother/others contribute to poor self-esteem, and difficulties establishing enjoyable and trusting relationships with others. As Mahler predicted in the early 1960s, Sara came to have a relationship of hateful dependency with her mother that carried forward into adulthood and defined her own experiences as a mother. Serena's early experiences of neglect and rejection contribute to lifelong interpersonal difficulties, extreme loneliness, persecutory preoccupations, and help-rejecting behaviors. Interestingly, both women exemplify the lack of memory, including poor specificity of autobiographical experiences, that characterize many Adult Attachment Interviews (AAIs) of dismissing adults (Main 2000).

With Sara and Serena, intervention focused on providing a space for each woman to reflect on her perceptions and expectations of others, gently challenging assumptions and asking "why" things seemed as they did, and "what" had indeed happened. In both cases there was a struggle to move beyond superficial descriptions of experiences, and create and sustain an account of the contents of therapy sessions, between sessions, and from one week to the next. Each woman was both invested in the process of self-exploration and also resistant/ambivalent to the therapeutic relationship and the challenges it presented to their existing narrative. In the therapy, transference represented a return to earlier attachments, one idealizing and one derogatory.

Case: Sara

Sara attended the MCC with her mother and sister for several years. Sara's early life has been studied in depth, and described in various contributions to writings on Separation-Individuation Theory, including a mixed-methods investigation into how the early experiences of babies observed in the MCC were represented in adulthood via the AAI and other measures (Blom 2009).

From infancy, Sara's mother expressed concerns about "spoiling her," and early on described her as stubborn, with a temper, and that she is "a good child except when she is cross." At the same time, she minimized her own role in infancy, emphasizing that not much has an effect as "there is no communication in the first year anyway." She took pride in Sara's early motor achievements, praising her independence while expressing frustration that Sara needed her so much. In over eighty pages of observations of Sara from the time frame that coincided with rapprochement, aggressive behavior is the most coded behavior, which was a unique feature of Sara's observations relative to the seven other children studied this way (see Blom [2009] for an explanation of coding procedures). Other behavioral patterns that stood out from that time included her tendency to seek out substitute adults more often when her mother was present than when her mother was absent. There were often frantic efforts at mastering various tasks, for example riding a tricycle. While Sara was observed engaging in behaviors that were directed at obtaining and maintaining contact with her mother, she was often not successful. Sara's aggression gave her mother the opportunity to stay close to her daughter and monitor her behavior, and gave Sara the chance to demonstrate her strength and keep her mother close and attentive in some way. While Sara's mother was observed at times to "enjoy" her daughter, and specifically to enjoy her aggressive nature, there was little indication that Sara derived pleasure from interactions. Her emotions were subdued within a restricted range.

When Sara was approximately 21 months of age Dr. Bergman described that her mother "commented in a sort of distant way about what Sara was doing . . . the mother talks about Sara rather than to Sara, or that maybe even when she talks to Sara, it seems as if she talks about her." Sara's mother was generally "pleased with her child's development" but exuded anxiety and lack of confidence in her daughter's presence, especially in the face of her daughter's "asking her to put limits on her" through acting out. Sara's mother could intellectually understand that Sara's oppositional behavior was an appeal for structure and attention, but putting this into practice did not come easily. This discrepancy between what she said and what she did was often described by the observers to whom Sara's mother would turn for help with Sara's difficult behavior at home and at the center; additionally, over the course of this time frame, Sara's mother was described as being surprised when Sara responded quickly and easily to other adults putting clear limits on her aggression. Sara's mother tried to "differentiate what she truly wanted for Sara and what she wanted for herself" but nonetheless put "a tremendous premium on reasoning behavior on the part of her child, in an effort to negate and deny and avoid her daughter's aggression." Thus Sara received mixed messages about the appropriateness of her behavior and about meaningful ways of relating. At one point Sara's mother told an observer that she wanted Sara to be a person who could stand up for herself and therefore did not want to suppress her aggression.

Sara's observations were coded with more "possible abuse" codes than the other children. While no clear abuse was described, aside from an occasional slap of her hand in punishment, her mother's poorly controlled frustration was a frequent topic of commentary. For example, one observer noted that "the tension in her body as she stands over Sara might lead one to wonder if she is not prepared to hit her rather than to help her." This blurry boundary between affection and aggression, real contact, and connection based in anger, was a prevalent aspect of Sara's early capacity for object constancy. Her main attachment figure was attentive and invested, but ambivalent about her parental role.

Many more details can be offered about Sara's early life, but these hopefully highlight a mother-child relationship that while close and attentive, was largely defined by maternal ambivalence that included overinvestment in achievement alongside fury at being depended on for so much, and uncertainty/concern for her capabilities that was masked by sweeping pronouncements. Sara worked hard to please her mother, and thankfully was an intelligent and capable child, but nonetheless developed rigid representations of self and other (object constancy) in which lovability was defined by achievement and negative affect was to be avoided, minimized, and externalized, with corresponding anxiety over safety, stability, and dependability.

As an adult, Sara's AAI was rated as dismissing, and her narrative was given high ratings on idealization and derogation, and maternal behavior was rated as highly rejecting and moderately loving. Thus, overall, Sara's interview was characterized by her use of strongly positive language to describe her relationship with her mother without much evidence to back it up. In fact, attempts at demonstrating the "close," "loving" and "warm" experiences of her childhood were marked by excessive dysfluences, and only one specific memory of being helped in college, which was meant to highlight her mother's "intuitive" support that was "always spot on." She was exceptionally anxious throughout the interview, clearly struggling with her wish to present a positive account of her attachment experiences. Nonetheless, in her interview she talks about "separation anxiety" as a child and adult, positioning it to reflect the strong bonds she has with her mother, and how hard she works to emulate her mother in her own relationship with her children. Sara calls her mother daily for advice on just about everything. Her mother weighs in on every major family decision, often staying in the family home for weeks on end on a whim. Sara experiences any family issues or difficult experience by her children as a reflection of her own difficulty living up to the gold standard set by her mother. Her relationship with her own children is fraught with conflict and fears of their underperforming or not living up to their intellectual potential. She has few relationships outside of her family, and has distanced herself from a high level of professional success. With her own entry into parenthood came a relinquishing of interests and activities that brought her into contact with the world beyond her family, a scenario that her mother had discussed with bitterness decades early, but nonetheless one that Sara seemed determined to replicate. Overall, Sara's follow-up material showed problems with separation that are self-reported and evidenced by inability to create a separate life, alongside problems with individuating, as specific aspects of her childhood experiences were reenacted between her and her own children.

Sara eventually sought treatment for help with strengthening family bonds. From one week to the next there is little carry over, as new ideas and insights seem to disappear in the service of sustaining a positive narrative of her own childhood experiences at the expense of her own agency, positive self-regard, interests, and abilities. After some time, with a lot of gentle questioning and encouragement, facilitated by an idealizing transference, Sara starts to entertain new ideas about her experiences and risk making her "own" choices and decisions.

Case: Serena

Serena first presented for treatment before her baby arrived. Therapy and psychiatry had long been a feature in her life, although most treatments and interventions had been unsuccessful at reducing symptoms and interpersonal distress in a meaningful way, and were experienced by Serena as unsatisfying if not dangerous. Serena reported that most clinicians did not get her, and she experienced them as reductionistic and hostile. Unsure of her own abilities and preoccupied with a sense of personal failure, Serena usually perceived others as stupid and opportunistic. As a member of a multiracial family, these experiences were often compounded by the systemic racism and prejudices of her day-to-day environment.

Depressive symptoms loomed large in daily life, including poor energy, lack of motivation, social isolation, and poor self-care. Serena was also easily irritated, although that was often masked with an impassive, almost frozen face, or a biting retort said with a smile. Serena recognized that there were aspects of her childhood that were not optimal, but either had "no memory" of specific experiences, or provided superficial and overly generalized responses to questions about relationships and events, whether major or minor. She could not name emotions or describe reactions to clearly distressing experiences—bullying, rejection, abuse—but these topics elicited experiences of being judged and rejected in the transference, along with increased irritability or tearfulness. Serena was adept at finding and obtaining new opportunities for personal and professional growth, but she experienced interactions with others in very black-and-white terms, and initially positive connections quickly turned into experiences of harassment and rejection.

Serena approached motherhood with excitement and trepidation, determined to provide her baby with a safe and secure experience that would "allow her to be her own person" while worrying that "my own issues will interfere." A clearly articulated motivation for treatment did not translate into thoughtful, reflective engagement in the tasks of therapy or the tasks of motherhood, however, as Serena often reverted to relying on extended family members for support and advice, even as they continued to disappoint her and she attempted to distance herself from her childhood experiences with them.

Serena came to therapy with her baby, who was adorably dressed, growing well, and generally meeting expected developmental milestones. In session, Serena attended to her baby in a perfunctory way if she fussed or sought contact, but otherwise would engage as she had before motherhood, as if we were the only two in the room. She read books and blogs on parenthood, but preferred those that advocated for minimal contact and "interference" with her baby. The idea of being needed sent her into a tailspin of intense self-criticism and emotional lability. Impressions and incidents of childhood rejection often jumped into her mind in session, and she could easily be preoccupied with the feelings of rejection and failure they evoked, disappearing into herself with a blank look and then lashing out. Furthermore, she minimized the value of therapy and often referred to the expertise of others while devaluing my own directly or indirectly. Periodic attempts to find ways out of therapy were nonetheless halfhearted and quickly abandoned.

There is much to explore in these brief vignettes of Sara and Serena, and the ways in which my understanding of Sara and Serena is defined by appreciation of separation-individuation processes, attachment, and intersubjectivity on the way from infancy to parenthood.

Sara and Serena are invested mothers. They made an intentional choice to become parents, with the goal of providing a safe and enjoyable childhood experience, and wanting their children to avoid the pitfalls of their own early experiences.

However, in becoming mothers, they have each been pulled back into memories and dynamics from their own childhoods in ways that feel inescapable, and sometimes frightening. Their felt experiences with their children are defined by the dynamics of their relationships with their mothers, and often thoughts, feelings, and decisions regarding interactions with their children are determined by what their own mothers did/did not do in the past and are/are not doing in the present. They struggle to think, act, and feel as separate from their mothers, as mothers in their own rights, with their own wishes, intentions, priorities, and beliefs. As parents, their own attachment systems are activated which lead them to seek safety and security from attachment figures who failed to adequately serve those functions in the first place and certainly fail in the present, making it seem impossible for them to engage with their own children, and establish a safe and secure base for them. Their object constancy/self-constancy was characterized by poorly integrated and conflicting representations in which self-sufficient mastery was valued over closeness and at the expense of pleasurable connections, and in the context of these new roles their sense of themselves and others is rigid, conflicted, and at odds with their conscious recollections and wishes for experiences with their children.

Sara and Serena worry that their children "hate them," that their children perceive them as inadequate and deficient. Likewise, they are on alert for signs of aggression or disproval in their children that would confirm their suspicions of themselves, and how they believe their mothers see them. What they perceive and how things are interpreted is shaped by how hyper-attuned they are to some things, and how well they defensively exclude other things from their awareness.

Furthermore, nonverbal communication was always at the forefront of interactions with Serena. In particularly stressful moments, she would perceive the other (clinician, coworker, partner) as making derogatory statements about her. Moving lips and minimal changes in facial expressions or gestures would be co-opted into these projections, that were often unbearably hurtful and insulting. These extreme projections—previously diagnosed as psychotic elements of a bipolar disorder—dissipated over time, but the tendency to experience important others as rejecting and judgmental did not.

Ultimately Sara and Serena find a space in treatment where these beliefs and experiences, about themselves and their mothers, can be examined and evaluated, albeit slowly and carefully. Treatment is often disrupted by life events, competing priorities, or anxiety or depression in some way. But they persist, and over time they continue to develop a clearer sense of themselves as separate from their mothers, and a stronger capacity to think, feel, and behave according to their present circumstances, with a better understanding of their experiences and ability to appreciate the thoughts, feelings, intentions, and behaviors of their children from a developmental perspective.

Discussion

The first year of life is a time of tremendous growth and development, and much of what happens sets the stage for subsequent growth, transitions, experiences in relationships and capacity to engage with the environment. "Good enough" separation-individuation and achievement of object constancy means a fundamentally positive view of oneself and others which allows for the flexibility of thinking and experiencing that permits subsequent growth and learning. Attachment security is discussed in similar terms. All of these achievements mean that the child/individual does not need to rely on defenses that exclude, minimize, or otherwise manage information from the environment to maintain a sense of security, closeness, and love.

The journey to motherhood is also a time of tremendous growth and transition, a time when childhood experiences and dynamics can reemerge in ways that can be experienced as exciting, comforting, discomfiting, and frightening. These days those involved in caring for women during pregnancy and women themselves increasingly recognize pregnancy as a time to engage in professional interventions, particularly psychotherapy, as using medication or other interventions to cope with changes in mood and anxiety are particularly complicated and often controversial. Nowadays mother-baby groups are a fairly common feature of the early postpartum period, as new mothers gather to compare stories and perspectives on childrearing. Forums can be community-based, offered by clinical settings, or some combination of both. Mommy blogs, podcasts, and social media offer a dizzying array of platforms for the latest "parenting" strategies and assertions on the right choices. I wonder what today's new parents would make of a time or place where mother's experiences were taken for granted and the idea of examining and evaluating parenting "practice" and "choices," of finding importance in the nuances of the mundane, was a revolutionary idea.

As Beebe (2005) notes, there are currently many good modalities for promoting psychological change during the perinatal period, including dyadic therapy, psychodynamic psychotherapy, cognitive-behavioral approaches for PMADs, and group interventions, that have demonstrated positive outcomes. She cites, among others, Brazelton (1994); Cramer et al. (1990); Fraiberg (1980); Hofacker & Papousek (1998); Malphurs et al. (1996); Murray & Cooper (1997). Women are often surprised to find themselves grappling with elements of their childhoods that seemed to be long gone, and thinking/behaving in ways that betray their intentions. Additionally, women are often unaware of the ways in which their engagement with their infants reflects limits or unresolved concerns of their childhoods. It is common for new mothers (new parents!) to feel torn between a sense of allegiance to the ways of their childhoods, to uphold the practices of their own caregivers even if they differ from the current values and priorities. In their classic article, Fraiberg, Adelson, and Shapiro (1975) wrote about the ghosts in the nursery that can intrude in very destructive ways, as happened with Serena. Serena's mother's voice, her words, her subtle and not-so-subtle forms of rejection intruded into her moment-to-moment experiences and actions; she could not function as a separate person. There are also less obvious ways in which elements of separation-individuation can complicate the experience of motherhood. As a smart, successful, middle-class professional, Sara too found herself pulled into old habits, compelled to uphold her mother's stated beliefs and replicate her actions. In the throes of motherhood, her difficulties with individuation became particularly apparent. Sara and Serena's internal world, the ways they processed information from their environment, and certainly their experiences of their children, were defined by qualities and problems in the separation-individuation processes.

As caregivers, their mental representations of attachment-related experiences—their capacity for object constancy—influenced how autonomously they functioned with their own children, and undoubtedly the extent to which they could attend to and respond to their own children. George and Solomon (2008) write about the caregiving system from a systems perspective, as a system that overlaps with but is also separate from the attachment system. They explore various things that contribute to caregiving and various influences on parental behaviors, while highlighting that caregiving is still an under researched area. Internal working models of attachment influence representations of caregiving and caregiving behaviors, as has been repeatedly demonstrated by the intergenerational transmission of attachment status. At the same time, there are transmission gaps, as when a child is found to have a different attachment organization from their parent, and when siblings demonstrate different attachment organizations (van IJzendoorn 1995). The specific ideas, experiences, or fantasies a mother can have toward her child, based on that child's temperament, biological sex, likeness, etc., along with social factors, and the quality of her other relationships, can all enhance or interfere with caregiving, in ways that adjust or reinforce attachment-related experiences and representations. Even the circumstances of childbirth can have a huge impact on a woman's transition to motherhood, independent of having a healthy baby, and the kinds of things from her past that get activated (Beck 2004). While childbirth and marital satisfaction appear to have minimal influence on attachment organization and specific caregiving behaviors, they can certainly influence a mother's experience and a child's experience of his mother. Serena's induction and ultimate c-section occurred in a context that reinforced her expectations of rejection and powerlessness in the face of authority, leaving her feeling helpless and humiliated. These were experiences that she referred to repeatedly in psychotherapy sessions, and in interactions with peers in various forums. These experiences intensified, at least in the immediate aftermath, her belief that her body was not fully her own, that it was the property of a spiteful and abusive other, and interfered with her ability to engage her baby with her own body in ways that she had intended to, for example through breastfeeding. The cacophony of voices weighing in on the innumerable decisions that arise in days, weeks, and months postpartum were invariably experienced as critical, and Serena had trouble knowing her own thoughts and feelings.

Likewise, the baby comes armed with his own inclinations and tendencies, and ability to flexibly engage with a mother and be satisfied, which influences and is influenced by his self-regulatory capacities. I am referring here to the concept of emotional refueling that occurs for both mother and baby, and concepts of self-contingency and interactive contingency that continue to be refined by Beatrice Beebe in the decades since Mahler and Bowlby did their groundbreaking work.

An essential aspect of entering parenthood is "making a shift away from *seeking protection and proximate care from attachment figures* (the function and goal of attachment for the child) to *providing protection, comfort, and care for the child* (the function and proximate goal for the parent)" (George & Solomon 2008, p. 4; italics in original). Separation-individuation thus influences the caregiving system, specifically the extent to which a new mother can focus on her infant, and engage fully with her mind and body according to her own inclinations, versus internalized aspects of her own separation-individuation experiences, when aspects were not achieved, unresolved, are complicated. Separation-individuation concerns reemerge as parenthood approaches, influencing the qualities of perceptions, behaviors, actions and decisions, affecting the flexibility required to accurately perceive and experience in the present, versus defend and exclude to maintain or preserve aspects of the past that were essential for adequate emotional adaptation. The qualities that define a parent's capacity for object constancy define a sense of self, the experience of the mind of the self (as separate from), the mind of the parent, and ultimately the mind of the baby—in other words, one's self-reflective or mentalizing capacity (Fonagy, Steele, & Steele 1991).

There are of course many more factors that influence the caregiving environment than the attachment system, and these other factors can serve to reinforce old ways of being or make space for new ones. Secure attachment tends to allow for the best possible scenario given the circumstances, simply because of the flexibility it permits, while insecure attachments are maintained by defenses that manage what is perceived and how experiences are interpreted. Although the mother has the greater capacity and range of resources, the infant is a very active participant in this exchange, bringing remarkable capacities to seek and avoid engagement (Beebe & Lachmann 2002; Beebe & Stern 1977; Stern 1971, 1985; Tronick 1989). This emphasis on the contribution of both partners to the organization of the exchange avoids the temptation to locate the source of difficulty in only one partner or aspect of the mother-infant, caregiving scenario.

In my work I hope to explore and demonstrate what Separation-Individuation Theory has to say about development and developmental process in adulthood. It also offers a framework for understanding and working with new parents. The Separation-Individuation Theory can also provide a language and framework for making sense, in a clinically useful way, of the unevenness of development, especially in suboptimal situations, and for bridging the concepts fundamental to Attachment Theory with the world beyond the attachment system. Attachment and Separation-Individuation Theory have fundamental underpinnings and goals in common (Coates 2004; Fonagy 1999; Steele & Steele 1998). Referring to Separation-Individuation Theory, Settlage and colleagues (1991) stated that "attachment theory research and psychoanalytic developmental research have thus come to share a focus on the process of psychic structure formation in the context of early parent-infant interaction" (p. 1006). Ongoing work into the important overlap between systems and psychoanalytic perspectives continue to yield important insights into development and clinical concerns. Certainly amazing things have been uncovered about the nuances and lifelong impact of early development and the intricacies of mother-child interactions, in the decade plus since I first sat in Anni Bergman's office and immersed myself in the thousands of pages of data from the MCC. Several times a year accomplished board members of the Margaret S. Mahler Foundation for Child Development gather to plan conferences, share ideas, and focus on supporting clinically important research and community initiatives. Hopefully there will continue to be a theoretically rich and clinically useful application of Mahler's, and her collaborators', years of painstaking attention to the moment-to-moment and day-to-day interpersonal and intrapsychic experiences of everyday families.

REFERENCES

Ainsworth, M. D. (1969) Object relations, dependency, and attachment: A theoretical review of the infant-mother relationship. *Child Development*, 40(4), 969–1025.

Beck, C. T. (2004). Birth Trauma: In the eye of the beholder. *Nursing Research*, 53(1), 28–35.

Beebe, B. (2005). Mother-infant research informs mother-infant treatment. *Psychoanalytic Study of the Child*, 60(1), 7-46.

———. (2014). My journey in infant research and psychoanalysis. *Psychoanalytic Psychology*, 31(1), 4–25.

Beebe, B., Jaffe, J., Lachmann, F., Feldstein, S., Crown, C., and Jasnow, J. (2000). Systems models in development and psychoanalysis: The case of vocal rhythm coordination and attachment. *Infant Mental Health Journal*, 21(1–2), 99–122.
Beebe, B. and Lachmann, F. (2002). *Infant Research and Adult Treatment*. Hillside, NJ: Analytic Press.
———. (2014). *The Origins of Attachment: Infant Research and Adult Treatment.* New York: Hove, Rutledge.
Beebe, B., Lachmann, F., Markese, S., and Bahrick, L. (2012). On the origins of disorganized attachment and internal working models: Paper I. A dyadic systems approach. *Psychoanalytic Dialogues*, 22(2), 253–272.
Beebe, B. and Stern, D. (1977). Engagement-disengagement and early object experiences. In N. Freedman and S. Grand (Eds.), *Communicative structures and psychic structures*, (pp. 33-55). NY: Plenum.
Bergman, A. and Fahey, M. (2005). Observations and representations of the earliest relationship: A view from separation-individuation and attachment. In S. Akhtar and H. Blum (Eds.). *The Language of Emotions: Development, Psychopathology, and Technique* (pp. 139–150). New York: Jason Aronson.
Bergman, A. and Harpaz-Rotem, I. (2004). Revisiting Rapprochement in the light of contemporary developmental theories. *Journal of the American Psychoanalytic Association,* 52, 555–569.
Blom, I. (2009). *A Longitudinal Study Evaluating Early Observations and Representations of Relationships: Separation Individuation Theory and Attachment Theory in a Qualitative Approach*. New York: The New School University.
———. (2017). Separation Individuation. In A. Wenzel (Ed.). *The SAGE Encyclopedia of Abnormal and Clinical Psychology.* Thousand Oaks: SAGE Publications, Inc.
Blom, I. and Bergman, A. (2013). Observing development: A comparative view of attachment theory and separation-individuation theory. In J. E. Bettman and D. D. Friedman (Eds.). *Attachment-Based Clinical Work with Children and Adolescents.* New York: Springer/Verlag.
Blos, P. (1967). The second individuation process of adolescence. *Psychoanalytic Study of the Child*, 22, 162–186.
Blum, H. (2004). Separation-individuation theory and attachment theory. *Journal of the American Psychoanalytic Association*, 52, 535–553.
Bowlby, J. (1973). *Attachment and Loss: Separation.* New York: Basic Books.
Brazleton, T. B.(1994). Touchpoints: Opportunities for preventing problems in the parent-child relationship. *Acta Paediatrica*, 83(39), 35–39.
Bretherton, I. (1992). The origins of attachment theory: John Bowlby and Mary Ainsworth. *Developmental Psychology,* 28, 759–775.
Coates, S. W. (2004). John Bowlby and Margaret S. Mahler: Their lives and theories. *Journal of the American Psychoanalytic Association*, 52, 571–601.
Colarusso, C. (2000). Separation-individuation phenomena in adulthood: General concepts and the fifth individuation. *Journal of the American Psychoanalytic Association*, 48, 1467–1489.
Cooper, P. and Murray, L. (1997) The impact of psychological treatments of postpartum depression on maternal mood and infant depression. *Archives of Disease in Childhood,* 77, 99–101.
Cramer, B., Robert-Tissot, C., Stern, D. N., Serpa-Rusconi, S., De Muralt, M., Besson, G., Palacio-Espasa, F., Bachmann, J., Knauer, D., Berney, C., and D'Arcis, U. (1990). Outcome evaluation in brief mother-infant psychotherapy: A preliminary report. *Infant Mental Health Journal*, 11(3), 278–300.
Fonagy, P. (1999). Points of contact and divergence between psychoanalytic and attachment theories: Is psychoanalytic theory truly different? *Psychoanalytic Inquiry*, 19, 448–480.
Fonagy, P., Steele, M., and Steele, H. (1991). Maternal representations of attachment during pregnancy predict the organization of infant-mother interaction at one year of age. *Child Development*, 62, 891–905.
Fotopoulou, A. and Tsakiris, M. (2017). Mentalizing homeostasis: The social origins of interoceptive inference. *Neuropsychoanalysis*, 19(1), 3–28.

Fraiberg, S. (1980). *Clinical Studies in Infant Mental Health: The First Year of Life*. London: Routledge.

Fraiberg, S., Adelman, E., and Shapiro, V. (1975). Ghosts in the nursery: A psychoanalytic approach to the problems of impaired infant-mother relationships. *Child and Adolescent Psychiatry and Mental Health,* 14, 387–421.

George, C. and Solomon (2008). The caregiving system: A behavioral systems approach to parenting. In J. Cassidy and P. R. Shaver (Eds.). *Handbook of Attachment Theory: Theory, Research and Clinical Application* (2nd Ed.). New York: Guilford Press.

Gergely, G. (2000). Reapproaching Mahler: New perspectives on normal autism, symbiosis, splitting and libidinal object constancy from cognitive developmental theory. *Journal of the American Psychoanalytic Association,* 48, 1197–1228.

Hofacker, N. G. and Papousek, M. (1998) Disorders of excessive crying, feeding and sleeping: The Munich interdisciplinary research and intervention program. *Infant Mental Health Journal*, 19(2), 180–201.

Jaffe J., Beebe B., Feldstein S., Crown C. L., and Jasnow, M. D. (2001). Rhythms of dialogue in infancy: coordinated timing in development. *Monographs on Social Research in Child Development*, 66(2), 1–132.

Kramer, S. (1992). Nonverbal manifestations of unresolved separation-individuation in adult psychopathology. In S. Kramer and S. Akhtar. (Eds.). *When the Body Speaks: Psychological Meanings in Kinetic Cues* (pp. 1–19). Northvale: Jason Aronson.

Lyons-Ruth, K. (1991). Rapprochement or approchement: Mahler's theory reconsidered from the vantage point of recent research on early attachment relationships. *Psychoanalytic Psychology,* 8, 1–23.

Mahler, M. (1971). A study of the separation-individuation process and its possible application to borderline phenomena in the psychoanalytic situation. *Psychoanalytic Study of the Child*, 26, 403–424.

———. (1981). Aggression in the service of separation-individuation: Case study of a mother-daughter relationship. P*sychoanalytic Quarterly*, 50, 625–638.

Mahler, M. S., and McDevitt, J. (1980). The separation-individuation process and identity formation. In S. J. Greenspan and G. H. Pollock (Eds.). *The Course of Life: Psychoanalytic Contributions toward Understanding Personality Development* (pp. 395–406). Bethesda: National Institutes of Mental Health.

———. (1982). Thoughts on the emergence of a sense of self, with a particular emphasis on the body self. *Journal of the American Psychoanalytic Association,* 30, 827–848.

Mahler, M. S., Pine, F., and Bergman, A. (1975). *The Psychological Birth of the Human Infant*. New York: Basic Books.

Main, M. (2000). The organized categories of infant, child & adult attachment: Flexible and inflexible attention under attachment related stress. *Journal of the American Psychoanalytic Association*, 48(4), 1055–1095.

Main, M., Kaplan, N., and Cassidy, J. (1985). Security in infancy, childhood and adulthood: A move to the level of representation. In I. Bretherton and E. Waters (Eds.). (2009). *Growing Points of Attachment Theory and Research (Monographs of the Society for Research in Child Development)*, (pp. 66–104). Hoboken: Wiley.

Malphurs, J. E., Field, T. M., Larraine, C., Pickens, J., Palaez-Noguera, M., Yando, R., and Bendell, D. (1996). Altering withdrawn and intrusive interaction behaviors of depressed mothers. *Infant Mental Health Journal*, 17(2), 152–160.

McDevitt, J. B. (1980). The role of internalization in the development of object relations during the separation-individuation phase. In R. F. Lax, S. Bach, and J. A. Burland (Eds.). *Rapprochement: The Critical Subphase of Separation-Individuation* (pp. 407–424). New York: Jason Aronson.

Murray, L. and Cooper, P. J. (1997). *Postpartum Depression and Child Development*. New York: Guilford Press.

Olesker, W. (1984) Sex differences in 2- and 3-year-olds: Mother-child relations, peer relations, and peer play. *Psychoanalytic Psychology*, 1(4), 269-288.

———. (1998). Conflict and compromise in gender identity formation: A longitudinal study. *Psychoanalytic Study of the Child*, 53, 212–230.

———. (2011). The story of Sam: Continuities and discontinuities in development. Transforming into and out of a perversion. *Psychoanalytic Study of the Child*, 65, 48–78.

Pine, F. (1994). Mahler's concepts of "symbiosis" and separation-individuation: Revisited, reevaluated, refined. *Journal of the American Psychoanalytic Association*, 52(2), 511–553.

Robertson, J. and Robertson, J. (1971). Young children in brief separation: A fresh look. *Psychoanalytic Study of the Child,* 26, 264–315.

Settlage, C. F., Bemesderfer, S., Rosenthal, J., Afterman, J., and Spielman, P. M. (1991). The appeal cycle in early mother-child interaction: Nature and implications of a finding from developmental research. *Journal of the American Psychoanalytic Association*, 39, 987–1014.

Slade, A. (2005). Parental reflective functioning: An introduction. *Attachment and Human Development,* 7(3), 269–281.

Smolen, A. (2017). Mothering without a Home: A psychoanalytically-informed approach. In T. Seitler and K. Kleinman (Eds.). *From Cradle To Couch: Essays in Honor of the Psychoanalytic Developmental Psychology of Sylvia Brody,* New York: IPBooks.

Steele, H. and Steele, M. (1998). Attachment and psychoanalysis: Time for a reunion. *Social Development*, 7, 92–119.

Stern, D. (1971). A microanalysis of the mother-infant interaction. *Journal of the American Academy of Child Psychiatry*, 10, 501–507.

———. (1985). *The Interpersonal World of the Infant*. New York: Basic Books.

Tronick, E. (1989). Emotions and emotional communication in infants. *American Psychologist*, 44(2), 112–119.

Tyson, P. (1991). Psychic structure formation: The complementary roles of affects, drives, object relations, and conflict. In T. Shapiro (Ed.). *The Concept of Structure in Psychoanalysis* (pp. 73–98). New York: International Universities Press.

———. (1992). The challenges of psychoanalytic developmental theory. *Journal of the American Psychoanalytic Association*, 50, 19–52.

———. (1996). Object relations, affect management and psychic structure formation: The concept of object constancy. *Psychoanalytic Study of the Child*, 51, 172–189.

———. (2005). Separation-individuation, object constancy and affect regulation. In S. Akhtar and H. Blum (Eds.). *The Language of Emotions: Development, Psychopathology and Technique* (pp. 69–82). New York: Jason Aronson.

Urdang, E. (2016). *Human Behavior in the Social Environment: Interweaving the Inner and Outer Worlds.* 3rd Ed. New York: Routledge.

van IJzendoorn, M. J. (1995). Adult attachment representations, parental responsiveness, and infant attachment: A meta-analysis. *Psychological Bulletin*, 117, 387–403.

van IJzendoorn, M. J. and Bakermans-Kranenberg, M. H. (1997). Intergenerational transmission of attachment: A move to the contextual level. In L. Atkinson and K. J. Zucker (Eds.). *Attachment and Psychopathology* (pp. 135–170). New York: Guildford Press.

Winnicott, D. W. (1956) Primary maternal preoccupation. In *Collected Papers: Through Paediatrics to Psycho-Analysis*. London: Tavistock, 1958.

Chapter Four

Gender Fluidity and Analytic Fluidity

Gabriel Ruiz

Defining "transgender" as a point of inception contextualizes how psychoanalytic theory can inform technique in the consulting room. *Webster's Dictionary* (2017) defines transgender as "someone who identifies with or expresses a gender identity that differs from the one which corresponds to the person's sex at birth." The National Center for Transgender Equality (2017) defines transgender as:

> A term for people whose gender identity, expression or behavior is different from those typically associated with their assigned sex at birth. Transgender is a broad term and is good for non-transgender people to use. "Trans" is shorthand for "transgender." (Note: Transgender is correctly used as an adjective, not a noun, thus "transgender people" is appropriate but "transgenders" is often viewed as disrespectful.)

In recent psychoanalytic literature, transgender is defined as "individuals who identify as a different gender regardless of any hormone treatments aimed at transitioning to the opposite sex" (Lament 2014). Beyond these anchoring yet concrete definitions is Judith Butler's work (1988), which sees gender identity as performative. In her words: "Gender reality is performative, which means quite simply that it is real only to the extent that it is performed"; and, ". . . an identity instituted through a stylized repetition of acts. Further, gender is instituted through the stylization of the body and, hence, must be understood as the mundane way in which bodily gestures, movements, and enactments of various kinds constitute the illusion of an abiding gender."

As can be inferred, Butler takes gender beyond the static and concrete to the dynamic and socially constructed. In this model how do we know our identity at any level, including gender? We do not know by looking in the mirror or by what a physician has designated on our birth certificate. We know by the nature (irony of this term) of how we act in and upon the world. Our series of actions creates a self-body-other relationship which constantly informs and reinforms our sense of gender identity. The dialectic of transgender as defined by the National Center for Transgender Equality and Judith Butler becomes a useful bridge to psychoanalytic thinking.

Additional analytic writers have discussed various issues of working with transgender patients. No conversation is more vibrant than when speaking of children and adolescents. While there exists intense debate over the use of hormonal treatments to block secondary physical characteristics for children identifying as transgender, it is beyond the scope of this chapter, which is focused on clinical psychoanalytic theory.

One central analytic model of gender identity development considers both a child's constitution and their lived history, including traumas endured, as crucial factors for clinical consideration (Coates, Friedman, & Wolfe 1991). Another quintessential thinker in this dialogue, Ehrensaft (2014), relies on Winnicottian (1965) concepts of self, creativity, play, and the facilitating environment. Fortuitously, these models guide Ehrensaft's thinking as she advocates "learning from the patient" and "not knowing" in order for the patient to consolidate a "True Gender Self." Perhaps Ehrensaft's most pithy statement on clinically working with gender nonconforming children comes when she says, "Like any other process of discovery, gender exploration is a long and careful endeavor, interweaving the conscious and the unconscious, the psychic and the social, the social and the cultural. This is not a one-person operation on the part of the child. Rather, it is a relational process between child and adult, interweaving thoughts and feelings." The purpose of this approach is to keep open and fluid the process of "gender creativity." In crystalline fashion Ehrensaft describes a model involving an in-depth and long-term process that includes ongoing parent sessions in the fostering of a child's optimal development of identity.

Knight (2014) adds complexity to gender theory, reminding us to keep a nonlinear model of gender identity development in the background, while holding the child's everyday reality in the foreground. Knight conveys that clinically we should consider issues from the child's neonatal medical/hormonal exposures to early familial dynamics, including how gender was thought about, engaged, and mobilized within the family system at both conscious and unconscious levels. Knight recommends analytic frequency and intensity to offer the appropriate and most ideal treatment for children who are working through "core self" identity, which is constantly in flux.

Most psychological models include both nature and nurture aspects of development, but Brinich (2014) extends this dialectic to prenatal and even preconception stages, all the way through death, when it comes to gender identity. This is in concert with Knight's model of development (2014), which suggests taking a nonlinear approach to both psychological development and analytic technique in our work with patients. One could say this is a modern-day Freudian version of "repeating, remembering, and working through" of gender fluidity that, like the depth of dreams, is infinite.

Perhaps the most evocative voice comes from Harris (2011), who sees dichotomizing gender as a defense against psychological loss of control akin to "some borderline structure." Harris's conceptualization of the "radical" level of psychoanalysis converges with Ehrensaft (2014) and Winnicott (1965) in terms of "not knowing" and listening to the Unconscious in subjective and social worlds.

Framed by "not knowing" and listening for the "inaudible," I now present a clinical case followed by psychoanalytic formulation of a transgender female patient over the course of ten year and twice per week psychotherapy (Harris 2011).

CASE OF LORI

Lori, in the beginning, went by the name "Lawrence." I will now refer to Lori as Lawrence, until the shift occurred and she began to self-identify as a transgender female. This allows me to present this case in "real time." Lawrence was referred to me by another therapist who had worked with him as a child doing cognitive behavioral therapy. The therapy was focused on helping him stay "on task" and complete school work despite testing at a high intelligence level.

Lawrence's mother contacted me reporting he had been in group therapy for attention-deficit/hyperactivity disorder (ADHD), as well as having sporadically been on psychiatric medication since age six. She was ambivalent and unsure about adding "another therapist," me. During my first in-person contact with both parents, they described Lawrence as a very smart and "nice" boy. Yet the parents described Lawrence as always seeming a bit "disconnected," at times finding him "odd." In the father's eyes, this was why Lawrence had very few friends. The mother, in particular, wished for Lawrence to have more social connections, be less awkward in general, and be more academically organized.

The first time I met Lawrence, he seemed anxious, walking with an awkward gait and sitting at the very edge of my couch. I even worried he would fall off as I began to listen. He immediately asked what the "goals and tasks" were to be accomplished. This felt rehearsed and ingrained, and I took great care to not answer specifically and keep the process open for my patient. Although Lawrence felt concern and anxiety over the "openness" of our sessions, over the initial year, he also seemed relieved and comforted that there existed a "place for my mental stuff" and a time to talk about being "out of rhythm." Lawrence gradually found in me an object that could be of "use," consciously and unconsciously, on his terms.

By the second year of treatment Lawrence had come out as being a gay male. He requested my help in coming out to his parents. We spent several sessions sorting through the various meanings and expectations about holding a family session where Lawrence could come out to them. Eventually, Lawrence and I concluded that such a family session was the best possible option, given it would provide a holding environment for all family members. Subsequently, we met with parents in a session where Lawrence told them that he was gay. Lawrence was twelve years old at the time. His mother was surprised, but relieved that this new information seemed to help "explain a lot" in hindsight. The father, however, became enraged and blamed me for "making" Lawrence gay.

During the third year Lawrence, now thirteen, began to explore his sexual attraction to boys, as well as connecting with other gay and lesbian students at school. I had continual contact with the school, which seemed supportive in dealing with gay and lesbian students and their families. During this year Lawrence worked through various transference issues, primarily seeing me as a "father" who would be judgmental, angry, and simply "not get it." The following session is representative of the issues being engaged during this phase of the treatment:

> L: Hi, I just talked with my advisor about dropping Phys Ed and maybe taking it this summer, but I don't know, if I do that then I have to take two classes this summer to stay on track, and I would like to work and finally make some money. You know, I met some more guys from LGBT today. They seem all right, and were all like welcoming and stuff.
>
> G: Must have felt pretty good.
>
> L: It did, yes, I remember going to other group things and feeling like, "okay, this is not my crowd," but with them it was okay, pretty good. I was thinking it was going to be all talking about being gay or something, but we just hung out in the art room and had pizza. Our sponsor did say we had to come up with some kind of project for the year. I don't think we got that far; kind of just wanted to socialize. The president said next time we have to get some ideas down for sure. I'm liking it, but still kind of weird because I came out a while ago and most everybody knows, but I am not going to go up to every single person at school and say that I am gay. So when they see me walk into the room, some people seemed surprised like they did not know already. I don't know.
>
> G: Part of you wonders what people think when they learn you are gay?

L: No, well maybe? I mean, who cares what they think right?

G: It would be okay if you did wonder.

L: I just want them to get it, and be cool about it. Not that anyone has not been at school. No one really gives me a hard time about it, and the kids who do, well I wouldn't want to hang out with them anyways. But still to have to announce or wear a sign that says I'm gay should not be what I have to do. I mean what would you think if you did not know I was gay and saw me go to the group?

G: How would it be helpful to know what I would think?

L: Well you have known me a long time and probably have an idea about me being gay? So come on what would you think? No question to my question, man.

G: I think you are struggling with whether I am really okay with it, like some of your friends where it makes no difference, or whether I am like some people in your life who judge you in their minds and don't see you for you.

L: I like the friends I've made this year. They mean a lot to me. I don't think I realized how much I care about them. It's the first year I feel I got a group, you know. I know you get it, get me. I know you helped me come out to my mom and dad, even if they don't like it. But then I think, you look like my dad sometimes. It's a little weird and I don't know.

G: You were going somewhere with my looking like your dad, but stopped.

L: Not that you have a look you give, you don't give looks at all actually if I think about it, but you're tall and dark like my dad, so it's weird sometimes. I don't talk to a lot of tall dark men in my life, so it's something I think like, shit this guy's cool with it?

G: You got it.

L: (laughing) I don't know why I doubt you.

G: Like you said, not too many men in your life who have had a positive view of you, especially you as gay.

L: I wish my dad could hear this. (begins sobbing). You really don't have a problem with it, do you? Sometimes it gets so bad, mom and dad fight about it, about me and I start to feel it's my fault. If I weren't gay they would be fine. Mom has been good, she talks to me about it and I can go to her with it but not with dad. I feel like he's sort of trying, he will still go places with me and wants to know what music I'm into right now, but I can't talk to him about anything that reminds him I'm gay. He knows I am but just doesn't want to really hear about it.

G: You're having to recognize your mom is available to you in this way that your father is not right now.

L: Maybe ever, Gabe.

Following this session Lawrence expressed concern that I was "hiding" in my own closet with a negative "judgment" of him. I understood this as a projection of his internalized father and gradually made interpretations organized by this understanding. Adding to the complexity of this case, for the first time I heard Lawrence talk about not knowing "how to be a man" and "who is a man I can be like?" Lawrence's father is a conflictual model, and he began to encounter my own masculinity as a "softer and gentler one."

Just prior to turning fourteen, Lawrence from a deeper level came out as having a long-standing feeling of not being a gay male at all, but in fact feeling he was always female. Further, Lawrence conveyed his frustration and despair that his body did not match his internal experience. Lawrence had worked through initial transference fears (me as father) in order to reach a deeper level of object usage. Our therapeutic relationship could allow for me to be an object to identify with and for the internalization of a benign and empathic early other, in order to explore his deeper gender identification as female.

Over the weeks following, Lawrence, now having identified as female, renamed herself as Lori. I shifted in referencing to Lawrence as Lori too, an adolescent young woman. Once again, Lori asked for assistance in coming out as female to both her parents. We explored and prepared for this type of session once again. When we held the family session, her parents expressed confusion, feeling disoriented, and clearly upset. Lori's mother over several months continued to meet with me to help process her feelings toward Lori. The mother was able to identify a sense of relief in that Lori identified herself as a transgender female. This made even more sense to the mother. In fact, she began sharing stories about Lori's discomfort with her own body at a very early age, reporting examples of Lori wanting to do and play more "traditional" girl games as young as age two. The father, however, became so enraged this time around that he stopped meeting with me for parent sessions altogether. It has been only in the last two years that he has returned to deal with various concerns, one involving being a father to a daughter.

In recent years, Lori has undergone hormonal treatments to block secondary male characteristics and develop more female features, with a wish to move toward eventual surgery for full transformation in the next few years. Lori is connected to a clinic specializing in transgender children and adolescents. Some of the current themes involve feelings of envy toward others whose physical body matches their gender identification. I have become both an object of envy and an object of developmental need simultaneously. The following session captures this issue:

> L: Yeah so I went to music practice today and it went alright I got to say. I had a new teacher but it was the one I wanted to get when I started there. She has been in all these huge bands that I even have on my phone. She's only there once a month and always booked, but I asked the director of the place to get me slot a few months ago.
>
> G: I know how much you have been wanting to work with her.
>
> L: For sure. It was cool because she showed me some good ways to get some beats going. It would be cool to do a show one day. There are some other kids there that I'm getting to know and we are thinking about getting together. I'm into different stuff than them, but I like some of their style too. I don't know, but we will probably do it at least to see if we can make some good stuff together. I've got all the recording gear I have been collecting for a while. It would be nice to use it. (small moment of silence) So last weekend I went to visit my aunt and uncle's. They were having a cookout for my cousin who just turned sixteen and I was looking at her, thinking, "I remember when we were like five or six and playing in her yard together, in her tree house." Well it wasn't really a tree house more like just a platform in a low tree, like the height of a bush or something. But to us it was so cool off the ground like that. Her dad built it for her birthday. I was just looking at her walking around and talking to some of her friends that she goes to high school with. She was wearing this cute skirt. Hmm.
>
> G: Something about her you were noticing.
>
> L: Well, I wanted to know where she got that skirt 'cause I want one. But well, this is kind of weird, but she has really nice full breasts now. I remember when we were kids and she didn't have them. Don't get me wrong, I am not saying that I was checking her out because I was attracted to her or anything, but I don't know.
>
> G: Wish you had breasts like hers?

L: Yes. Sucks, you know. She was just born with them. Well, she wasn't, but they just grew like that. She looked good, like a woman. So unfair, I have to put these on and sometimes it's a pain (referring to a bra with synthetic breasts that she wears everyday).

G: Betrayed by your body.

L: Seriously, but how would you know? You were born the right way. What do you know about your body not being you? You say that like you know something, but you haven't been there. You wanted a penis and have it. I don't want mine but it's stuck to me. I want to grow my own breasts.

G: You feel it's hard for me to help you, if I have not gone through it myself.

L: Sometimes I look at my mom and wish I had her body. She looks good for her age. Once I walked in on her in the bathroom. The lock sticks sometimes and doesn't work. I felt bad and said sorry to her. She understood and was good about it. But I saw her sort of with pants down. I mean I couldn't really see anything but I could see more of her body than I have before. She looked like a woman. Well, I mean I know she is a woman.

G: How could you not feel envy?

L: I never put it that way, but I sort of am jealous of her. It's hard you know. It's my mom and she's been great about me being trans. But she was born with a body to match who she is and I wasn't, so it doesn't feel fair. When I first got my forms, I remember how good they felt, to have them on and people just took me for a girl automatically cause I had the shape now. Sometimes I would sleep in them and it felt really kind of good to feel them up against me as if they were another girl's but also mine too at the same time; kinda weird, but cool. You know as cool as my mom is about it all, I can't really tell her this. I think she would kind of freak out and not know what to say.

G: You are finding ways to have and talk about those things, those feelings here.

L: Yeah, I think so.

CASE FORMULATION

To conceptualize the work Lori and I have done over the years is to consider many aspects of what it means to be a person intrapsychically, in relation to one's body, and in relation to the outside world. When Lori first came in as Lawrence, she was an eleven-year-old boy who, up until that point, had been in mental health treatments which artificially divided her into parts, addressing only one level of psychological life such as "behavior" or "cognitions." When the parents brought Lori in, finding her "odd, distracted, and lacking friends," Lori herself was concerned with anxiety and feeling "out of rhythm, off balance." This reminds me of Freud's 1923 view that the first ego is the body-ego. From the first moment Lori came in as Lawrence, she expressed her "out of rhythm" through her body in her awkward and uneven gait. In my countertransference, I identified with the "out of rhythm, off balance" feeling. In reaction, I searched to regain my analytic footing as an internal anchor. Unknowingly, at the time, this "anchor" and "footing" seemed to represent a missing developmental aspect in Lori's psychological structure. Through my initial analytic listening, reflection, holding, and containment, Lori came to discover what she had always known but not yet allowed to come fully into thought about her identity. This runs parallel to Bollas's concept of the "unthought known" (1989), and contrasts with her parents' difficulty in empathizing with and holding Lori's internal world throughout her development. While the parents wished the therapy would make Lori less socially awkward and academically competent, they struggled with a deeper thoughtfulness about Lori's emotional life. I imagined this reflected the parent's own parental early environment which also lacked an overall psychological mindedness.

In the second year of treatment, Lori first comes out as a gay male, still by the name of Lawrence at the time. In the session where I assisted Lori in communicating this to her parents, we saw her mother express slight relief in integrating this new reality, while her father regressed in his blaming me for "making" Lori gay. Possibly, the father was having deep anxieties about his own sexuality and gender identifications, which made it difficult to engage in a process of accepting Lori fully.

At age thirteen, Lori, still Lawrence at the time, began to explore her sexual attraction to males, which represents a developmental achievement both for Lori individually and in the therapeutic process. From a psychic foundation built through early developmental functions and served by me as a new object, there sprouted an era of Lori engaging her deeper internal conflicts, played out in the transference. I had to tolerate and interpret Lori's transference to me as a "father" who would be angry, critical, rejecting, and unempathic. We had to work through this transference to make me enough of a usable object, gradually allowing for Lori's unfolding of old and new identifications. Her father is a conflictual model, while I offer, in Lori's words, a "kinder, gentler" option. It is this identification and internalization in the treatment which serves as a way station on the road to deeper levels of her internal world, levels which allow for Lori to come out as Lori, a female.

Again the challenge of helping Lori let her parents know she is Lori (and not Lawrence) arises. Here we are again. At this juncture in the treatment Lori's father fragments to the point of completely removing himself from the treatment. His unconscious rage overwhelms his capacity to maintain an alliance with me for the sake of his child. I continue to think and ask whether my own empathic limits with the father interfered with maintaining an alliance throughout this period of time. Lori's mother, admirably, continues to work through her feelings of having a daughter, and even mourning a son. The father eventually returns, in spite of his anxieties and vulnerabilities. In the end he wishes to have a connection with his, now, daughter. This case is a reminder to me of the analyst's holding of many empathic levels within the family unit's various subjectivities, which can be at complete odds with one another.

This case raises a set of striking questions in relation to parents of a transgender child. What level of loss do parents experience? How does grieving unfold for each individual parent as well as the collective couple? Taking a leap here: does the transgender child present a new developmental potentiality not only for the child, but for the parents' internal world too? These questions and others continue to develop as I work with Lori. In the final process I reported, we see Lori's use of me as a new object, meeting previously sequestered developmental yearnings. We also see Lori's dilemma in using me at the new object level when it is diametrically opposed to her painful envy at my gender experience matching my anatomy. This is both a transference and a reality, the transference of the envy she experiences from the reality of her everyday world, where she sees others go about life without the dysphoria of their bodies being at odds with their sense of gender identification.

Having one's gender match one's anatomy is something most of us take for granted, as we take for granted the child's use of a parent's selfobject function, or the experience of the transitional space a primary caregiver provides to suspend reality: all for the sake of a child's solid psychological foundation (Kohut 1971; Winnicott 1953) . How does the transgender child develop a sense of self-continuity when from the beginning there has already existed a body and mind discontinuity that cannot be symbolized until much time has passed?

One moment in the final process I presented stood out to me upon reflection and led to a realization of my deeper countertransference. Informed by analytic temporality, this countertransference elucidates the history of the treatment, its current state, and a potential future (Cairo 2017). This occurred when Lori in her stream of associations said, "Sometimes I would sleep in them" (referring to her synthetic breast forms) "and it felt really kind of good to feel them up against me as if they were another girl's, but also mine too at the same time; kinda weird, but cool."

Although I responded with an observation of her capacity to use the therapy for elaboration of her internal world, there seemed to be another level of meaning to her association and my resulting countertransference. This meaning was implicit in Lori's prior associations of her questioning my capacity to understand what it is like to not have anatomy match gender experience. In vivid description, Lori expresses sleeping in her breast forms and the pleasurable sensation within a particular transitional space between her own body and that of another's. Is this her memory of the early mother breast? Does this convey something about her identifications?

On another level, it seems to me that there was an unconscious communication from Lori of her need that I not only imagine, but actually feel the sensation of my anatomy as both mine and someone else's. This serves as an empathic bridge to Lori's experience of connection and disconnection between anatomy, gender identity, and an other.

Several authors speak to what it means to function psychoanalytically with the transgender child. Ehrensaft (2014) offers a model of "true self gender" therapy where children are the "ultimate anti-essentialists." In other words, we may define gender, like psychoanalysis, as a fluid, dynamic process and not as a static, predetermined position. This allows us to see gender as not necessarily anatomical, but as psychologically determined. In Ehrensaft's view the transgender child is "gender creative." This hearkens back to Winnicott's concept of the spontaneous gesture finding its true self expression in the world (1965).

However, the question of providing a facilitating environment needs to be considered at the level of deciding what we are facilitating: Are we facilitating a space between fantasy and reality, between merger and separation? Or are we facilitating a gender transition? While these questions are not mutually exclusive, I wrestled with them at the level of not wanting to impinge on Lori's process while facilitating a deeper introspection via holding, containing, and interpretation. This framework kept the process open for Lori to go where she was intrapsychically compelled.

In a sense, I came to make conscious that my analytic focus was on the development of Lori's psychological capacities to experience and reflect on her experience. Further, that these internal capacities support an overall psychic process. Consequently, Lori's identity, including gender, will forge itself out of her internal way of working, which is deepened and elaborated by analytic therapy. This model coincides with Brinich's (2014) thoughts on seeing the fluidity of a nonlinear process of development, where we can conceptualize the transgender child as having a "currently adaptive self."

This provides greater freedom in terms of gender fluidity, allowing us to follow the child to where they are at any given time, while continuing to "not know" and be "surprised." This is what I aimed for, at first unconsciously, and now consciously with Lori. In essence, identity formation is a complex process involving many levels of experience from physical, sensory, affective, and cognitive factors, to relational, social, and cultural factors. I anticipate this chapter will evoke a conversation in the clinicians' individual and collective minds regarding the challenges a transgender child and family endure at both conscious and unconscious levels.

REFERENCES

Bollas, C. (1989). *The Shadow of the Object: Psychoanalysis of the Unthought Known*. New York: Columbia University Press.

Brinich, P. M. (2014). Discussion of Diane Ehrensaft's "Listening and learning from gender-nonconforming Children." *Psychoanalytic Study of the Child*, 68, 71–78.

Butler, J. (1988). Performative acts and gender constitution: An essay in phenomenology and feminist theory. *Theatre Journal*, 40(4), 519–531.

Cairo, I. (2017). It's about time: Temporality in analysis. *Journal of the American Psychoanalytic Association*, 65(2), 317–326.

Coates, S., Friedman, R. C., and Wolfe, S. (1991). The etiology of boyhood gender identity disorder: A model for integrating temperament, development, and psychodynamics. *Psychoanalytic Dialogues*, 1(4), 481–523.

Ehrensaft, D. (2014). Listening and learning from gender-nonconforming children. *Psychoanalytic Study of the Child*, 68, 28–56.

Freud, S. (1923). The ego and the id. In J. Strachey (Ed.) (1961). *The Standard Edition of the Complete Psychological Works of Sigmund Freud, Volume XIX (1923–1925)* (pp. 19–27). London: Hogarth Press and the Institute of Psycho-Analysis.

Harris, A. E. (2011). Gender as a strange attractor: Discussion of the Transgender Symposium. *Psychoanalytic Dialogues*, 21(2), 230–238.

Knight, R. (2014). Free to be you and me: Normal gender-role fluidity—commentary on Diane Ehrensaft's "Listening and learning from gender-nonconforming children." *Psychoanalytic Study of the Child*, 68, 57–70.

Kohut, H. (1971). *Analysis of the Self: A Systematic Approach to the Psychoanalytic Treatment of Narcissistic Personality Disorders*. Chicago: University of Chicago Press.

Lament, C. (2014). Conundrums and controversies: An introduction to the section. *Psychoanalytic Study of the Child*, 68, 13–27.

Transgender, adj. (n.d.). *Merriam-Webster.com*. Retrieved May 8, 2017, from https://www.merriamwebster.com/dictionary/transgender

Transgender. (2017). The National Center for Transgender Equality. Retrieved May 8, 2017, from http://www.transequality.org/issues/resources/transgender-terminology

Winnicott, D. W. (1953). Transitional objects and transitional phenomena: A study of the first not-me possession. *International Journal of Psychoanalysis*, 34, 89–97

———. (1965). *The Maturational Processes and the Facilitating Environment: Studies in the Theory of Emotional Development*. The International Psycho-Analytical Library, 64, 1–276. London: The Hogarth Press and the Institute of Psycho-Analysis.

Chapter Five

Severe Emotional Disturbances in Childhood

Theodore Fallon Jr.

INTRODUCTION

In discussing children with severe emotional disturbances (SED), I might have used any one of a number of other labels, such as childhood schizophrenia (Bender 1956), autism (Kanner 1943), Asperger syndrome (Asperger 1991), childhood psychosis (Tustin 1995), children with sensory integration difficulties (Ayres 1973), the vulnerable child (Anthony, Koupernik, & Chiland 1978), pervasive developmental disorder (Fombonne 2009), nonverbal learning deficits (Rourke 1989), the severely traumatized child (Knafo 2016; Read, van Os, Morrison, & Ross 2005), and children with thought disorder (Fallon 2014). Each of these terms carries with it an entire history of its own, its own literature, diagnostic criteria, published cases, treatment recommendations and continuing questions. Of course, within each of these literatures, there are considerable disagreements, controversies, and unknowns.

SED is terminology that comes from education (Forness & Jane Knitzer 1992) and work with public mental health systems of care (Knitzer 1982; Schlenger, Etheridge, Hansen, Fairbank, & Onken 1992). In the context of education and systems of care, SED has been given explicit definitions, has its own history, literature, and so on. In the psychoanalytic literature, there is one reference (Zapparoli & Gislon 1999), which never actually defines the term, but does use the words "psychotic" and "serious psychopathological disorders" (p. 23) to describe the child with SED.

In comparing and contrasting the various terms listed above, one finds much to think about; and despite the differences and unknowns between and within each of these terminologies, the similarities are quite remarkable. The discussions focus on children whose psychological development and functioning are severely impaired or have altogether ceased. Those times might be episodic moments, as with out-of-control tantrums in a fourteen-year-old, or prolonged periods during which interpersonal interaction and cognition do not function. For purposes of this chapter, I will make use of SED as a descriptive placeholder, bringing all of the above literature to bear on a phenomenon that all of these terms share.

AN EXAMPLE: THE CASE OF WALLACE

Although one might point to some diagnostic differences among the entities mentioned above, children in this spectrum frequently fulfill overlapping criteria, as can be seen in the following case. Wallace presented as a six-year-old boy following an incident in his first grade classroom at the beginning of the year. After an altercation with another child, Wallace had retreated to hide under a table, yelling, "You're wrong! You're wrong!" When the teacher reached under the table to retrieve him, he bit the teacher's hand and yelled even more loudly, now saying, "Get away, get away!" It took several teachers and the principal to safely subdue him until the parents could come to pick him up. Even before this incident, he had regularly struggled with getting along with peers, was not keeping up in his academic work, and frequently whined in school that he missed his mother.

Wallace's mother recalled that as a newborn he had been very cuddly, perhaps even hypotonic, and had slept through the night at three months of age. However, at times even as an infant, he would be willful, and would stiffen and scream inconsolably. This got worse as he got older. When he began feeding himself, he would shove food in his mouth, at times having so much in his mouth that he was not able to swallow it, and would spit it out. He was slow to sit up, walk, and learn language. When he did learn to speak, he would frequently speak gibberish, at other times singing nonsense syllables.

During his preschool years, Wallace had occupational therapy to help him with his eating as well as with a delay and dyscoordination in walking. He also had speech therapy for delayed speech, but when he did begin to talk, he quickly developed a remarkable vocabulary, at times sounding like a fifty-year-old man. When tested just prior to entering first grade, he was found to have a remarkably high verbal score, but was below average nonverbally. As a preschooler, his free play often included mixing various liquids together, or taping and gluing objects together as he talked about "inventing" things. Sometimes he would get out of bed at night to pursue these activities.

At home, he frequently got into altercations with his older brother, who was remarkably tolerant of Wallace's provocations. His parents were exhausted, constantly chasing him around, trying to get him to do what was needed. For example, meals were constantly disrupted, as he would repeatedly get up from the table to look at something outside, or to return to his play. His parents commented that despite his excellent vocabulary, and negative consequences for his behavior, he did not seem to learn. His father later revealed that he became so frustrated that he would yell at Wallace, who often would respond by cowering, curling up in a ball, and holding his ears. His mother also revealed later that she and Wallace would watch television and movies together, after which he would have nightmares and become anxious, sometimes developing fears and phobias.

During the initial evaluation, Wallace was quite curious to meet the therapist, and easily engaged in a lively conversation, much like one would experience with a brilliant high school student involved in a fascinating project. However, when the therapist mentioned feelings, Wallace began throwing toys off the shelves, knocked over an easel, and attempted to overturn a coffee table. When he returned for another visit, he was very reluctant, and announced that he hated the therapist because the therapist had opened up his mind. Then he suddenly got off the couch where he was sitting beside his parents, and came at the therapist forcefully, intending to stab the therapist in the eye with a ruler. He yelled, "I will kill you," and he certainly seemed to mean it. When restrained, he screamed loudly, kicking, flailing about, spitting, and attempting to bite.

In this presentation, we see various developmental delays alongside accelerated growth. For example, his advanced vocabulary and engagement in intelligent lively conversation appeared in conjunction with his poor social development. We also see simultaneous sensitivities and insensitivities: he did not appear to have much oral sensitivity while stuffing food in his mouth, but at the same time became overwhelmed at simply mentioning his feelings. We also see a complete disruption of his overall functioning, both in the incident described from school and in the first two office visits.

This child's development unfolded under the watchful eye of the parents, who brought such resources to bear as they were able to find. These resources successfully addressed the developmental deficits, such as the walking and his delayed speech. With less attentive parents, his difficulties might not have been noticed, and without occupational and speech therapy, he would likely have fallen further and further behind in his development. But even with those interventions, there was something challenging his forward movement in maturation.

MOVING FORWARD

With the vast array of literature to call upon, it may seem odd that a case such as Wallace's would befuddle many therapists. Perhaps, however, it is because such cases are so befuddling that therapists have put forth successful cases and numerous ideas in an effort to offer possible solutions to the challenges in working with this population of children. However, at the end of each skillful, resourceful presentation, we have to ask: How can this case help the next such child move forward in his development? And the broader question: With all of this information and experience, how can we move the field forward?

It would be difficult to review all of this literature in less than an entire volume. We would need to compare and contrast the diagnostic criteria, consider how each of the cases in the literature fulfills each set of criteria, then consider the treatments and outcomes, and try to match children fulfilling each set of criteria with the success of each types of treatments. An endeavor using this array of literature is daunting if not impossible.

However, even with a quick broad overview, we can glean three interconnected motifs that reoccur throughout. One motif is a sense of out of control chaos at the outset. The second is deficits in psychological development. The third is deficits in sensory integration.

In doing this broad overview (below), I make certain assumptions which I have found helpful in bringing order into the chaos. I approach this material with an assumption that all children's functioning, both behaviorally and emotionally, has valid meaning. That is, for example, whatever the neurobiology, the child has a subjective experience that can be understood in terms of meaning. Another way of putting this would be to say that I am, as Sigmund Freud was, focused here on the mind.

I mean to leave out the neurobiology not because we cannot learn valuable things from it. Other chapters in this book amply demonstrate its usefulness. However, there is a usefulness in considering a person for what they think, say, do, and feel without invoking normal or aberrant biological processes behind these experiences. It is also not to say that there are no differences in how the world is experienced by different particular children, and that these differences are not important and not due to neurobiological differences. It is to say that we can study and understand these disturbances and differences in perception without referring to neurobiological processes.

This chapter demonstrates the usefulness of considering children with SED from the perspective of the functioning mind. This perspective allows the integration of disparate terminologies since it goes to the source rather than depending on theoretical structures and narratives, or leaps from neurobiology to the mind. It also considers the child from the perspective of present processes and functioning rather than postulating latent attributes of the child or hypothesizing connections with the past. That is not to say that past experiences have no connection with present functioning, only that present functioning cannot be determined by past experiences.

At the same time, considering the child with SED from the perspective of the mind gives precedence to the child's subjective experience, which is the bedrock of psychoanalytic thinking. Furthermore, this perspective points the way to a focal point in attempting to understand and treat children with SED and moving them forward in development rather than considering the child's difficulties as an intrinsic, unchangeable attribute of a child.

To restate all of this another way, the perspective being put forth in this chapter considers what are the present psychological, cognitive and emotional capacities and processes of a child in the present moment. This is the same perspective as Bion's recommendation that one begin each analytic session with a patient afresh, open to the possibilities (W. R. Bion 1963, p. 69; 1970, p. 107). This perspective keeps the focus on the present and on the possibilities for development and interventions, rather than on some condition the child is sentenced to have for the rest of his/her life. It is different than the traditional one and offers advantages that are clarified throughout this chapter.

HISTORICAL PERSPECTIVE

Let us think how each of the diagnostic entities might inform us about this case and about the development of children with SED in general. Keeping in mind the commonality of all of these disorders, let us consider each of the terms mentioned above in their approximate historical sequence.

The psychoanalytic literature contains a number of papers dating from 1941 describing childhood schizophrenia. Hinsie and Campbell define childhood schizophrenia as "a clinical entity occurring in childhood, usually after the age of one and before the age of eleven, characterized chiefly by disturbance in the ability to make effective contact with the environment and by autistic thinking" (Hinsie & Campbell 1976). Lauretta Bender (1947) formulates childhood schizophrenia as having pathology "at every level and in every area of integration or patterning within the function of the central nervous system, be it vegetative, motor, perceptual, intellectual, emotional, or social." Some descriptions vividly describe murderous fantasies (Mahler 1944). In the case of Wallace, we do see murderous fantasies enacted and deficits of functioning at many levels.

Hertzig and Walker (1975) hypothesize that the clinical symptomatology of childhood schizophrenia can be understood in terms of the child's incapacity for processing information due to a failure in the development of intersensory integration. In other words, the information received by the various sensory modalities remains dissociated and unconnected, with the resultant effect of profound sensory conflict and "adaptive" sensory deprivation. This can be seen in the comment by Wallace's parents that "despite his excellent vocabulary and the negative consequences he has suffered, he does not seem to learn."

There are many descriptions of treatments in the literature. An extensive literature review of the many documented treatments suggest that work with this population takes great patience and skill, but there is not a clear sense of any particular formula or formulation of these cases that tell us about how to treat the next case. However, part of the formulation of childhood schizophrenia talks about the "development of intersensory integration." For Wallace, development is quite inconsistent, with advanced functioning alongside significant delays.

Next in historical appearance is autism. By 1943, Leo Kanner had provided a systematic organized account in which we again find the concept of delayed development of psychological processes (1943). Kanner's cases demonstrate abnormalities, especially aloofness from birth. He contrasts this with earlier identified cases of childhood schizophrenia in which the children are born without any peculiarities but later, as early as two years of age, regress. Although Kanner is clear that whatever is happening is due to innate problems with the child, it also becomes clear in this literature that the child's supportive nurturing environment is an essential ingredient for the child's developmental success.

However, as Martin noted, "there is a further form of deprivation. The child may be deprived of his mother's care and the full stimulus of a warm and loving environment because he is neurologically incapable of making sense of the world around him. Through no fault of his mother, there results severe and prolonged insufficiency of interaction" (Martin 1971, p. 294). Singletary further elaborates this using clinical examples, and Norian (1978) attributes it again to sensory integration deficits.

Hans Asperger, working under the Nazi regime in Germany, described a population of children similar to Kanner's autistic group. His description gave examples of children with high intelligence who could possibly make a contribution to society (Asperger 1991) but who had sensory integration difficulties (Ayres 1973). However, Asperger did not provide much in the way of diagnostic criteria, and there is little information regarding the children's development, treatment or outcome (Harris 2016). In this regard, Asperger's work is of little help to us.

Next historically is a broadening of the concept of childhood schizophrenia to childhood psychosis. In 1995, Tustin published *Autism and Childhood Psychosis*. She felt that Kanner's autism "misses the point that pathological autism seems to be an arrest at, or regression to, an early developmental situation which has become intensified in a rigid form." Here Tustin is putting autism squarely in the context of development, saying that this state is a normal phase of development, something that Mahler had said two decades earlier (Mahler, Pine, & Bergman 1975). It is only when the child "remains in, or regresses to, a sensations-dominated state" due to the child's inability to make use of the nurturing environment that she saw "pathological autism."

There is much in Tustin's book that attempts to make distinctions between various types of autism and childhood psychosis, concluding with a chart that lists twenty eight points of difference, liberally referencing the literature of case studies (Tustin 1995, p. 136). These observations echo Kanner's comparison between autism and childhood schizophrenia with the main emphasis on age of onset–autism being at birth and childhood psychosis after two years of age. Just as with the criteria for Kanner's autism (1943) and Bender's childhood schizophrenia (1947), it is clear we are talking about children with significant disturbances.

However, clinical presentation and outcomes rarely fit neatly in any category. In the case of Wallace, going through Tustin's checklist (1995), we can identify elements on both sides of her psychosis/autism ledger. For example, as a newborn, Wallace was willful, with screaming and tantrums, which is characteristic of autism; but otherwise he was easy, which is more characteristic of schizophrenia. He also clearly has fantasy play, inventing things, which is not considered consistent with autism where there is no fantasy play, and identifies him on the schizophrenia side. And yet the play focused on mechanical objects, which would move him to the autism side of the ledger. In the end, this distinction, at least for Wallace, is not particularly helpful. In addition, there is no treatment or outcome data to suggest any distinction between autism and childhood psychosis.

There have been other attempts to identify diagnostic criteria that might assist in differentiating children with SED. A recent study (Fombonne 2009) considered pervasive developmental disorder as an overarching diagnostic category, identifying 0.6–0.7 percent of children. This study was useful in that it included defined and tested diagnostic criteria. In *DSM-III* (American Psychiatric Association 1980), pervasive developmental disorder is divided into two major categories: infantile autism and childhood onset pervasive developmental disorder, which might be more akin to childhood schizophrenia or psychosis. The criteria differ, primarily in the age of onset. Fombonne (2009) studied 129 patients who had received diagnoses of pervasive developmental disorder or a related disorder and found only five cases of apparent childhood psychosis. These would have been children that Bender and Tustin would have identified. However, these five patients with childhood psychosis were behaviorally indistinguishable from those with other diagnoses. In addition, age of onset may be more appropriately termed "age of recognition," and its use as a major diagnostic criterion for such disorders may not be justified (Volkmar, Stier, & Cohen 1985).

In the case of Wallace, date of onset is not a particularly useful criterion, as there seems to be interference with the developmental process early on, but then some correction with treatment. And even still there seemed to be interference in his maturation as development moved on. Diagnostic criteria might be useful as they might point to delay in particular areas of psychological development of the mind. However, criteria in DSM list only behaviors and symptoms. There is no mention of processes going on in the mind.

Another classification for the population of SED children was proposed by E. James Anthony in *Vulnerable Children* (Anthony, Koupernik, & Chiland 1978). In this book, Anthony, a psychoanalyst, identifies innate attributes of children that lead to SED. His focus is on the child's psychological functioning and processes of the mind. Theodore Cohen, also a child analyst, extends the understanding of the vulnerable child to include external factors as well, such as poverty, abuse, and neglect (Cohen, Etezady, & Pacella 1993). In identifying children's vulnerabilities to SED in this way, we are annexing another population of chaotic, difficult-to-treat children, those with histories of external trauma, abuse, and neglect. And if we look at that population of children with SED as a result of external factors, we recognize the same clinical presentations, diagnostic and treatment challenges as well as outcomes (Knafo 2016; Read et al. 2005).

SENSORY INTEGRATION DYSFUNCTION

So far, we have talked about childhood schizophrenia, autism, childhood psychosis, and the vulnerable child. A common criterion among these classifications is developmental delay. Age of onset, once thought to be useful, seems to have more to do with the sensitivity of the child's caregivers (usually parents) in identifying abnormalities. Another commonality identified has been sensory integration dysfunction. The concept of sensory integration was introduced in 1972 as a significant factor in the etiology of learning disorders (Ayres 1973): "The results of sensory deprivation appear similar to the clinical picture of the child with sensory integrative dysfunction. In both cases, there is a lack of organizing, structuring and relating of self to objects and of objects to objects. In the child with poor neurological organization, the stimuli are usually available, but there is inadequate processing of them."

Another related aspect of deficits in sensory processing can be seen in children with nonverbal learning differences (Rourke 1989). Children identified with such learning difficulties appear similar in presentation to the other children we have been describing. In fact, some studies suggest that nonverbal learning difficulties are one of the contributors of autistic spectrum disorders (Ames & Jarrold 2009; Gavilán, Fournier-Del Castillo, & Bernabeu-Verdú 2007). If we consider that nonverbal processing is a part of sensory integration, then Rourke's children are an extension of Ayres's children. Although Ayres approaches the child from a learning disability perspective, she is also pointing to the deficits suffered by Kanner's, Bender's, and Tustin's children. Shortly after Ayres's publication, others approached the sensory integration problem as a way of considering autism (Norian 1978, p. 68). Norian found that "autistic children do indeed have perceptual deficiencies; deficiencies which render them incapable of cross-modal transfer in the visual, haptic, and kinesthetic senses." Just as the child with blindness and deafness has sensory deficiencies, some children have difficulty taking in and/or integrating sensory information. This sensory information that these children are not able to take in deprives them of the basic data that we all need to build up a model and understanding of the world. This sensory data also allows us to take in supplies that are needed at the psychological level the same way we need food at the physical level. These psychological supplies include a sense of feeling loved, understood, cared for, safety, and a sense of not being alone. Being deprived of access to these supplies at the psychological level leaves them without nutrients for emotional growth, hence the delay in development.

Ornstein emphasizes that empathic surroundings are imperative for the development of a stable and healthy self (A. Ornstein 1976). Children who have a disturbance in being able to take in that environment are at risk for SED (Anthony et al. 1978). This disturbance in taking in may be a hyposensitivity or a hypersensitivity to the sensory input. Let us consider auditory input, for example. If a child cannot hear the input, such as in deafness, or even attentional problems preventing the child from attending to the input, the nurturing information is not received. But likewise, if the child is hypersensitive to the input, it would be like a loudspeaker with the volume turned up. The sound would be painful and distorted and the child might avoid the sensory information, or the sound might be too distorted to be understood.

Parents unaware of a child's sensory integration difficulties are ill-equipped to effectively help their child. Parents who are aware of their child's sensory integration and nonverbal learning deficits are much better prepared to support the attachment and security bonds that are so essential for these children (Rass 2003). In a parallel way, children who experience a neglectful, abusive, or traumatic environment are deprived of or overloaded with sensory input and do not have parents that provide those same attachment and security bonds. A more detailed examination of environmental factors and processes that support and inhibit emotional growth (Parens 2011) also contributes to our understanding of how to evaluate the developmental environment that parents provide, and also how to provide parental guidance to enhance that developmental environment.

Ayres (1973) also presents empirical evidence that sensory integration deficits can be corrected with exercises. Like the physical exercises that

Ayres suggests for promoting improvement in sensory integration, fortifying the developmental environment is extremely important in creating stronger, more robust sensory signals for children with SED so that they can more firmly experience the loving, growth promoting developmental environment that is so essential for their continuing forward growth and maturation. In addition, the therapist of the child with SED will exercise the child's mind in preparation for development. I will say more about this below.

We now have an hypothesis of the etiology of a child with SED: The child has difficulty taking in and/or integrating sensory information. This deficit of taking in and integrating data from the outside world leads to deficits in constructing a working model of how the world, and others in the world, work. It also leads to deficits in constructing a model of how one's own mind works. In addition, the child will be deprived of the psychological nutrients that are so necessary for emotional growth, hence the delay in emotional development that is at the core of the child with SED. Note that the deficit may be due to either the child's innate difficulty in taking in and/or interpreting sensory data, as is the case in children with autism or childhood psychosis, or the environment may not have provided the child with the sensory information needed, as is the case with children of trauma, abuse, or neglect.

For children with innate sensory integration deficits, increasing the strength/volume of those sensory signals is like giving enriched psychological nutrients for children who have difficulty absorbing those nutrients. Similarly, for children who have suffered trauma, abuse, and neglect, providing those nutrients in a nutrient poor environment promotes growth and maturation. As we are talking about sensory integration dysfunction, it is important to clarify what we mean. Observing children with sensory integration deficits is an exercise in viewing oddities that do not make sense at face value. Why should Wallace want to poke out the therapist's eyes and kill him at the mere mention of feelings?

Another example is a case (Fallon 2014) in which it took several months for a three-year-old child to enter the therapist's office. In that case, it became clear that this child was extremely sensitive to space and distance. This sensitivity was expressed in a number of symptoms, including: 1) the inability to tolerate another child in the room as he "knew" the other child would violate his space; 2) the exquisite sensitivity to the therapist's proximity to the child, seen in the child's response to the slightest movement from the therapist; 3) the child's extreme difficulty with his parents restraining him when he became out-of-control (such attempts at restraint would lead to hours of tantrumming which only came to an end with sheer exhaustion and falling asleep); 4) the child's fascination with planes flying through space; and 5) the child's advanced ability to fold at least 50 different paper airplanes, including his own designs before the age of 5 years. What this child's subjective experience was in each of these circumstances was difficult to say. However, his hypersensitivity to space may be similar to the experiencing of a very bright spot light being shined directly on one's face. He clearly communicated his discomfort.

Returning for a moment to the case of Wallace, there are numerous hypotheses and questions that are generated in thinking about nonverbal learning deficits and sensory integration issues. Wallace's sense of self, his possible sensitivities to his own internal states and at the same time insensitivities to his own bodily states, become fertile areas to explore with Wallace himself, as well as his history and his parents' experiences in working with him and providing for him.

In the recent literature there are many examples of excellent treatments of children with SED, all highlighting how one can approach and work with SED children (Franchi 2015; Green, Fazio-Griffith, & Parson 2015; Kawai 2009; Knafo & Selzer 2015; Singletary 2015). Although these are sensitive and skillful treatments, it is important to ask what they tell us so that we have a better idea of what to do with the next child and family who needs our help. Looking at these cases, it is sometimes explicit and sometimes only implicit that these children need not only a sensitive and skillful therapist who becomes aware of the child's sensitivities and insensitivities, but also a developmental environment at home, in school and in their community that provides an enriched growth-promoting form of support. With this enriched support, despite their sensory integration and nonverbal learning deficits, these children can then experience an empathic attunement they so badly need (Rass 2003). In short, they require multimodal treatment (Zapparoli & Gislon 1999). I add here that those responsible for the milieu also need to learn to be sensitive to the child.

CHILDREN WITH SED FROM A DEVELOPMENTAL PERSPECTIVE

So far in this chapter, we have considered diagnostic criteria and sensory and nonverbal learning deficits, topics that have arisen and have been addressed historically. We can also see from the recent literature that children with SED can be successfully treated. Although not always explicit in these descriptions of treatment, there is at least an implied understanding that successful treatment means the child is moving on in development, a principle that Anna Freud made explicit for the goal of successful analytic treatment (A. Freud 1963; Miller 2002). If we consider moving on in development as success, and Kanner's and Tustin's idea of delay in development as a marker of the child with SED, then we need to look more closely into the process of development itself. There are arguments that suggest that a diagnosis of autism or childhood schizophrenia is a life sentence, and that if a child improves, then that is evidence that the child did not have one of these diagnoses. From an historical perspective, that argument is baseless. Certainly Kanner could not have known the lifelong outcome of the population of children with whom he was working.

In the argument that autism is a neurobiological disorder, I would help the reader realize that a neurobiological deficit is a concept in search of an actual brain lesion. I would, in addition, pit that argument against the repeated demonstration in the literature of the neuroplasticity of the mind to reconstitute after actual physical injury to the brain. In addition, we have over a half century of understanding and experience in working with these children and are in a much better position to be sensitive to their needs and deficits, now particularly in terms of sensory integration, the same way we are in a better position to work with children with nonverbal learning deficits now compared to fifty years ago. We can also conceptualize that children with SED have their difficulty precisely because they are delayed in development. That is, because these children are delayed in their development, they do not have the psychological equipment to address the psychological demands that they might be expected to address given their chronological age. For example, with Wallace, there is every reason to believe that he had poor object constancy as described by Mahler et al. (1976). Because of this, he was not prepared for school hours away from his mother. He also did not have the social development to support peer-to-peer interaction that is expected of a school-aged child. If he had the psychological capacity of object constancy and the social development of a school-aged child, he would not have suffered as he did.

The challenge in treatment of these children, then, is the same as the challenge in their development: What is the core of the problem that is interfering with meeting the developmental challenge at hand?

In classical analytic thought, the interference lies in unresolved conflict. The oedipal boy feels conflicted about taking his place as a child within the family in which mother and father have a relationship exclusive of him. Conflict indeed may play some role in children with SED. For example, with Wallace, his father's yelling at him may be so overbearing, with no sense of love, that all Wallace can think of is revenge and killing. Certainly we can imagine an environment in which a child's experience of a father's aggression more closely matches the reality of the situation. However, in Wallace's case, although the father's yelling was not helpful, it was easy to see and understand the father's frustration, which became intolerable. And in addition, when Wallace's experience with yelling was explained to his father, the father understood and quickly modified his responses to Wallace's constant disruptions.

The idea of development itself suggests an alternative conceptualization, one of deficit. That is, in development, initially something is missing in the psychic structure, process, or model of the world and in oneself. Then with growth and maturation, something new is added. For example, with Wallace in therapy, initially seeing the therapist was experienced as all bad. However, with repeated experiences of support and caring from the therapist, there came an idea that there was something good. For a time, the bad and the good were side by side like oil and water. When it was bad, Wallace wanted to kill the therapist. When it was good, he wanted to stay with the therapist forever. Gradually, something new began to emerge. He was able to delay his "kill" response longer and longer, until one day he allowed the therapist to talk about the two feelings side by side. After that Wallace himself was able to talk about his two feelings of loving and killing, not needing to enact either. What happened? Initially, there was no capacity to tolerate his feelings and delay his response. That was the deficit. Then he had the capacity. Development happened. How did it happen? Perhaps one way to conceptualize this process is to consider Ayres's empirical success (1973) with sensory integration deficits: exercises. Instead of exercises of the body, we are providing exercises of the mind.

In the example of Wallace, he was able to repeatedly experience a sense of wanting to kill the therapist. Gradually he learned to tolerate that feeling. Finally, in a moment he had never experienced before, he was able to resist the force to respond which came from the inside. In further work with Wallace, it became clear that he had been hypersensitive particularly to his aggressive feelings. With his father learning to accept his aggressive feelings at home, and with his learning to tolerate these feelings with his therapist, suddenly in one moment he went from doing to not doing. In another moment, he went from not doing to talking. One could then see in his talking how he magnified his internal stimuli. For example, he would experience tiny little bugs as threatening. In this way, one could see the hypersensitivity sensory integration difficulty. But even with his sensory integration dysfunction, Wallace moved on in his development. New properties emerged.

THE MOMENT OF DEVELOPMENT

We have established that children with SED, no matter what the flavor, have delays in their development. These delays, we have hypothesized, are due to sensory integration difficulties. There is much empirical evidence for this. There is also empirical evidence for the fact that with "exercises," these sensory integration deficits can be addressed, although I would say from experience that the exercises may not always be successful. However, I do not think we can predict who will respond to our treatment and who will not.

There are cases where there are clear brain abnormalities such as no corpus callosum, where the plasticity of the brain has overcome deficits imposed by the lesion (Fallon 2014, pp. 69–72). We can see in the literature, as well as in the case of Wallace presented in this chapter, that despite these sensory integration difficulties, development can and does progress.

How does development happen? Fallon conceptualized development in the context of nonlinear systems theory (Fallon 2014). Development, as evolution, begins with a steady state of the personality. In that state, the person, be they infant or wise elder, has a working model of reality and responds to challenges based on that model. For example, an infant's model of reality usually includes crying when challenged with hunger. A toddler's model of reality usually includes seeking and finding a parent when anxious. At some point in a single moment, the person meets a developmental challenge. For example, the toddler, driven by a growing curiosity, begins to explore beyond the bounds of the parent and is pulled between her curiosity and anxiety of exploring the unknown. It is likely that the child will meet that challenge many times and retreat. But at some point, if all goes well, in a single moment, the child strikes out on her own as she never has before. That child is now forever changed. Her world will never be as it was before. There is a newfound independence that has emerged. Another example that parents can readily relate to is having a child. Once a person becomes a parent, they are forever changed. If all goes well, we will say that person has matured. Their model of reality will have expanded to include responsibility for another human being.

Of course there are other possible outcomes to developmental challenges. Sometimes stepping back from the challenge is not an option, as for example, becoming a parent or being sent off to school. In those cases, the person may meet the challenge successfully, or the person may continue to operate using a model of reality that is not up to the challenge. In that case, overwhelming anxiety likely ensues, leading to decreasing function, which leads to increased anxiety, and finally a breakdown of the mind. Wallace's response at school is an example of this outcome. He managed as best he could but it was clearly not adequate, and eventually led to a complete breakdown, with him under the table defending himself like a cornered animal. This is the process we see in children with SED.

What can we understand about that moment of development that will allow us to usher forward a child who is stuck there? To begin with, such moments are filled with chaos. We see this empirically described in the literature and in cases. We can also imagine the chaos as being the moment when one recognizes that the old model of reality is not working, but a new one is not in place. It is being lost with an old map that you know is incorrect. But this is no ordinary map. It is the map that feels like it keeps you alive.

The affect that one experiences in that instant is likely something between terror and annihilation anxiety. One's psychological existence is on the line. It is so terrifying that although we all have experienced it many times, few of us ever remember it. It is not a place one wants to be. That is the place that children with SED experience frequently and many times for long periods. That is also the experience that you as a therapist will have if you want to assist such a child. Therapists who do this work need to be competent in assessing the external safety of everyone involved while at the same time experiencing and containing the annihilation anxiety, all the while gathering the data and pondering how it all fits together. The good news is that in working with children with SED, if you miss it on the first or the fiftieth time, you will have another opportunity to see the crisis. In fact, you will likely have all the opportunities you need until you figure it out. Because of the chaos, it will take time, reexperiencing it, and multiple tries to have any sense of orientation, let alone get any purchase on reality. During this time, you need to recognize that you as the therapist will not be able to do anything except survive and make sure the child is safe physically. In this regard, if you try to do anything, you risk becoming the object of projections, which will likely be all bad and difficult to undo.

Once you have collected enough data and had an opportunity to experience enough meltdowns, gradually pieces will begin to fall into place. Having sat with the child and many times the parents also, and weathered these storms, if all goes well, the child and the parents, perhaps for the first time in their lives, will not feel alone. They will have an attachment and trust with you. With that experience, you will be able to track the chaos and begin to anticipate when the child will be able to tolerate it and when it will lead to meltdowns. At some point, you may begin to have an idea about what material or issues lead to meltdowns. You can use these ideas to formulate tiny "bits" you might offer to the child, verbally or nonverbally, that might provide a nidus for organizing a new model.

You will have to experiment in offering your "bits," knowing that you will likely need multiple tries to get it right. If there is an acceleration in the meltdown you are likely on the right track, but it is too much. If the child reconstitutes, you got it close enough; if the meltdown occurs as usual, then you completely missed the mark. You want to provide enough that the child grabs on to it, but not so much that the child chokes on it, or feels invaded by what you offer. When you are able to consistently provide just the right amount of organization and support with the "bits" that you provide, there will be an increasing sense of an alliance. The child will have an increasing sense of security, trust, and feeling understood. This is the condition that addresses the sensory integration difficulties and provides nutrients at the psychological level for the emotional development. At the same time, the

Penelope's internal pubescent pressures were too loud, and had been overwhelming her ability to work through her developmental challenges. Her sensory integration difficulty was a hypersensitivity to her internal developing sexual experiences. The therapy allowed her to bring her chaos to the consulting room first in the form of silence, then in the disorganized flute playing, then in the meandering stories, and finally it coalesced into an intense romance. Bit by bit, the therapist provided the organization which turned out to be a proxy for a model of reality that met the challenges of her world at home and at school.

SUMMARY

This chapter has considered those children who, at some point in their development, cease to function psychologically. As a somewhat nebulous term, we dubbed these children as having SED. We considered the vast array of different literatures and the different designations that describe these children, including childhood schizophrenia, autism, childhood psychosis, and vulnerable children. Historically, the criterion which has primarily distinguished these designations one from the other, age of onset, has not been found to have much validity. What does tie these designations together is that they describe developmental delays and are likely caused by sensory integration deficits, including nonverbal learning disabilities. A model of development was formulated that put the developmental delays and sensory integration deficits in the context of nonlinear systems theory. Using this theory as a foundation, a framework for therapy was offered that addresses the developmental challenges that children with SED face, with strategies to help usher these children through the places in development where they get stuck, assisting them in their maturation.

REFERENCES

American Psychiatric Association (1980). *DSM-III: Diagnostic and Statistical Manual of Mental Disorders.* Washington, DC: APA, 205–225.

Ames, C. S. and Jarrold, C. (2009). Identifying symbolic relationships in autism spectrum disorders: A deficit in the identification of temporal co-occurrence? *Journal of Autism and Developmental Disorders,* 39(12), 1723–34.

Anthony, E. J., Koupernik, C., and Chiland, C. (Eds.). (1978). *Vulnerable Children.* New York: Wiley.

Asperger, H. (1991). Autistic psychopathy in childhood. In Frith U. (Ed.). *Autism and Asperger Syndrome* (pp. 37–92). Cambridge: Cambridge University Press.

Ayres, J. (1973). *Sensory Integration and Learning Disorders.* Los Angeles, CA: Western Psychological Services.

Bender, L. (1947). Childhood schizophrenia. *American Journal of Orthopsychiatry,* 42, 40–56.

———. (1956). Schizophrenia in childhood: Its recognition, description and treatment. *American Journal of Orthopsychiatry,* 26, 499–506.

Bion, W. R. (1963). *Elements of Psycho-Analysis.* London, UK: Heinemann.

The affect that one experiences in that instant is likely something between terror and annihilation anxiety. One's psychological existence is on the line. It is so terrifying that although we all have experienced it many times, few of us ever remember it. It is not a place one wants to be. That is the place that children with SED experience frequently and many times for long periods. That is also the experience that you as a therapist will have if you want to assist such a child. Therapists who do this work need to be competent in assessing the external safety of everyone involved while at the same time experiencing and containing the annihilation anxiety, all the while gathering the data and pondering how it all fits together. The good news is that in working with children with SED, if you miss it on the first or the fiftieth time, you will have another opportunity to see the crisis. In fact, you will likely have all the opportunities you need until you figure it out. Because of the chaos, it will take time, reexperiencing it, and multiple tries to have any sense of orientation, let alone get any purchase on reality. During this time, you need to recognize that you as the therapist will not be able to do anything except survive and make sure the child is safe physically. In this regard, if you try to do anything, you risk becoming the object of projections, which will likely be all bad and difficult to undo.

Once you have collected enough data and had an opportunity to experience enough meltdowns, gradually pieces will begin to fall into place. Having sat with the child and many times the parents also, and weathered these storms, if all goes well, the child and the parents, perhaps for the first time in their lives, will not feel alone. They will have an attachment and trust with you. With that experience, you will be able to track the chaos and begin to anticipate when the child will be able to tolerate it and when it will lead to meltdowns. At some point, you may begin to have an idea about what material or issues lead to meltdowns. You can use these ideas to formulate tiny "bits" you might offer to the child, verbally or nonverbally, that might provide a nidus for organizing a new model.

You will have to experiment in offering your "bits," knowing that you will likely need multiple tries to get it right. If there is an acceleration in the meltdown you are likely on the right track, but it is too much. If the child reconstitutes, you got it close enough; if the meltdown occurs as usual, then you completely missed the mark. You want to provide enough that the child grabs on to it, but not so much that the child chokes on it, or feels invaded by what you offer. When you are able to consistently provide just the right amount of organization and support with the "bits" that you provide, there will be an increasing sense of an alliance. The child will have an increasing sense of security, trust, and feeling understood. This is the condition that addresses the sensory integration difficulties and provides nutrients at the psychological level for the emotional development. At the same time, the

child will use the bits you offer as scaffolding for organizing a new working model of reality.

In this process, it is also important, if possible, to help the parents to understand their child in the way that you have come to understand the child. This is particularly true for younger children, but less critical for adolescents who, with the therapist's support, will eventually negotiate a relationship with their parents themselves. In the end, the child will come to a new working model of reality that is up to the developmental challenges they face. At this point, it may be useful to talk with the child, and perhaps the parents, about your understanding of the sensory integration differences, the way these differences contributed to the presenting symptoms and the possible risks they may pose in the future. Some of these sensory integration difficulties may fade with development and maturation, others may persist. Some of these differences may even become strengths, such as the adolescent who studied human protocol the way he studied computer protocols and now is a very successful aerospace engineer. If this description of how to do this work with children with SED seems to be more about affect than information, I would confirm that from my own experience. Much of what is happening to the child is felt by the therapist rather than arriving in the therapist's mind articulated in words. Initially, the therapist may respond without any articulated understanding, such as when the therapist restrained Wallace when he tried to lay waste to the office. Eventually, however, it is good to put these feelings into words and formulations. In the end, the formulations will only be shadows of the feelings and will not contain all that went on; in fact, if one is able to reflect back on the feelings of a case, it will be a wellspring for new understanding for years to come.

THE CASE OF PENELOPE

To illustrate this process, I present a final, very different case of a thirteen-year-old girl whose parents brought her against her will. She appeared as a slight, young looking prepubescent child. She had secluded herself in her room, refusing to go to school or to participate in any family or other outside activities, and had stopped eating. Instead, she was silent in her room, punctuated only by what her parents described as "weird" noises. The history that the parents provided had little else that seemed relevant to this sudden withdrawal from the world. The therapist sat with Penelope alone in silence for a number of sessions until finally she made eye contact. Without asking any questions, the therapist then wondered about what Penelope's parents had been talking about when they mentioned "weird" noises. In the next session, she brought a wooden flute, and the therapist wondered how it was to play the flute.

In the following session, Penelope brought a beginner music book, opened it, and began to play. The therapist studied Penelope as she played, and eventually figured out that she knew nothing about music or about this instrument, but that she had taught herself to play, removing a finger from a covered hole when the notes ascended the staff and covering a hole in line when the note descended. There was no sense of timing, accidentals, and no knowledge of the instrument's proper fingerings. After a few sessions of listening to her play and learning how she played, the therapist asked if he could bring in his wooden flute and play along with her. She consented.

In the next few sessions, Penelope and the therapist played in perfect unison. Penelope seemed delighted. Occasionally, the therapist would play a "wrong note" and ask for guidance from Penelope, in response to which she began to talk for the first time. After a time, the therapist wondered why one note was solid, but another was not filled in. She did not know and the therapist wondered if they might agree that the one with the hole in it might be held two counts while the solid looking one be just held for a single count. Likewise, gradually, accidentals, proper fingerings, rhythms were all introduced until Penelope was now playing the recorder the way others might play it. Finally, after playing in unison for several weeks, the therapist suggested they might play a duet. Penelope agreed and after some practice, it sounded wonderfully pleasant to hear. In the meantime, Penelope had come out of her room, began attending family meals, and returned to school.

Next in her sessions, Penelope began to bring in stories she had written. These stories were about gnomes and wood elves who would lose themselves in looking at a sunset through a drop of water as it expanded to fill the sky, and would jump from leaf to leaf in the great forest, meandering about without a sense of purpose or direction. It was easy to see that something was missing, but impossible to know what was missing. Penelope brought these stories on a thumb drive and transferred them to the therapist's computer, where they would read them together. One day, she let the therapist know that there was a story on her thumb drive that she did not want to talk about, and then handed the thumb drive over.

The mystery story, which was no doubt written by Penelope, was an intense romance between a common girl and a prince, a shadow of the missing piece. The missing piece was her pubescence. Her breakdown occurred under what Penelope had experienced as an intolerably intense pubescent development. With her story, she was revealing her inner world. It became clear that she could only think in the silence of her room and in the silence of the therapist's office. She then learned to think when she was in unison with the therapist; and with practice, she could think in harmony with others. This is when she returned to her life in the world, where she had to think in harmony and in the presence of others.

Penelope's internal pubescent pressures were too loud, and had been overwhelming her ability to work through her developmental challenges. Her sensory integration difficulty was a hypersensitivity to her internal developing sexual experiences. The therapy allowed her to bring her chaos to the consulting room first in the form of silence, then in the disorganized flute playing, then in the meandering stories, and finally it coalesced into an intense romance. Bit by bit, the therapist provided the organization which turned out to be a proxy for a model of reality that met the challenges of her world at home and at school.

SUMMARY

This chapter has considered those children who, at some point in their development, cease to function psychologically. As a somewhat nebulous term, we dubbed these children as having SED. We considered the vast array of different literatures and the different designations that describe these children, including childhood schizophrenia, autism, childhood psychosis, and vulnerable children. Historically, the criterion which has primarily distinguished these designations one from the other, age of onset, has not been found to have much validity. What does tie these designations together is that they describe developmental delays and are likely caused by sensory integration deficits, including nonverbal learning disabilities. A model of development was formulated that put the developmental delays and sensory integration deficits in the context of nonlinear systems theory. Using this theory as a foundation, a framework for therapy was offered that addresses the developmental challenges that children with SED face, with strategies to help usher these children through the places in development where they get stuck, assisting them in their maturation.

REFERENCES

American Psychiatric Association (1980). *DSM-III: Diagnostic and Statistical Manual of Mental Disorders.* Washington, DC: APA, 205–225.

Ames, C. S. and Jarrold, C. (2009). Identifying symbolic relationships in autism spectrum disorders: A deficit in the identification of temporal co-occurrence? *Journal of Autism and Developmental Disorders,* 39(12), 1723–34.

Anthony, E. J., Koupernik, C., and Chiland, C. (Eds.). (1978). *Vulnerable Children.* New York: Wiley.

Asperger, H. (1991). Autistic psychopathy in childhood. In Frith U. (Ed.). *Autism and Asperger Syndrome* (pp. 37–92). Cambridge: Cambridge University Press.

Ayres, J. (1973). *Sensory Integration and Learning Disorders.* Los Angeles, CA: Western Psychological Services.

Bender, L. (1947). Childhood schizophrenia. *American Journal of Orthopsychiatry,* 42, 40–56.

———. (1956). Schizophrenia in childhood: Its recognition, description and treatment. *American Journal of Orthopsychiatry,* 26, 499–506.

Bion, W. R. (1963). *Elements of Psycho-Analysis.* London, UK: Heinemann.

———. (1970). *Attention and Interpretation: A Scientific Approach to Insight in Psycho-Analysis and Groups*. London: Tavistock.

Cohen, T., Etezady, H., & Pacella, B. (1993). *The Vulnerable Child*. Madison, CT: International University Press.

Fallon, T. (2014). *Disordered Thought and Development: Chaos to Organization in the Moment*. New York: Jason Aronson.

Fombonne, E. (2009). Epidemiology of pervasive developmental disorders. *Pediatric Research*, 65, 591–598.

Forness, S. R. and Jane Knitzer. (1992). A new proposed definition and terminology to replace "serious emotional disturbance" in Individuals with Disabilities Education Act. *School Psychology Review*, 21(1), 12–21.

Franchi, V. (2015). The gaze, the mirror and representation of a self in the treatment of a young boy with pervasive developmental delay and marked autistic features. *Journal of Child Psychotherapy*, 41, 41–56.

Freud, A. (1963). The concept of developmental lines. *The Psychoanalytic Study of the Child*, 18, 245–265.

Gavilán, B., Fournier-Del Castillo, C., & Bernabeu-Verdú, J. (2007). Differences between the neuropsychological profiles of Asperger's syndrome and non-verbal learning disorder. *Revista de neurologia*, 45(12), 713.

Green, E. J., Fazio-Griffith, L., & Parson, J. (2015). Treating children with psychosis: An integrative play therapy approach. *International Journal of Play Therapy*, 24(3), 162–176.

Harris, J. (2016). Leo Kanner and Hans Asperger: Setting the historical record straight. *Journal of the American Academy of Child & Adolescent Psychiatry*, 55(8), 728–735.

Hertzig, M. E. and Walker, H. A. (1975). Symptom formation as an expression of disordered information processing in schizophrenic children. *Journal of Autism and Childhood Schizophrenia*, 5, 13–24.

Hinsie, L. E. and Campbell, R. J. (1976). *Psychiatric Dictionary*. New York: Oxford University Press.

Kanner, L. (1943). Autistic disturbances of affective contact. *Nervous Child*, 2, 217–250.

Kawai, T. (2009). Union and separation in the therapy of pervasive developmental disorders and ADHD. *Journal of Analytic Psychology*, 54, 659–675.

Knafo, D. (2016). Going blind to see: The psychoanalytic treatment of trauma, regression and psychosis. *American Journal of Psychotherapy*, 70(1), 79–100.

Knafo, D. and Selzer, M. (2015). "Don't step on Tony!" The importance of symptoms when working with psychosis. *Psychoanalytic Psychology*, 32(1), 159–172.

Knitzer, J. (1982). *Unclaimed children: The failure of public responsibility to children and adolescents in need of mental health services*. Washington, DC: Children's Defense Fund.

Mahler, M. S. (1944). Schizophrenia in childhood: The Nervous child, I, 1941, pp. 137–250. *Psychoanalytic Quarterly*, 13, 131–133.

Mahler, M. S., Pine, F., and Bergman, A. (1975). *The Psychological Birth of the Human Infant: Symbiosis and Individuation*. New York: Basic Books.

Martin, J. A. M. (1971). Sensory disorder in the autistic child and its implications for treatment. In M. Rutter (Ed.). (1971). *Infantile Autism: Concepts, Characteristics and Treatment* (p. 21). London, UK: Churchill Livingstone.

Miller, J. M. (2002). Anna Freud: A view of development, disturbance, and therapeutic techniques: Rose Edgcumbe. *Psychoanalytic Quarterly*, 71(1), 139–142.

Norian, P. (1978). *Sensory integration impairment in autistic children* (Master's thesis, Chicago School of Professional Psychology). Retrieved from ProQuest Dissertations and Theses (EP40086).

Ornstein, A. (1976). Making contact with the inner world of the child: Toward a theory of psychoanalytic psychotherapy with children. *Comprehensive Psychiatry*, 17(1), 3–36.

Parens, H. (2011). *Parenting for Emotional Growth: A Textbook, Workshops, and Curriculum for Students in Grades K-12*. Philadelphia: Jefferson Medical College.

Rass, E. (2003). Chapter 13: Making contact with the perception world of a child: Undetected disabilities in sensory motor integration and the effects on the development of self-esteem. *Progress in Self Psychology*, 19, 287–308.

Read, J., van Os, J., Morrison, A. P., and Ross, C. A. (2005). Childhood trauma, psychosis and schizophrenia: a literature review with theoretical and clinical implications. *Acta Psychiatrica Scandinavica*, 112(5), 330–350.

Rourke, B. P. (1989). *Nonverbal Learning Disabilities: The Syndrome and the Model*. New York: Guilford Press.

Schlenger, W. E., Etheridge, R. M., Hansen, D. J., Fairbank, D. W., and Onken, J. (1992). Evaluation of state efforts to improve systems of care for children and adolescents with severe emotional disturbances: The CASSP initial cohort study. *Journal of Mental Health Administration*, 19(2), 131.

Singletary, W. M. (2015). An integrative model of autism spectrum disorder: ASD as a neurobiological disorder of experienced environmental deprivation, early life stress and allostatic overload. *Neuropsychoanalysis*, 17(2), 81–119.

Tustin, F. (1995). *Autism and Childhood Psychosis*. London, GB: Karnac Books.

Volkmar, F. R., Stier, D. M., and Cohen, D. J. (1985). Age of recognition of pervasive developmental disorder. *The American Journal of Psychiatry*, 142(12), 1450–1452.

Zapparoli, G. C. and Gislon, M. C. (1999). An integrative approach to severe emotional disorders. *Psychoanalytic Psychotherapy*, 13, 19–30.

Chapter Six

Narcissism

How It Develops and How It Appears

Mary Davis and M. Hossein Etezady

The concept of narcissism is a universal feature of all mental life, but is complex and difficult to discuss clearly. It becomes even more complicated when we consider the many different ways in which the term is used. In popular discourse, it is used to accuse people of being self-involved and selfish, and this emotional resonance imbues our thinking sometimes even when the intent is to be nonjudgmental in professional contexts. In psychoanalytic thinking, we use it most commonly to discuss issues of self-esteem and its maintenance; "the overall well-being of the self, including feelings of aliveness, initiative, authenticity, coherence, and self-esteem" (Auchincloss and Samberg 2012, p. 162); narcissistic pathology; or narcissistic defenses. The term was generally used primarily in pejorative ways until Heinz Kohut (1971) introduced self psychology and the idea that there can be a normal developmental line of narcissism.

Because the phenomenon of narcissism is central to our psychological functioning, it can be identified in any developmental discussion, whether that discussion focuses on biology, separation-individuation, psychosexual development, or epigenesis. When we focus on narcissism, all other psychic resources and experiences can be (but are not necessarily) seen as operating in the service of self- and mutual regulation. When we focus on other elements of personality, consideration of narcissism supports and illuminates the discussion. Structural, functional, and neurocognitive perspectives all intertwine with the issues of normal narcissism. We cannot clearly discuss notions of self-centeredness, self-regulation, self-esteem, and self-reliance, or self- and object relations, without also discussing normal narcissism; whenever we consider the relationship of self to self, we consider narcissism.

DEFINITIONS OF NARCISSISM

References to narcissism ideally will include, for clarity, a description of the ways in which the term is being used in the discussion at hand. Multiple definitions representing different levels of abstraction, as well as different views of how narcissism exists within the full character structure, have been used in the professional literature in the past. Freud (1914) set the stage for the confusion by himself using narcissism in a variety of ways and at varying levels of abstraction. He used it to refer to a sexual perversion, as it was used prior to the beginnings of psychoanalysis; to the self as a libidinal object; to a developmental stage that precedes object ties; to primitive, omnipotent, and magical aspects of thinking and feeling; to a type of object relationship; to a mode of relating to the environment (characterized by withdrawal of libidinal cathexis, as in "narcissistic neuroses" or psychoses); and to self-esteem.

Today we include the concept of normal narcissism, which depends on the development of self- and object constancy; the structural integrity of the self-concept; the ability to maintain an equilibrium between libidinal and aggressive drive derivatives; harmony between the self and superego structures; the capacity for ego-syntonic expression of impulses; and the capacity to receive gratification from external objects. It can be strongly affected by the presence or absence of a state of physical well-being. In the presence of normal narcissism, we can see a sustained, realistic, and resilient self-regard, with mature aspirations and ideals and the capacity for deep and satisfying object relations.

PATHOLOGICAL NARCISSISM

When we consider the ways in which narcissism goes "wrong," we find different levels of pathology: narcissistic defenses, narcissistic character or personality disorders, and pathological narcissism, all of which exist in a spectrum ranging from fully adaptive to severely maladaptive. Van der Waals, in 1965, was the first to suggest that "pathological narcissism" did not represent a fixation at an early stage of normal development, but was a reflection of distorted object relations, arising from other, earlier fixations or disruptions of development. Rosenfeld, in 1964, suggested that in narcissistic pathology the separateness of self and object is denied as a defense against depression and envy, but that behind the defensive structure are rich but primitive object representations. He distinguished between libidinal narcissism, in which the defense is against experiencing separateness from others and envy of others, and destructive narcissism, which he saw as a manifestation of the death drive.

Narcissistic defenses are those which attempt to preserve an idealized view of the self, denying any limitations. They tend to be rigid and uncompromising, and include omnipotence, idealization, devaluation, and splitting; all are used to ward off challenges to the omnipotent sense of self.

The *Psychodynamic Diagnostic Manual* (PDM Task Force 2006) suggests that there are two types of narcissistic personality disorder, the "arrogant/entitled" type and the "depressed/depleted type." Both exhibit a lack of cohesion of the self-concept; intense dependence on the opinions of others, with driven perfectionism or maladaptive altruism in an attempt to gain positive acclaim from others; vulnerability to shame, rage, and humiliation when positive acclaim from others fails (with the shame and rage often followed by depression); and impairment in empathy and concern for others, with resultant maladaptive object relations. The individual with an arrogant/entitled narcissistic personality disorder will exhibit defensive grandiosity and a tendency to sadomasochistic object relations. The depressed/depleted narcissist is the individual in whom attempts to maintain a positive sense of self have failed, resulting in a turn to envy and a search for people to idealize as the individual attempts to find a stable way to feel acceptable to others and to him- or herself.

Pathological narcissism describes an individual in which defensive splitting, used to defend against envy and aggressive wishes, has distorted the basic structure of the self, putting a grandiose view of oneself in place of a balanced view of self with integration of good and bad aspects. In this defensive position, the self is viewed essentially as "all good," while others are viewed as "all bad," hostile, malevolent, and perhaps unreal or inhuman in some way. The consequences of such pathological narcissism include an inordinate dependence on acclaim by others; unstable and unsatisfactory object relations; and an impaired capacity for concern, empathy, and love for others.

NORMAL NARCISSISM

We encounter narcissism in three different contexts: in normal development, in pathological development, and in treatment settings. In normal development, normal narcissism is present with splitting and the operation of the pleasure ego. In the course of development, the split between negative and positive is fused at the point when the child recognizes that mother and child are separate individuals and that mother can go away: what those who follow Mahler (1972) would call "rapprochement resolution." As this occurs, primary narcissism develops into the object-related secondary form of narcissism. Organic, environmental, or intrapsychic factors may cause deficits, deviations, disruptions, arrests, or fixations, so that pathological development occurs. In treatment settings, narcissism contributes to adaptive coping, symptom formation, resistance, pathological defenses, and certain forms of transference and countertransference. "Malignant narcissism" is the arrested primary form of narcissism, characteristic of the pre-rapprochement individual, who has not yet achieved self and object constancy.

In everyday life, what we term "normal narcissism" is the ability to maintain a positively toned and stable sense of self and of relative internal comfort throughout the vicissitudes of daily life. This sense of internal comfort is described variously as a sense of OK-ness, sense of contentment and harmony, competence, emotional equilibrium. People with adequate normal narcissism are able to acknowledge failure, disappointment, or conflict with others, and to recognize the impact on their lives. Because they can maintain a positively toned sense of self, however, they have the emotional resilience and resources to persist in a difficult task when failure is possible, and to venture onto new and untried ground knowing that the response from others may be negative. Narcissistic equilibrium makes it possible to say to oneself, "I think I can do this, and I'll try. If I fail, I may feel awful, but life will go on and I'll be OK." The individual continues to function in daily activities, to risk future failure, disappointment, or conflict, and to be able throughout to return after temporary setbacks to an overall sense of OK-ness, contentment, and satisfaction. An individual with normal narcissism will be able both to find this narcissistic equilibrium and to support it or reestablish it through intrapsychic mechanisms and through interactions with others.

In early life, approximately the first nine months, the infant exhibits a monadic mode of functioning which is primarily oral and narcissistic. Children may have some sense of relatedness as early as possibly the first few days of life; for instance, an infant whose mother has read out loud daily during the pregnancy will respond differently to mother's voice than to the voices of other women. The early stages of relating can be seen from very early on, with affective reactions and affective reciprocity (Trevarthen and Grant 1979), suggesting some early awareness that others exist. However, representations of the libidinal object are still partial, and very early object relations are internalized only in fragments of part objects, not distinctly differentiated from self-representations. One might suggest that the infant begins to recognize that the other is not-me, but does not yet recognize that the other is an Other.

At about nine months, the infant generally has moved to the dyadic mode of relatedness, which can be described as anal, sadomasochistic, and mostly preverbal. Primary process thinking and primary narcissism, with infantile omnipotence, dominate the first three years, and they live on in the unconscious in later life. In the second and third years of life, the years of transition, we see significant events that prepare the ground for the emergence of self-constancy and normal narcissism in synchrony with the emergence of object-libidinal constancy. The emergence of these two capacities are indispensable for the development of a triadic mode of relatedness and oedipal conflict resolution. The gradual and progressive transition from primary narcissism, in the monadic mode of relatedness, to a dyadic and later a triadic mode of relatedness, along with the transition to a dyadic and later a triadic mode of secondary narcissism, occurs in these years.

Sometime around thirty-six months we begin to see the third mode of functioning, which is triadic, genital, verbal, oedipal. Followers of Mahler (1979) would describe this as "post object constancy" (implying that the rageful upheaval of momentary separations no longer overruns and eradicates libidinal ties to the primary object) and would say that rapprochement resolution has occurred. Even though (with the attainment of object constancy) the child knows that mother still exists, the absence of mother is anxiety provoking and acutely disorganizing, and in normal development toddlers go through a phase of increased clinginess and closeness to mother as they struggle to reach the "resolution" that allows them to better tolerate their own ambivalence toward the mother or the mothering figures. Rapprochement resolution is facilitated by and facilitates (in synchronous development for the normative child) the healing of the split in good and bad object representations on the way toward increasing self and object constancy. As this psychological development occurs, we see also the development of secondary narcissism (in which libido, or emotional energy, previously invested in the idealized symbiotic object is withdrawn and invested in the ego and the sense of self) and secondary process thinking (in which reality-processing rather than emotion and wish-fulfillment is preeminent). Later in this paper, as we discuss the vicissitudes of early development and their effects on narcissism, we will address these issues in more detail.

RECOGNIZING NORMAL NARCISSISM

Let us examine what normal narcissism looks like in practice. Susan is a successful middle-aged professional woman who exhibits a good supply of healthy narcissism. When she was turned down for promotion recently, she was angry and sad but talked with her supervisor about what had gone wrong, and worked to remedy the holes in her experience so that she could be promoted the next time. When her daughter married, she excitedly took part in planning the wedding, but didn't take over completely, and gave up her own fantasied wedding so that the daughter's wedding could be hers and not Sue's. When she lost her father to heart disease, Sue was briefly unable to work due to her grief. Later she returned to work, successfully coped with a major new project, and found some relief from grief in her work. Her marriage has had its ups and downs, and she was estranged from her husband briefly after he had an affair. Now however, they are back together, have been working on their relationship in therapy, and each of them feels that they are closer than ever. Because of her early development, she can maintain a positive sense of self despite narcissistic blows. She can face and work through the griefs and triumphs of life without losing her balance more than temporarily, and can find ways both to minimize the impacts of the negatives and to fully enjoy the positives. This is healthy narcissism in an adult.

Individuals who lack this healthy narcissism are unable to maintain or restore internal well-being. They must resort to various maladaptive intrapsychic or interpersonal mechanisms in order to feel less ashamed, guilty, rageful, or helpless, and to rid themselves of their internal discomfort. The strategies they use are primitive, and include idealization, denial, omnipotent fantasy, grandiosity, primitive paranoid projection, and splitting. Susan's colleague, for instance, was turned down for the same promotion that Susan lost. The colleague, however, began talking with co-workers about his perception that he had been discriminated against because he was a white man, when the individual actually promoted was a black woman. He encouraged others to resist the direction and to interfere with the work of the newly hired woman; eventually he was sanctioned and ultimately lost his job because of his narcissistic rage and his inability to keep it from interfering with his daily work. We use the term "pathological narcissism" to describe people who react in similar ways.

In children we look for different capacities. Susan's grandson, Tim, has just turned four. His early years were difficult, as he had some physical problems that required many visits to the doctor. Although he often cried when blood was drawn, he allowed mother to comfort him and is now proud of being a "big boy" who cooperates with the doctor. He is in a preschool class where he is learning to share his toys. Usually he can do so without conflict, but if he is ill or upset he may have a small tantrum when required to give up a favored toy. He likes his teacher and has no trouble leaving mother to be with her. He listens better to her than to other staff at the preschool, and he lets her comfort him when upset. Tim's relationship with his father is relatively good, though Tim prefers mother's company and at times tries to exclude father from activities. Tim often objects to going to bed, but is developing a routine of bath, story, and lights out that he insists on. He exhibits normal narcissism in his ability to use important relationships for comfort and emotional equilibrium. This helps him to negotiate the stresses of growing up and to tolerate limits as he learns to deal with the world on his own. This is normal narcissism in a young child who is just developing early object constancy.

Children whose development is going awry will not be able to use the presence of others to comfort themselves and to tolerate the stresses of daily life. They may have severe separation anxiety and be unable to attend school;

they may become enraged and aggressive when other children try to share their toys, or to join in their play; they are often bossy and coercive with peers and with family; and they are generally unable to soothe themselves in order to go to bed in the evening, to go to sleep easily, and in other aspects of daily life.

THE DEVELOPMENT OF NORMAL NARCISSISM

A reminder at this point as we deal with the first three years of life: we must often refer to the role of the primary caretaker for the children we discuss. For the sake of simplicity we have used the term "mother" in that context, but it should be remembered that the "mothering figure" role in the child's life is not gender specific, and that the concept "mother" may refer to multiple caretakers at the same time.

Foundations of Early Development Prior to Birth

To understand how children develop their ability to maintain a healthy narcissistic balance through adulthood, we must begin with pregnancy, since prenatal events certainly affect development in many ways. Mother's attitudes toward and fantasies about the child and about her relationship to the child, as well as about her own life, may determine in part whether the infant will be born with an optimal opportunity for normal development of narcissism, as well as other characteristics. Pleasure in the pregnancy certainly increases the likelihood of adequate prenatal care, so that possible medical problems are more likely to be detected early. Pleasure in the pregnancy also makes it easier for mother to cope with the physical discomfort of the pregnancy, affecting her attitude toward the infant when born. Although the evidence is not yet compelling, we suspect that stress or anxiety in mother may affect the intrauterine environment and physiology, changing the neurotransmitters in the intrauterine fluid. This may in turn affect the developing brain and compromise the infant's innate, biologically determined capacity for self-soothing. Such disorders as schizophrenia, bipolar disorder, and anxiety disorders, which clearly have a biological substrate and which affect the infant's experience of living in the world, also will have a major impact on development and will modify the infant's capacity for self-soothing.

In addition, because the child's early ability to regulate his or her sense of self is heavily dependent on the relationship with mother, we should consider the recent research data that suggests that children whose mothers read aloud daily during the pregnancy show differential responses to mother's voice as versus the voices of other women in the first few days after birth. This certainly suggests that some rudimentary capacity for relatedness is present almost from the first moment, as the nidus for a later crucial ability to use mother's presence to soothe, as the child learns to self-soothe.

Whatever the child experiences in the womb, and whatever the physiological effects of prenatal stress, mother's psychological state matters. The child is born into an environment largely shaped by mother's psychology, and her emotional capacities shape the development of the child's emotional capacities. Mother's own object constancy, with self-reflection, empathy, and tolerance for ambivalence, allows her effectively to contain, mirror, and reflect a view of her baby as a feeling and intentional being. Fonagy and colleagues (2004) has described how the self is formed from the reflection in the eye of the mother, and he has shown, at nine months and six years of age, that a self-reflective capacity in mother strengthens her ability to attach and to foster the child's development of secure attachment (where secure attachment is understood as the ability to know that mother will return, so that the child can manage the anxiety of separation). Secure attachment, in turn, helps the baby to use mother's presence, and the memory of mother's presence, to maintain an emotional equilibrium, the core of normal narcissism.

Early Infancy and Parental Roles

In pregnancy and early infancy, the child has a set of inborn capabilities and traits. In response to their own conscious and unconscious wishes and needs, the parents selectively respond to and encourage trends and tendencies that fit their expectations or wishes. Children whose parents are enthusiastically athletic, for instance, may be encouraged to explore their body and the bodies of others, and may be played with in more physically active ways. The same child, born to parents who are less physical and more intellectual, may be sung to, read to, encouraged to be attentive and alert but if vigorously physical may be told to "settle down," or to "be quiet," discouraging the activity. In general, the child's first seeds of knowing what and how he or she is germinate in the interactions with mother: the "gleam in the mother's eye" teaches a child how to be, as mother mirrors the tendencies that fit her needs. The child's ability to be what mother sees and what mother wants strengthens the attachment, and mother's pleasure in the infant conveys the pleasure of normal narcissistic balance.

Some parents are so needy that the selective encouragement of some behaviors over others becomes extreme and they cannot recognize the child's realistic endowment because it does not fit their wished-for reality. Examples might include the child who is excessively idealized, who is a disappointment due to birth defects, or who is seen as a possession and not an individual. These children become vulnerable to narcissistic pathology because they are not able to see themselves reflected both realistically and positively in the parents' eyes, and so cannot develop a sustainable positive view of who they are. Although the development of healthy narcissism does not come to fruition for years, the foundation is laid with the pregnancy and birth and the parents' ability to value the child highly and realistically, for who he or she is and can be, rather than for what parents want that the infant is not. Any time the parents' needs are allowed to overwhelm the needs of the child, the child has difficulties in maintaining and improving an already tenuous (because newly forming) capacity for narcissistic balance.

0–2 Months

In the early months, cognitive development, primordial ego formation, and development of precursors to later psychic structure are all occurring in synchrony. The foundations for the development of a self and for individuation are laid as the infant's endowment interacts with the expectations and wishes of parents. The neonate makes many adjustments to the environment, first physiologically and later psychologically, in an effort to reduce unpleasure and return to the quiet alert attentiveness that takes in the external world. Children are initially unable to maintain physiological homeostasis without mother's interventions, and respond to excessive stimuli with crying and undifferentiated negative affect. Most likely they do not distinguish mother's help—diapering, feeding, rocking—from their own crying, urinating, defecating. All, most likely, are experienced as unpleasure relieved, and the first affective differentiation in an infant's experience of the world is "pleasure vs. unpleasure," "good vs. bad." The child who is difficult to soothe, or who is easily overstimulated to the point of undifferentiated distress, is likely to have later problems with self-regulation and with maintaining a narcissistic equilibrium.

Children show evidence of perceptual, cognitive, and mnemonic differentiation from birth. Soon after birth, it can be demonstrated that they differentiate mother's voice from that of other women reading pieces that mother read out loud during the pregnancy (DeCasper and Spence 1986). By six weeks they recognize mother's face; by two months they respond differentially to mother's presence in other ways. With this early awareness of the need-satisfying object, the child is absolutely dependent on mother for survival. Mother is in turn only relatively dependent on the child, as she experiences Winnicott's primary maternal preoccupation (1960).

As mother "libidinizes" the dyadic interaction by her pleasure in it, the child's overall positive affective experience gains continuity as a gestalt of well-being. When this is interrupted, the discontinuity is experienced as unpleasure. The interruption might be due to injury, mother's distress, loss of attunement with mother's ability to soothe and contain the infant's distress, or other factors. As the mother-child dyad restores and maintains the infant's experience of well-being, adaptive mechanisms which are precursors to ego (based on internalizations of mother's ability to soothe and contain distress) will develop and foster resilience. The capacity of the mother-child dyad to maintain the infant's experience of well-being is affected by many factors, both internal and external. They may include neurophysiological integration at birth, overall evenness of maturity, or innate activity level. The excitability and reactivity of sensory modalities make sensory overload more or less likely. The child's response to ministration or need for holding will affect the child's ability to use the dyad for self-regulation. The need to experience and explore external reality, cognitive abilities to focus, concentrate, and discriminate, and potential for anxiety also affect the overall experience as the mother-child dyad interacts with external reality.

Normal narcissism is reflected in the ability of the mother-child dyad to respond to physiological or environmental stress with soothing, comfort, and settling back to alert attention. Mother's ability to tolerate and regulate affect, to be attuned to the infant and to soothe and mirror the infant, enhances the possibility that the child's precursor adaptive mechanisms will succeed in adaptation to the environment. Children contribute to the narcissistic equilibrium by working actively to adjust themselves to mother, and by eliciting soothing maternal behavior. If mother ignores or is irritated by whimpering, for instance, some children will cry lustily to bring mother for help. If the child does not cry, or elicit maternal soothing in other ways, there likely has already been some disturbance in the development of normal narcissism, either as an inborn inability to behave in ways that elicit soothing or for some environmental reason.

The rhythms of daily life, as hunger becomes satiety, dry becomes wet and then dry again, involve both baby and mother, and provide sensations that the baby begins to understand as coming both from within and without. The infant discovers regularities in the world and works actively to adjust to the mother in order to achieve physiological homeostasis and to stop unpleasure. With recurring regularities in one's physical state, a sense of the body develops, and the child begins to make a rudimentary, incomplete distinction between models of inside and outside. He or she creates a primitive model of how the world works, and begins to develop patterns of repetition, experience, gratification, and modes of attachment which define how he or she will deal with the world. All of these primitive patterns of interaction, including the pattern of how we restore homeostasis and affective equilibrium, move the individual toward what much later becomes a mature ability to establish and maintain self-cohesion.

2–9 Months

At about two months, the child has some dim recognition of the mother as a need satisfying object but not as a fully recognized Other, with internalized fragments of the libidinal object (the mother). The child likely has differentiated the part-objects from self but may not yet have recognized mother as an object in her own right. Children still function as if the mother-child dyad is a "dual unity with a common boundary" (Mahler 1979, p.78) that they control. Ego precursors and the primordial narcissistic equilibrium are developing simultaneously, and the developing ego takes part in shaping healthy narcissism; the baby, for instance, learns that if the "unpleasure" of hunger is present, crying often brings some relief as mother brings the breast or the bottle to feed. Developing capacities for narcissistic equilibrium, in turn, shape the developing ego by providing stronger pleasurable response to some ego functions than to others. Eventually there is some beginning recognition of one's existence, what Stern (1985) calls the emergent self, and a primordial self-regulatory equilibrium that can be upset, such as when the infant must wait longer than usual for a bottle. When children confidently expect that their hunger will be relieved imminently, they can maintain themselves with minimal unpleasure. Once they have waited longer than their primitive models of the world say is expectable, they lose their sense of OK-ness, and may experience organismic distress and primitive rage. Repeated brief experiences of unpleasure followed by relief, when mother feeds/changes/comforts the distressed child, build the beginning of trust that comfort can be restored and that the balance of pleasure over unpleasure can be regained. These repeated experiences also build the beginning of an understanding that the child can exert some control over the environment, by crying and thus stimulating the response that relieves the distress.

These early experiences of relief of unpleasure, and the growing belief that one can rely on that relief, also represent the beginnings of the development of trust, the "very first essential developmental task of early life, particular to the nature of human object relations" (Etezady 2017). It is indispensable in the development of secure attachment, self and object constancy, and self-cohesion, and the structural complexity of the personality (as well as phase-specific advances) in all subsequent development depends on the achievement of this very basic task. It is the "sustained background of safety created by the caregiver(s) that allows the incremental and multilayered internalization of the selfobject functions that meet the requirements of internal regulation of the budding self" (ibid.).

By 4–5 months, if all has gone well, the child's facial expressions are increasingly complex and communicative. If early experiences have been predictable, safe, and not usually overwhelming, with mother attuned enough to provide relief from overstimulation or other unpleasure, the child's quiet, alert attentiveness has become active interest and scanning of the surround, and searching for preferred stimuli like mother's face.

Mahler (1972) called the child's interest in the world "hatching," and felt that it occurred when pleasure in outer sensory perceptions and maturational pressures joined with an optimal level of "safe anchorage," within the experience of the mother-child dyad, to foster venturing out to the world. In some children, the maturational pressures are insufficient to stimulate that venturing out. For such children, mother's own pleasure in the dyadic interaction (libidinization) woos them out of the "safe anchorage." The child's basic endowment, including the strength of the drives, continues to make a variety of different behaviors possible, and mother and others in the environment continue to respond preferentially to those behaviors that match their wishes and expectations for the child. The developmental patterns of repetition, experience, gratification, and modes of attachment become elaborated over the first year of the child's life, and create internal models of the world, the early nuclei around which the personality coalesces, so that the child becomes that particular child of that particular mother in that particular family and society. For instance, a child who is born an extrovert and has not been impeded by the environment may smile at everyone, with a special smile for mother, and grab for everything in reach. Those who are born as an introvert, or with a risk averse temperament, or who have not been allowed self-expression by caregivers, may be more somber, smile mostly or only at mother, and be less eager to reach out for things. The former child not only has a basic endowment that includes higher levels of energy and a more intense need to observe and experience the environment, but likely also has experienced fewer disruptions of safety and pleasure. This child does not expect interactions with the environment to be aversive, and so has no primitive anxiety to suppress interest.

By 6–7 months children are generally actively exploring mother and mother's body, as we see the peak of face-patting, hair-pulling, grabbing jewelry. They are visually exploring an awareness that mother's face, the face that accompanies comfort, food, and safety, is different from other things in the world, and they check the unfamiliar against the familiar in a "customs inspection" (Brody 1966).

Even this early we see the split between healthy and disrupted narcissism. With a background of predominantly positive experiences within the mother-child dyad, the confident expectation of safety has developed and children can feel sure of their ability to return to harmony. They are able to feel safe and secure within themselves and in relationships with others. The more stable the consistency and predictability of caregiving, the more the child has internal representations of empathic attunement and libidinal availability from the parent; and the more the child is then able to use these internal representations for maintaining internal harmony and a sense of well-being, or "normal narcissism." This normal narcissism is reflected in the child's ability to restore his or her own harmony and physiological homeostasis more easily, to stop crying and return to alert attentiveness to others. Children with normal narcissism use mother's comfort more easily, and are less easily frustrated to the point of disintegration. They can let themselves be soothed as long as mother provides her part of the process, and may be able to soothe themselves with a thumb or a nipple.

If mother's interaction with her child has been unpredictable, unstable, distant, anxiety-ridden, rejecting, hostile, or otherwise unsatisfactory, children will be unable to (re)create the experience of a safe, predictable stable mother-child dyad. Without that safe harbor, primitive precursors of self are less able to develop, and the child's as yet incomplete ability to maintain a narcissistic equilibrium is compromised.

Early signs of disrupted narcissism may include more intense or prolonged stranger anxiety, reluctance to leave mother's arms or side, or easy frustration to the point of disintegration into tantrumming or tears. A more subtle sign may be seen in a lack of *any* anxiety at separation, an indiscriminate attempt to attach to any adult that appears. Basic trust in the predictability and safety of the world is unavailable, and the child often feels overwhelmed and helpless. Whether the failure of containment by the dyad is due to environmental trauma, poor parental functioning, excessive stimulation, or inborn higher-than-usual levels of tension, the outcome is the same. Primitive ego precursors are inadequate to the task of maintaining the child's sense of OK-ness, harmony, and safety, so that he or she uses whatever intrapsychic mechanisms are available to foster a sense of being OK. If the failure of containment is due to excess stimuli, the infant may not turn his attention as readily to the world, trying to delay hatching in favor of the safety of the mutual mother-child preoccupation, of having more trustworthy, reliable, confidently expectable interactions with a nurturing mother. Alternatively, if mother has been unable to provide enough safety and soothing, either because of environmental stresses or because of her own lack of emotional equilibrium, the child may move more quickly to find ways of coping that do not require mother's presence, and may prematurely enter the next developmental stage.

9–18 Months

From 9–18 months, development proceeds rapidly. The child has begun actively to brace himself against mother's body, to move away, and is crawling. He has discovered that the sounds that mother makes are somewhat predictable and attached to specific events, and he is developing early language. He has established that his body is different from mother's by experiences such as sucking on mother's thumb, which feels different in totality from sucking on his own, or by crawling or walking away from mother. Before the development of language, he creates primary process juxtapositions of ideas that then become hypotheses about how the world works and what is expectable. These hypotheses are checked by experimentation and observation of continuing experience. The child's striving, experimenting, and integration of a schema of the world drives the development of psychic structure, and secondary process begins to grow, first within the mother-child dyad and then independently within the child.

At this stage, the child is in a "love affair with the world," impervious to falls or bumps, "intoxicated with his own faculties and with the greatness of his world" (Mahler 1979, p. 128). As the child explores the world in the confidence of mother's presence, with the coming and going a recognition grows that mother does not experience the same things that the child experiences. The toddler will try to restore a sense of well-being even when mother is not available for checking and joint looking. When he or she shares the experience with mother, the focus of attention is shared, but different for each. The mutual focus allows the child to reestablish the emotional state that fuels exploration, the confidence of mother's presence and the belief in one's own abilities, and so the child can again turn to an outward focus.

Mother's ability to allow exploration while being ready to prevent danger, her belief that her baby is wonderful and can succeed in the world, allows her to let the child explore the world, to fall and recover without distress. Since mother is not distressed, the child can recover and, after only brief tears, return to elated exploration. When mother can take pleasure in the child's exploration without being less available for his return to home base, when both going out and coming back are equally welcome, the emotional equilibrium of normal narcissism grows and deepens.

At times this need to tolerate being apart is necessitated by mother's coming and going, rather than the child's. When the child recognizes that mother is not available to him, through mother's preoccupation or absence, often he or she reacts with "low-keyedness," an inward-turned attention. If this inward attention can be maintained, and the internal image of mother can be sustained until she returns to the shared focus, the child's narcissistic equilibrium is not disrupted and all is well. If that ability to maintain the image of the good mother fails, the child will be unable to sustain a sense of OK-ness and likely will cry. On mother's return, he or she will regain the equilibrium with varying degrees of resilience, but the recognition that mother is not always available to share experience—that she can be lost even temporarily—adds impetus to the developing sense of separateness. The experience of feeling the sadness and anger at mother's absence, and bouncing back either independently or with mother's help, teaches the child how reliably to restore the narcissistic balance.

As development continues, with the transition from the dyadic mode of relatedness, the internal representation of the object is becoming more complex and more cohesive. Early in the dyadic mode, however, the object's independent presence is "stripped of its subjectivity. It is used, controlled, dominated, and subjected to destruction" (Etezady 2015). Mother's continuing libidinal constancy and concern allows for the continuing repair of disruptions in the mother-child relationship, and thus allows for continuing "micro-internalizations" (Tolpin 1971) that contribute to growth of an internal representation that is more complex. The object's subjectivity can be recognized as separate from but similar to the child's subjectivity. "With the dawning recognition of transgressive damage inflicted upon the object and fear of loss of the object, attempt at repair of the damage and recovering the lost object," (Etezady, ibid.) the child is increasingly more able to recognize and accept the subjectivity of the object. In healthy secondary narcissism, the object's subjectivity is allowed, respected, and accommodated to, as self and object constancy move closer to completion. Triadic relationships and triadic conflict resolution become possible, allowing for ambivalence in a sustained relationship that "ties the self to an other, as well as to a second other, while at the same time tolerates, respects, and values the relationship between those two others to the exclusion of one's self" (Etezady, ibid.). This oedipal resolution allows for a sense of safety and connectedness and value—for healthy secondary narcissism—in complex relationships that involve multiple others, and allows for concern for the other, empathy, conscience, and other essential elements of the healthy adult.

Contributions of Language Development

The development of language supports this process. Language has many intrapsychic functions in toddlerhood, and among other things it serves to support the process of understanding how the world works, through naming, labeling, and categorizing. It also supports and drives the complexities of relationships, as the child learns to communicate one subjective self to another self that can be recognized as separate and different. The child needs mother to help in the reorganization of previous experiences and models of the world as he or she learns to put new experiences into words. Verbal skills enhance the capacity to deal with the external world, when mother tells the child what is going to happen and they plan for upcoming events, including separation and reunion. The need for plural and singular pronouns strengthens the recognition of separateness as well as the possibility of "me" and "you" coming together as "us." As the child's language develops, the developing internal world begins to shift from nonverbal to verbal, and the dyad must be reorganized and seen in a new way, moving toward secondary process.

Language also assists the child in maintaining a narcissistic equilibrium with the beginning turn from mother to the outside world. Mother's interaction with the baby initially included communicative babbling, which helped to establish the prosody of speech in the reciprocal noises that precede true language. As the child vocalizes and mother responds, mother's support becomes available from a distance. The ability to recognize mother both visually and vocally from a distance allows the child to know that mother is present even when not close by, lengthening the time for which he or she can maintain the internal image of mother and sustain the dyadic "safe harbor." The child begins to be able to create the experience within the developing self, with less reference to mother's capacities and contributions.

All along, mother's ability to think about her baby as an intentional and feeling Other has helped her with her own narcissistic equilibrium. When she could know that her baby was crying from hunger, or because of the discomfort of a wet diaper, she was able also to know that she could remedy the problem, and so did not have to feel that she had failed to be "good enough," but could be proud of her parenting abilities. With language, she can talk to the baby about that thinking, describing what she is doing, predicting that changing the diaper will make the baby more comfortable, encouraging the baby to wait as mother prepares the bottle or the breast. This ongoing monologue, likely present from the first days of the infant's life, fosters development of the child's ability to recognize his or her independent existence. Mother reflects on her child's inner world ("Oh, you are so mad! But here's your binky"), in order to stay attuned, but this also helps the toddler learn to reflect on himself, on the world, and on possible causes of his internal distress and its relief. Mother's reflection on the toddler's inner world fosters the toddler's ability to do the same. He then can use that reflective capacity to try out new coping mechanisms, to understand what has happened outside himself, and to regain his narcissistic equilibrium.

As mother and child reflect together on the toddler's inner world, they again share a joint focus of attention, and language enhances their union through shared meaning (Stern 1985). Again, however, the very existence of union implies the possibility of its absence, and language also serves as a contradiction to wishes for magical union, through the possibility of being misunderstood. The back and forth of union and separation through language within the relationship echoes the back and forth of union and separation through physical movement, and reinforces the growth of psychic structure and capacity to tolerate separation from mother. Naming affects and describing one's inner state to the Other (mother to child and child to mother) prepares one to know both one's own mind and the mind of the Other, in an early move toward full intersubjectivity. It also helps with self and mutual regulation and promotes abstract thought.

The child must now begin to work consciously to make the world suit him, and he uses language to get mother to care for him. A part of his growing mastery of the world is the ability to say "I want" to the primary caretaker, and to have the "want" satisfied. Spitz's third organizer (1965), the word "no," is another step toward mastery of the external world. It emphasizes that mother and child are separate, and fosters self-assertion. A successful "no" teaches the child that separateness can be acceptable. When the mother-child unity is reestablished after the no, in the recurring to and fro of that dyad, "no" becomes again an experience of disunity that can be repaired.

18–24 Months

When the early omnipotence of the mother-child dyad is no longer available—when mother is not there to "kiss it and make it better," or when mother cannot make it not-hurt—the child experiences it as mother's fault, and experiences mother as useless, the bad mother who makes him feel bad. If mother is able to contain (understand and accept) the child's rage at loss of the good mother, to survive without retaliation, and to stay libidinally available—to still be loving and caring and not punitive—the child can use his own primitive mechanisms for affect regulation and can experience success in restoring the dyadic "safe harbor." Repeated cycles of this disruption and repair facilitate ego growth, structure formation, and an increased capacity for self-regulation, as well as an increasing sense of mastery, and as the child repeatedly experiences this disruption and repair, his ability to repair the disruption becomes more sturdy. Pleasure in this mastery, enhanced by mother's pleasure and belief in it, becomes an important source of narcissistic supplies.

As development continues, ego functions become secondarily autonomous: the abilities that originally grew in order to please mother now exist for their own sake, because they are useful and pleasurable. The child's new ability to maintain a mental representation of mother allows for a sense of connection even if mother is absent, unavailable, disappointing, or angry. Mother's continuing libidinal availability supports a positive relationship that fosters mastery and increases the child's confident expectation of loving and being loved even in the face of his anger. He begins to move from idealization to realistic assessment of mother, and from grandiosity and infantile omnipotence to acceptance of his own vulnerabilities and shortcomings. As he learns to tolerate his ambivalence with healing of the split, he moves toward the establishment of self and object constancy.

At around eight months, the child developed object permanence (Piaget 1926), and knew cognitively that even when he could not see mother, she still existed. His ability to know *emotionally* that mother is still there, to know that she can come back, and to use that knowledge to sustain his emotional equilibrium, is a reflection of libidinal object constancy, and waxes and wanes until about thirty months, at the mercy of the toddler's moods and dependent on the tone of the mother-child situation at the moment. This is the developmental stage that Mahler (1972) labeled rapprochement, and there continue to be multiple trends in development. The child is less preoccupied with locomotion because he has mastered it, is more aware that he can be physically separate from mother, and is less oblivious to her presence even when he is busy. There tends to be constant concern with mother's whereabouts, and lots of active approach behavior, sharing of discoveries, showing of treasures, giving of gifts. Refueling—returning to mother to reestablish the internal feeling of safe harbor—is eventually replaced by the quest for continuing interaction, at a higher level of symbolization, by talking. The child wants conversation, not just being beside mother, and wants to play.

Late in this developmental period, the child is solidifying his recognition that he is different from mother and that mother cannot always make it right. He elaborates his primitive early models of who mother is and how she behaves, and of who he is and how he behaves; the internalized part-objects are becoming more complex and closer to becoming whole internalized objects. The differentiation between these self and object representations strengthens, and as rapprochement continues the child recognizes fully for the first time that he must manage in the world on his own, as a relatively helpless, small, separate individual. This is the first appearance of self as defined by Kohut (1971). The challenge to the infantile omnipotence, and the resultant anxiety about survival in a hostile world, stimulate the early beginnings of narcissistic defenses.

Rapprochement Resolution

The child's recognition of separateness results in increased active wooing of mother, and a demand for mother's presence in order to regain the internal dyadic "safe harbor." The increased clinginess is often puzzling to parents, who may respond with dismay or irritation. At the same time as the child needs mother's presence more, he is also more individuated and more aware of his separateness, and resists returning to the dual unity that was so pleasurable before. He can now no longer rely on everything going OK just because that's how the world works for an infant in a healthy family. The conflict typical of rapprochement includes the child wanting to be soothed by mother in ways no longer possible, and pushing mother away in disillusionment. The increased demand for mother's presence is fueled by the ambivalence that arises in the back and forth from rage and loss, to soothing by mother's continued libidinal availability. The child's persistent attempts to re-create the lost and longed-for blissful symbiotic state inevitably end in frustration, disorganizing rage, and experiencing mother through the fog of his own projected destructive and unbearable negative emotions. When mother's empathic attunement and reflective function allow her to tolerate her own frustration and confusion about her child's unpredictability, she can sustain her libidinal availability and respond to the destructive upheaval with consistent holding, containing, and tolerant mirroring, which can lead to repair of the disrupted relationship. Repeated cycles of this disruption and repair gradually and progressively succeed in neutralizing the primitive aggression, in turn taming and converting its destructive energy into generative fuel for ego growth and crystallization of positively toned introjects of good self and object representations, supporting the growth of the positive normal narcissism that allows for emotional resilience.

This process, called rapprochement resolution by Mahler (1972), allows the child to learn to tolerate frustration and to accept failure without giving up, but also allows the child to learn about the value of persistence and self-assertion. Healthy children begin to experience and establish boundaries between self and object, wish and reality, pretending and "for real." They can begin the process of accepting loss, tolerating ambivalence, accepting imperfection and vulnerability in self and others without rage or emotional collapse, relinquishing omnipotence and grandiosity gradually, in tolerable increments. When rapprochement resolution fails, and the cycles of disruption and repair in the mother-child dyad are not successful in neutralizing the primitive aggression, omnipotent defiance, rage storms, and sadomasochistic, coercive modes of interaction dominate. Idealized part objects, and the grandiosity of the primary narcissism, dominate, and ambivalence and loss cannot be tolerated. The child cannot segregate reality from fantasy, and the difference between self and object, wish and reality, pretending and "for real" are lost.

During the second and third years, the child's characteristic methods of dealing with the world become more complex and can accurately be termed forerunners of characteristic defense mechanisms. These elements of personality will echo through his development for the rest of his life. If his experience brings him to this stage with basic trust and a general sense that he can manage the world even without mother present to help, as well as a general sense that there are lots of good things to be experienced, he will be cheerful, resilient, and his response to the developmental push toward self and object constancy will be generally adaptive and positive. He will believe in his capacity to master difficulties, and will be able to persist at efforts toward mastery. Disruptive and distressing experiences will not usually overwhelm him, but will stimulate responses that restore equilibrium. He may ask for help in managing his distress, may find something else to occupy himself, or may manage to accomplish the task himself. A toddler asked to wait while mother talks on the phone, for instance, may hold mother's skirt as a way of being with her, may find a toy to occupy him, or may pull the tablecloth to get a cookie or to get mother's attention. Successful coping provides further experiences of mastery, enhances self-esteem, strengthens healthy coping mechanisms, and strengthens his capacity for healthy narcissism.

If the toddler's experience has been that mother is unable to help him feel good, and he has learned that the world is a dangerous place where you are never safe and you can never predict what bad thing will happen, he is likely to be irritable, coercive, tantrumming, refusing to accept limits or disappointments. He will be less able to use redirection or substitutes when he cannot get what he wants, and will omnipotently behave as if he is the boss in the family. He may become quite skilled, in a two-year-old way, at getting mother to break family rules for him. He is unlikely to believe in his ability to master the world around him, will be unable to persist at a task, and will be quick to respond to failure with frustration and anger. These behaviors are remnants of primary narcissism, defensively preserved through fixation or reactivated in regression: rage, grandiosity, omnipotent fantasy, denial, mastery in fantasy, splitting, and primitive projection. They allow him to believe that he still can manage everything, that he need not face the reality of being neither big enough nor smart enough to prevent frustration, disappointment, or danger. As these mechanisms of restoring narcissistic equilibrium are used excessively or predominantly, they come to dominate the personality of the child and he moves toward a personality organization that would be seen in pathological narcissism.

In the early months of life, the tie to the libidinal object is the primary key to maintenance of normal narcissism. During the toddler years, with the development of self and object representations, the stability and constancy of the mental representation of the object are the crucial elements. Early in infancy, narcissistic equilibrium or OK-ness is impossible without mother's caretaking, which manages physiological needs and affect regulation. As the child begins to separate and individuate, increasing mastery brings with it a concomitant awareness that mastery is finite, and that there are dangers in the world. He uses refueling in the relationship with mother to restore his narcissistic equilibrium, to renew the conviction that mother approves of his activity and his moves to master it, and to reassure himself that mother believes he is able to master the world. Children with transitional objects are able to use them as a sort of portable mother, to carry the internal image of mother with them for support. Transitional phenomena act as reservoirs of self-soothing, control, and self-affirmation, thus supporting and strengthening the capacity for normal narcissistic balance. Transitional phenomena, at this stage and through life, include fantasy, play, art, creativity, and faith, as well as concrete transitional objects such as blankets. They allow us to feel even when alone that we can access the original sense of safety, cohesion, and regained equilibrium.

In cultures that have a stronger emphasis on extended family than is seen in Western culture, the mothering figure tends to be multiple, so that the child may turn to another adult for sustenance and comfort when biological mother is absent; the multiple caretakers offer a different experience of internalizing of the sense of safe harbor and of the caretaking role, and likely make transitional objects less necessary: when there is always some one of the multiple mothers present, the "portable mother" is not needed to sustain internal comfort and equilibrium.

24–36 months

The second and third years of life coincide with the subphases of Mahler's separation-individuation process (1975): practicing subphases, early and late, from 12–16 months; rapprochement, from 18–24 months, followed by a year of consolidation; leading to the rudimentary beginnings of libidinal self and object constancy. An optimal resolution of the rapprochement crisis is crucial to successful negotiation of pregenital, interpersonal, and interactive conflicts of the oral and anal phases of psychosexual development. In this period (the "terrible twos"), the toddler's persistent assertion of his will and omnipotent wishes for unconditional dominance and instant gratification are frustrated by daily events and the demands of reality, resulting in rageful reactions and the stirrings of negative emotions that threaten to annihilate the self, the object, and the libidinal object tie. By about twenty-four months, however, the child has learned to use mother for help and guidance; to comfort himself or to seek comfort from mother when necessary; to assert his initiative or opposition without fear of rejection. Previously established patterns of mutual affect regulation between the child and parent now assist in taming the rage at being frustrated, and allow the child to integrate his own initiative into the relationship while maintaining the warm mutuality of late infancy.

After about thirty-six months, as the child continues "on the road to object constancy," the affective experiences which have so far been split into good and bad begin to be fused, as the representations of the self and the object, merged until this point, become increasingly and more distinctly separated. The child learns to tolerate and contain his anger and disappointment at the failures of both himself and his mother to re-create the magical bliss of a symbiotic union. The internal maternal image, now more consistently recognized as different from the self, is becoming reliably available for positive emotional (libidinal) sustenance and for the maintenance of a narcissistic equilibrium. Aggressive impulses, arising from the failure to have the world exactly as the child wants, have been tempered by the recognition that mother-that-he-wants-to-destroy (because she failed to re-create the symbiotic union and make everything perfect) is the samc person as mother-that-he-loves (because she makes things at least better, if not perfect).

As the separation between self and object grows, and the split between good and bad self, and good and bad object, begins to heal, the intensity of affective reactions are modified and so can be modulated more adaptively; this allows the child to tolerate ambivalence and a more realistic appreciation of the internal and subjective states of both self and of object. Affects begin to serve as signals which mobilize ego resources for defense, adaptive or creative solutions to reality problems, and compromise formation for internal conflicts. Repression, in place of splitting, becomes the predominant mode of defense and conflict resolution, and the new capacity for affect regulation allows enhanced self-regulation. As the child attains libidinal self and object constancy, oedipal triangulation and the emergence of triadic modes of conflict regulation become possible. Primary process thinking begins to give way to reality-based secondary process thinking, object related secondary narcissism takes precedence over pre-objectal monadic and dyadic modes of primary narcissism, and the depressive position emerges, with its capacity for concern and a reparative sense of guilt. By the beginning of the fourth year, the capacities for narrative formation, abstraction and symbolic thinking, reality processing, and verbal communication usher in the so-called oedipus complex and its momentous structural implications for identity, character formation, ego and superego consolidation.

36 Months and On

Up until this time, primary narcissism has predominated, although it has been slowly waning. With this developmental achievement, however, and the move into the oedipal stage, secondary narcissism emerges. With the achievement of ambivalence, energy for the expansion of ego resources and ego growth has been freed up, and the capacity to maintain an affectively positive state of self is now (during and after the oedipal stage) mediated by the rapid expansion of the ego and all its functions, both within and without the sphere of neurotic conflict. If development has gone awry, and the individual is unable to maintain narcissistic equilibrium, the ego will be easily overwhelmed by affect that cannot be tolerated or managed. Compromise formations, allowing partial gratification of wishes to be accepted as "good enough," are more difficult to find because the affect associated with internal neurotic conflict is less easily contained.

As development continues, the child reaches school age, with associated emotional challenges and rewards. The child with healthy narcissism will be able to tolerate the separation from family during the school day, and will be able to take some pleasure in learning and the rapidly growing assortment of new skills and new knowledge. He will have more practice with learning to share, to tolerate waiting for having his needs met, and for learning to deal with strangers, both adults and children. In addition, the ability to find ego-syntonic solutions to internal conflict allows for sublimation, the substitution of teachers and peers as objects for wish fulfillment, and the beginnings of an emotional turn toward the outside world, away from the intensity of the family relationships. Showing off new skills at soccer, football, or other physical skills, as well as showing off knowledge about dinosaurs, or storms, or other things learned in school, become sources of pleasure and pride, as the child enlists his parents in helping him to engage more fully in negotiating the exciting new world with all the new choices for ego gratification and growth.

For the child who has not successfully negotiated this transition, in the absence of an optimal resolution of rapprochement and the achievement of relative self and object constancy, attachment cannot be fully secure. The child is not able to feel safe enough within himself to negotiate the move to the world outside the family, and self and object representations continue to be split into good and bad, rather than ambivalent and complete. Archaic remnants of primary narcissism and omnipotent grandiosity interfere with a realistic assessment of object relations, preventing the utilization of available personal resources, or of the resources of others who might provide self-object functions. The self-object, as described by Kohut (1971), is an individual whose presence in our lives makes it possible for us to maintain an internal sense of stability and "OK-ness" that allows for continued functioning even in the face of stress or trauma. Without the ability to utilize our own resources or self-object resources, object relations become coercive and sadomasochistic; but the individual's experience is still unable to satisfy his grandiose expectations, either for himself or for the other. He is unable to maintain the sense of safety, security, and mastery—his narcissistic equilibrium—that allows him to continue to function. Without the ability to maintain a stable narcissistic equilibrium, later developmental surges result in disorganization and regression, and those later developmental tasks cannot be negotiated successfully.

Adolescence

This becomes apparent perhaps most obviously in adolescence, when the individual must yet again face the prospect of moving away from the containing family to establish an independent existence as an adult. Adolescence places great demands on the individual's ability to manage internal affects, to tolerate uncertainty and conflict, and to maintain a sense of ability to be competent and capable even when faced with entirely new experiences. Without the stable, realistic, and resilient belief in one's own capacities to face the world independently, and the ability to turn without resentment or narcissistic injury to family and friends for support when needed, the "launching" from adolescent dependence to adult independence becomes troubled and may be an insurmountable obstruction.

REFERENCES

Auchincloss, E. L. and Samberg, E. (Eds.). (2012). *Psychoanalytic Terms and Concepts.* Yale Univ. Press.

Brody, S. and Axelrad, S. (1966). Anxiety, socialization, and ego formation in infancy. *International Journal of Psycho-Analys*is, 47, 218–229.

DeCasper, A. J. and Spence, J. M. (1986). Prenatal maternal speech influences newborns' perception of speech sounds. *Infant Behavior and Development,* 9, 133–150.

Etezady, M. H. (2015). Conclusion: Change is us. In M. Nayar-Akhtar (Ed.), *Identities in Transition: The Growth and Development of a Multicultural Therapist* (pp. 164–165). London: Karnac.

———. (2017). Trust, faith, and transcendence. In S. Akhtar (Ed.), *Mistrust* (p. 132). London: Karnac.

Fonagy, P., Gergely, G., Jurist, L., and Target, M. (2004). *Affect Regulation, Mentalization, and the Development of the Self.* New York: Other Press.

Freud, S. (1914). On narcissism: An introduction. In J. Strachey (Ed.). (1971). *The Standard Edition of the Complete Psychological Works of Sigmund Freud, Vol. XIV (1914–1916): On the History of the Psycho-Analytic Movement, Papers on Metapsychology and Other Works*, pp. 67–102.

Kohut, H. (1971). *The Analysis of the Self: A Systematic Approach to the Psychoanalytic Treatment of Narcissistic Personality Disorders.* New York: International Universities Press.

Mahler, M. S. (1972). Rapprochement subphase of the separation individuation process. *Psychoanalytic Quarterly*, 41, 487–506.

———. (1975). On the current status of the infantile neurosis. *Journal of the American Psychoanalytic Association*, 23, 327–333.

———. (1979). *Selected Papers of Margaret Mahler, Vol. 2: Separation-Individuation.* Lanham, MD: Jason Aronson.

Mahler, M. S., Pine, F., and Bergman, A. (1975). *The Psychological Birth of the Human Infant: Symbiosis and Individuation.* New York: Basic Books.

Piaget, J. (1926). *The Language and Thought of the Child.* London: Routledge & Kegan Paul.

PDM Task Force. (2006). *Psychodynamic Diagnostic Manual.* Silver Spring, MD: Alliance of Psychoanalytic Organizations.

Rosenfeld, H. (1964). On the psychopathology of narcissism: A clinical approach. *International Journal of Psycho-Analysis,* 45, 332–337.

Spitz, R. A. (1965). *The First Year of Life: A Psychoanalytic Study of Normal and Deviant Development of Object Relations*. New York: International Universities Press.

Stern, D. N. (1985). *The Interpersonal World of the Infant.* New York: Basic Books.

Tolpin, M. (1971). On the beginnings of a cohesive self—An application of the concept of transmuting internalizations to the study of the transitional object and signal anxiety. *Psychoanalytic Study of the Child*, 26, 316–352.

Trevarthen, C. and Grant, F. (1979). Not work alone. *New Scientist*, 81, 566–569.

Van der Waals, J (1965). Problems of narcissism. *Bulletin of the Menninger Clinic,* 29, 293–311.

Winnicott, D. W. (1960). The theory of the parent-infant relationship. *International Journal of Psycho-Analysis*, 41, 585–595.

Chapter Seven

A Developmental Perspective on Trauma

The Analysis of a Severely Traumatized Adolescent

Ann G. Smolen

BRIEF LITERATURE REVIEW

Early Understanding of Trauma

The term "trauma" is often used in a vague manner that can be confusing. Cumulative trauma is confused with massive trauma, and adult trauma is confused with early trauma. While these different traumatic experiences possess diverse characteristics, they are also interconnected in profound ways (Amir 2012).

Ferenczi and colleagues (1921) understood trauma as an experience in which the adult failed the infant through action or the inability to act. The result was the death of the self, causing a split. According to Ferenczi et al. healing is possible within the therapeutic relationship, where a safe environment provides the setting in which the traumatic memory may be transformed into a coherent narrative. Winnicott coined the term "impingement," that could be either strengthening, if the infant has a good-enough environment, or traumatic. Winnicott explains that if the impingement occurs too early in life or if it overwhelms the developing ego, the result will be traumatic. If gross impingement is cumulative, the result is fragmentation and the threat of annihilation (Winnicott 1953). Masud Khan (1964), in agreement with Winnicott, states that cumulative trauma results in the individual's inability to sustain emotional stability, which results in character distortions and symptoms (Khan 1964).

It is known that cumulative/strain trauma (Kris 1956), which is frequently silent, often goes unnoticed by all. It is only in retrospect that we are able to view it. Strain trauma promotes the development of rigid ego defenses, but in addition, it renders the person more vulnerable to shock trauma (Krystal 1978). When an infant lives with strain trauma (such as an ill mother who is emotionally unavailable), an acute trauma becomes magnified because the infant does not have the ego defenses, self-structures, and actual relational and social support necessary for flexible adaptation to challenges from the environment. It is known that an acute trauma can change the brain's pathways for mood regulation (Van der Kolk et al. 1996), however it is also thought that inadequate caregiving can have comparable effects. Van der Kolk contends that traumatic events are remembered vividly and are resistant to integration.

Parents who have unresolved traumatic histories often find their children's emotional needs overwhelming. As a result, the child's needs and fears may be misinterpreted and distorted (Fraiberg 1982; Lieberman 1997). Fonagy points out that trauma interferes with the parent's capacity for reflective functioning, which then adds to distortions and misattribution of the child's affects (Fonagy et al. 1995, 2002). "At a most basic level, the defensive processes enlisted in the face of trauma fragment the development of stable, coherent representations of the self and other" (Slade et al. 2006, p. 77).

Infants who experience maltreatment are more likely to develop insecure attachments (Bacon & Richardson 2001). Attachment researchers connect maltreatment with the formation of the disorganized pattern of attachment, arguing that this occurs when there is a "collapse of behavioral strategy" by the infant. This happens when the infant is unable to integrate conflicting behaviors on the part of the attachment figure that is both the supplier of closeness and the cause of extreme distress. These children often display contradictory behaviors, such as approaching their caregiver asking for comfort while simultaneously turning away. These infants may also exhibit a frozen, trance-like expression (Main 1996).

A child who is securely attached to his or her primary caretaker usually develops flexible emotional relationships and, if all goes well, the preoedipal and oedipal stages of development proceed smoothly as the child individuates and acquires a strong sense of self. When the mother is emotionally unavailable or rejects and ignores her child's emotional needs, the child is unable to develop an efficient and adaptive method of communicating his or her needs. Very quickly a system of gross misattunement is set up, setting the stage for dysregulation and distress (Stern 1985; Slade 1998).

As the mother recognizes and finds meaning in her child's affects, the child is then able to see herself as a thinking, feeling, separate self. When the mother is unable to contain and reflect her infant's affects, the infant becomes unable to self-regulate and normal development is at risk (Slade 1998). The mother's ability for attunement is crucial to an infant's development. In order to be properly attuned to her child the mother must be able to differentiate her infant's needs from her own. The mother must provide a "holding environment" (Winnicott 1974), "wherein the mother is sensitive and responsive to her infant's needs which will gradually promote the child's slow internalization of the maternal soothing function to help organize beginning ego functioning and modulate the intensity of the drives" (Beebe & Sloate 1982, p. 601). This, in turn, affects all future development.

Stern defines attunement as the "intersubjective sharing of affect" (Stern, p. 141). Several developmental and attachment theorists (such as Bowlby, Ainesworth, Winnicott, Stern, Karen, Fonagy, Beebe, and Steele to name a few) all consider attunement to be critical to the psychological and physical development of the infant. As the infant cries and demands to have his needs met, the mother responds and thus gives meaning to the infant's signals. Eventually the infant begins to know what he wants and how to signal with intent. This harmonized mother/infant pas de deux is a form of mutual regulation, and as a result the infant learns to regulate himself. In addition, between birth and five months of age, the face-to-face interactions between mother and infant where affective signals are exchanged are key in the baby's development of self-representation of affect (Fonagy & Target 1997).

First, the infant is able to self-regulate biological functions such as sleep patterns, elimination, and eating. Gradually, as the mother/infant dance continues to develop, the baby learns to self-regulate on a psychological level as well. Shared social experiences, such as playful interchange and mirroring, give the child a sense of being appreciated and cared for. His emotions and affects are accepted and validated. He feels approval. These early social experiences usher the child into the richness of object relations and what it means to relate to another person.

A parent who does not have the capacity for self-reflection is unable to reflect on the inner states of her infant. This child will, in turn, be unable to relate to his or her own inner world. Attachment research has shown that insecurely attached adults tend to persist in strategies and schemas that they first learned from their own rejecting parent. In an effort to avoid an empty inner world devoid of objects, people incorporate malevolent inner objects. This loyalty to the early depriving caregiver causes a parent to continue rejecting patterns in her own interaction with her own children (Eagle 1995; Karen 1998). The infant who does not experience attunement and mirroring may experience his emerging preverbal self as defective. He is left to feel empty, helpless, and perhaps even without hope.

Infant researchers and clinicians who observe the earliest interactions between mother and baby describe the delicate dance between the two, the finely tuned rhythms that develop between the couple as the tiniest nuances of nonverbal communications take place. When misattunement occurs, when the beautiful pas de deux falters and the mother is unable to accurately respond to the baby's affective signals, the child has no choice but to resort to defensive behavioral strategies. It is important to note that mother-infant relationships constantly oscillate between attunement and disruption, which causes dysregulation, followed by repair. These disruptions are part of all normal relationships. It is the repair that leads to hope and the expectation that differences can be negotiated and disagreements and misunderstandings repaired. Beebe has demonstrated in her infant-mother research that maternal impingement is highly anxiety-provoking for the infant and contributes to "defenses of dissociation, fragmentation, and, in extreme instances, a disruption of the very capacity to think itself" (Beebe 2000).

Neurobiology and Attachment

The neuropsychoanalytic perspective of attachment theory adds a neurobiological component. The affective interactions between infant and caregiver "provide a foundation for neurological development and lead to the creation of neural networks (particularly in the right hemisphere) that will influence the infants' personality and relationships with others throughout life" (Hardy 2007, p. 28). It is interesting to note that the right hemisphere is vital in the communication and reception of emotion. Optimal performance in this area of the brain is crucial for empathic interpersonal experiences.

Schore states that attachment constitutes "*synchronized dyadic bioenergetic transmissions*" (Schore 2002, p. 444) between caregiver and infant. This is the capacity of the caregiver to "modulate and process affective states and provide this structure to the infant" (Hardy 2007, p. 28), and it is vital to the infant's early brain development. The attunement of the mother to her infant provides maintenance of "homeostasis and equilibrium in the infants' central and autonomic nervous systems" (Schore 2002, p. 445). When this homeostasis is disturbed the baby's nervous system must work very hard to maintain equilibrium on its own. If this fails, the right brain is "unable to maintain coherent neural connections and goes into a state of shock that leads to dissociation and stalls normal development. When both internal and external regulatory systems fail, a sense of helplessness and hopelessness could result" (Schore 2002, p. 445).

In order for the infant to be able to develop a symbolic representational system of mental states that includes the ability to mentalize, the infant needs to bond to another person. When these affectional bonds are disrupted, maladaptive attachment patterns develop which challenge further social development (Fonagy et al. 2003). Infant researchers (Stern 1985; Morton & Johnson 1991; Meltzoff & Moore 1977, 1989; Trevarthen 1979; Brazelton & Tronick 1980; Beebe 1985; Tronick 1989; Jaffe et al. 2001) have demonstrated that infants can tell people apart from birth. They are able to recognize their mother's voice and imitate facial expressions from birth. There is a "turn-taking" structure to infant's interactions with their caregiver, and the "mother and infant are engaged in affective communication from the beginning of life in which the mother plays a vital role in modulating the infant's emotional states to make them more manageable" (Fonagy et al. 2003, p. 422).

The contributions of Meltzoff and Moore (1998) demonstrate that the newborn infant's imitation, such as opening his mouth or sticking out his tongue, is the infant "comparing his own action . . . against an internal memory, schema, or representation of the action" (Beebe et al. 2003, p. 810) that he saw the adult make. "By six weeks, the infant can observe the model one day and then return 24 hours later and imitate action" (Beebe et al. 2003, p. 810). It is speculated that this capacity may be based on mirror neurons.

There seems to be a connection between mindfulness and attachment. "The caregiver's mindfulness about the child's mental states appears to be a significant predictor of the likelihood of secure attachment" (Fonagy et al. 2003, p. 430). There is evidence that secure attachment is necessary for the optimal development of cerebral structures supporting mentalization (Schore 2002). "The right hemisphere is specialized for emotion and social cognition, and the right hemisphere is dominant in the first three years of life, providing an opportunity for attachment relationships to participate in the sculpting of the cerebral substrates of socioemotional behavior and emotional self-regulation" (Fonagy et al. 2003, p. 432). When the attachment relationship is poor, the development of cortical structures may become compromised. "These are the same structures that are essential to the activity of mentalizing. Thus, we have potentially interlocking, vicious developmental circles in which attachment disturbance, affective hyperarousal, and failure of mentalization are all intertwined" (Fonagy et al. 2003, p. 434).

Early stress and maltreatment inflicted on the infant causes multiple neurobiological events that could produce lasting changes to the developing brain. Structural consequences of early stress and maltreatment include "reduced size of the midportions of the corpus callosum and attenuated development of the left neocortex, hippocampus, and amygdala. Major functional consequences include increased electrical irritability in limbic structures and reduced functional activity of the cerebellar vermis" (Teicher et al. 2003, p. 33). In addition, early maltreatment and chronic stress affect "neurogenesis, synaptic overproduction and pruning, and myelination during specific sensitive periods" (ibid., p. 33). The above neurobiological events play a significant role in the later development of psychopathology. It is known that we are hard-wired to respond to threat with a readiness to attack or retreat. The amygdala sounds the alarm, cortisol is released and the body springs into action. When the individual has a history of trauma, help is often needed to regulate once again (Cooper 2012).

Incest and Sexual Abuse

The trauma of incest is devastating and overwhelming: it "is an act of unmodulated aggression against a helpless child" (Fischer 1991, p. 48). Nothing the little girl has known can prepare her for it and nothing she can do can make it go away. She is unable to self-protect and she is left without the protection of another adult. She has no one upon whom she can depend for her safety and well-being. One of the most destructive outcomes of sexual trauma is the disruption of thinking. This intrusion upon the unconscious and conscious thought processes results in the inability to symbolically represent the trauma. When conscious and unconscious processes are disrupted, "cognitive structure, sign recognition, symbol formation, syntax, discrimination and the availability to use these capacities to formulate and organize language are either absent or are present but ineffectual" (Nachmani 1995, p. 423). When incest occurs there is a blurring of boundaries, which informs the child that her environment is unsafe. She is left vulnerable and defenseless in the face of danger. When the environment is experienced as having caused pain from neglect and abuse, there is a "radical break between trauma and expectation, victims often cannot find categories of thought or words" (ibid., p. 424). Another consequence of severe boundary violation is that there is a "formidable destruction of the capacity to 'make sense,' to make and preserve order, to sustain a fundamental sense of the order of relatedness through the use of symbols and language and the trustworthy reliance upon others" (ibid., p. 425). These humiliating, shameful and pain-ridden violations can cause the cessation of mental growth. In addition to a defect in symbolic thinking, reality testing is also compromised (Kramer & Akhtar 1991).

When child/parent incest occurs, *betrayal* becomes a trauma in its own right. A child is dependent on a parent for care, love, and safety. When the parent uses the nature of this dependent relationship for exploitation and harm, it undermines the meaning of dependency. "In betrayal, a pseudodependency is created by deceit based on trust. Betrayals are traumatic because trust is broken, while the need to depend on others remains" (Nachmani 1995, p. 425). When incest occurs the child is being deceived and meanings become confusing. What does it mean to have privacy? How is trust understood? When this terrible betrayal transpires, object constancy ceases to develop and the separation-individuation process becomes impaired (Nachmani 1995).

Another traumatic outcome of the incestuous relationship is the child's not being seen as a separate person. Nachmani describes this phenomenon as "when people act 'as if' one were absent" (Nachmani 1995, p. 429). The abuser denies that his child has a "self" or a mind of her own. Many victims of father/daughter incest experience feelings of emptiness as if they have no self. Their needs have been ignored and denied. However the child is trapped and must keep that parent available to avoid annihilation anxiety and total abandonment. Many children make use of dissociation in order to keep the parent "good." The child cannot tolerate the fear of family disintegration and at times incest is seen as keeping the family together (Cohler 1987). Children who are the victims of their parent's unmitigated rage are overwhelmed and rendered helpless by their own feelings of fury. "But this rage must be denied in order to maintain the sense of the good parent" (Fischer 1991, p. 53). It is also important to note that some semblance of self is sought, because "being misrecognized feels so much more secure than being unrecognized and unknown. 'As if' is better than 'no if'" (Nachmani 1995, p. 430).

Cohler agrees with Nachmani that, as a result of incest, self-identity and self-representation may be damaged. As a result a narcissistic disturbance may occur and masochism and passivity also abound. Cohler explains how many female incest victims become male-identified. "There is the growth of a complex fantasy system involving destruction of the mother, identification with father, securing of his powerful phallus. In this regard a female incest victim becomes male in her self-representation; this, too disturbs the development of identity and object relations" (Cohler 1987, p. 606).

When incest occurs early the separation-individuation process is disturbed, and thus "abused children manifest a great vulnerability to separation problems, depression, and splitting of good and bad self and good and bad object" (Kramer & Akhtar 1991, p. 4). These children also experience intolerable sexual excitement that becomes unmanageable, tremendous anger, and an overwhelming sense of helplessness and powerlessness. When an abused child reaches adolescence there is a tendency for masochistic behaviors such as eating disorders and cutting. Kramer also notes that "[g]irls molested by their fathers may become homosexual as a defense against their strong heterosexual stirrings or as an angry response to their father's sexual abuse" (Kramer & Akhtar 1991, p. 6).

When sexual abuse takes place the abuser commits *Soul Murder* (Shengold 1999). Soul murder is the malicious abuse and neglect of children by adults. When a child is traumatized in this way, her consequent emotional development is profoundly negatively affected and severely compromised. For sexually abused children, their childhood innocence is lost, never to be recovered. These children become deadened; their fragile developing selves have been murdered. When a relatively helpless child is physically and/or sexually abused she becomes extremely overstimulated, which in turn evokes traumatic anxiety and rage. If the child's abuse comes in the form of neglect, this understimulation may result in rage and intense sexual longing. Every child deserves, needs, and expects good-enough parenting. Children cannot survive without parents, and they need to believe that the adults will protect them and keep them safe. Abused children have no choice but to look to be rescued by the same person who committed the abuse. This is mind-splitting and causes sadomasochistic impulses such as perverse sexual excitement and murderous wishes. When this happens the child must guard against these traumatic feelings by developing massive defenses, which include dissociation, again, a splitting of the mind. These girls must defend against the rage they felt toward the abusing adult, so they become dead inside, what Shengold calls "emotional zombies," or they cannot control their impulses and may become drug addicts. Abused children grip tightly to whatever benevolent parenting exists and cling to the delusion that their parents are loving and caring. This is actually one of the most destructive effects of child abuse, the need to hold onto the abusing parent or parental figure. Children must deny what has taken place as if it did not happen.

THE CASE: SUSAN

Susan experienced physical, emotional, and sexual abuse as well as neglect. I would like to ask you to hold in your minds, while reading, a few points: 1. This is an adolescent who experienced severe and chronic physical, verbal, and sexual abuse for almost her entire childhood. 2. In addition, perhaps worst of all was the level of emotional neglect. It was as if she were invisible to her parents, teachers, and the world. 3. In working with this patient, together we have weathered and survived both external as well as intrapsychic storms. 4. I have presented this patient and I have become aware that it is extremely difficult for many to listen to her story. Her affects are often unbearable and her pain is difficult to be with in the space we created together. As in any analysis and psychotherapy you have to work with, understand, and tolerate multiple transferences and countertransferences within the intersubjective matrix. Understandably, and as expected, these were often extremely intense. I ask you to be aware within yourselves what countertransferences and feelings you may experience to the patient herself and also to me as the analyst. 5. In addition, she dissociated and was often unable to find the words to communicate with me. My natural style with her was quite active. Within our traumatic transferences and enactments I was constantly aware, on the one hand, that my activity might be repeating the trauma, as some of my interventions and interpretations might appear intrusive. On the other hand, if I remained silent and static I would be repeating the silence that surrounded her trauma, and she would continue to feel invisible in my eyes. And lastly, I wish to emphasize that she has done beautifully. While Susan's story is tragic and the vignettes you are about to read are difficult to metabolize, she is functioning at an extraordinary high level as an adult.

I will give a brief history, and then move on to clinical vignettes.

Brief History

I wish to preface this brief history by stating that the following facts were gathered over a period of several months. Conversations with my patient and her father were so difficult that I often misunderstood information with which I was provided. This was very confusing. There were times when I questioned my listening ability and even my hearing. In retrospect, my confusion reflects the chaos of the inner life of both my patient and her father.

Susan, an only child, was born six weeks prematurely to a chronically ill mother, who died when Susan was eleven years old. She was cared for by a nanny for her first eighteen months. When Susan was eighteen months old her mother's condition improved and she was able to take on the care of her daughter; the nanny was let go. Throughout Susan's childhood her mother was absent frequently and for long periods of time. Subsequently, Susan's father became a stay-at-home dad when Susan was four years old.

Over a period of a year it came to light that Susan witnessed domestic violence and was emotionally, physically, and sexually abused by her father. Susan was left with her mentally unstable and abusive father when the mother was away. Shortly after her mother died, when Susan was eleven years old, she befriended an older teenage boy who quickly became her mother-substitute. He introduced her to heroin and she remained addicted for the next two years. She remained a chronic drug user until her analysis. It is important to emphasize that nobody suspected her drug use or, if it was suspected, no interventions were attempted by her private school, her highly educated family members, or friends of the family. In fact, it was not until four months into our work together that I became aware of her addiction.

Susan was referred to me through a former friend of the mother's when Susan was fifteen years old. Her presenting problem was school failure. The referring adult expressed concern and confusion, because Susan was gifted intellectually and nobody could fathom why she was failing at her highly competitive private school. After a short evaluation period Susan gave me an ultimatum stating that she would only attend therapy if I referred her father for treatment. I thought her request showed strength and insight. I referred her father to a colleague and we worked together to help him put his daughter into in-patient rehab. When she returned to her father's home after six weeks of rehab, Susan began her analysis. To help keep the time-line easier to follow, when we began her analysis I had seen Susan in a three times per week psychotherapy for an eight-month period. At this point she was sixteen-years old. We started five sessions a week, and we met once a week in family work with the father.

To summarize, Susan had experienced chronic severe abuses throughout her life beginning with her premature birth and spending her first six weeks of life in a neonatal intensive care unit. Once well enough to go home she was delivered into the arms of a nanny, her own mother too ill to care for her, her father too disturbed and angry. At eighteen months her nanny was taken from her. Her father reported that Susan was a quiet, good toddler who never had a tantrum. She kept to herself. It is possible that Susan experienced an anaclitic depression from the loss of her primary object, her nanny.

Susan learned very young that her world was not a very safe place. At eleven years old her mother died, her father blamed her for the death, and the abuse worsened. She found refuge in a drug-induced nirvana. Nobody noticed that this little girl was a heroin addict. She became invisible.

Susan described how she came to use heroin for the first time:

> *I begged for a skateboard, which my mom would never let me have because she thought they were too dangerous, but right after my mother died my father bought me one. I would hang out at this parking lot where all the skaters hung out. An older boy was so nice to me. He became my best friend. He injected me for the first time and all my worries evaporated.*

Susan remained addicted to heroin for two years. With the help of her drug addicted "family," she went cold turkey off of heroin. She described how ill she became, but was tenderly cared for by this boy who had become like a mother to her. Susan remained an active drug user until four months into our relationship. It is important to note that nobody ever acknowledged her drug use. She took drugs with her to summer camp, family visits, and on a summer vacation with her paternal grandmother. As she seemed to be invisible to her parents, she remained unheard and unseen to everyone around her, including me because I was totally unaware of her drug use.

Beginning Treatment

Susan expressed from the onset of treatment that she and her father had a poor relationship. She made it clear that she thought her father was "crazy" and gave him (and me) an ultimatum, stating she would not attend therapy unless he went into therapy also. I promptly referred the father to a colleague. Susan also told me that she did not trust adults and would not like an "intrusive therapist."

A month into our work Susan began to relate some of the physical abuse she had experienced. She began by telling me of an incident that had occurred two years earlier. It was extremely difficult for her to verbalize. Her words came out in segments and were barely audible. Eye contact was visibly painful for her to maintain and she began to dissociate in her sessions. She spoke of the emotional abuse inflicted on her by her father. He told her she was responsible for her mother's death and often threatened to send her away to boarding school or give her up to foster care. He often threatened to kill both Susan and himself. She lived in fear that she would come home from school and find him dead.

Four months into our work she confided to me that she was a lesbian. She was afraid to tell me, fearing I would reject and abandon her. It was also at this time that her drug use slowly came out. She began to describe wild weekends filled with dangerous, uninhibited use of multiple combinations of crack, cocaine, ecstasy, and assorted prescription drugs. With Susan's permission, I met with her father and his therapist, attempting to help him set limits and keep his daughter safe. He was unable to do this, which he demonstrated by continuing to allow her to leave the house and go to a part of the city that was unsafe. Susan overdosed, was hospitalized, and spent six weeks in rehab. In consultation with all the professionals involved it was decided that Susan should go back to live with her father. I need to be clear here, that Susan had not yet told me (or anyone) about her sexual abuse. Her father continued in his therapy and Susan and I began a five-session/week analysis plus one session/week with her father. It is important to note that I (and the father's therapist) were forthright and made it clear that he was not to physically or emotionally abuse his daughter. He wanted help to be a better father and Susan also wanted to remain at home (there was no other place for her to live). Another valid and important point is that all the professionals involved, including the physicians from the in-patient facility, knew of Susan's past physically abusive relationship with her father.

When we began the analysis Susan still had a difficult time speaking. She was able to tell me that if I was silent it caused her overwhelming anxiety and she would dissociate. Susan showed her anxiety in her body. In every session she would grab a toy of some sort to fiddle with. It seemed to help her if her hands were busy. In many sessions one or both of her legs would shake. As I got to know her better I was also able to read the tiniest change of facial expression, tightening of her jaw, sadness in her eyes, or even the reddening of her skin. I began to use her body language as a way of helping her acknowledge what she was feeling and begin to express it verbally.

She tried very hard to tell me about a gang rape she had suffered when she was twelve and on heroin. She began by telling me parts of dreams and alluding to something dreadful that had happened to her. Finally she was able to tell me about the rape as she sobbed, and even her sobs were silent. As weeks turned into months she spoke more about her relationship with her father and memories of her childhood. When she was little she kept a box next to her bed where in the middle of the night she would hide. She spoke of the nights she crept into her closet to a back shelf behind all the clothes and would curl up to finally be able to sleep. She described how she would sit up late into the night, surrounding herself with her stuffed animals and planning an escape route through her second floor window.

Disclosure: One Year Later

Susan entered my office and sat down. I noticed how sad she looked. She did not speak. Within this very long silence she seemed to disappear from the room. Her silent fight within her mind began. I could see it on her face and in her eyes. I asked her if she was fighting with herself about telling me something. She nodded her head "yes," and in an almost inaudible whisper told me the unthinkable. [In telling you this, I notice that I too remain silent . . . I do not tell you what the 'unthinkable' is.]

The next day she told me she felt relief in the telling but remained terrified of her father. She was afraid he would kill her or himself or both of them. Now she had told, but she remained responsible for him. Her drug urges returned with a severity she had not previously experienced, but she withstood them.

I sought consultation with a colleague as well as with Susan's father's psychiatrist as I labored over what to do. Should I report my knowledge to the child welfare system? Would that benefit Susan? I have had dealings with our city's child welfare system and had been disappointed and appalled repeatedly. In most cases, situations were worsened by their involvement and the child was traumatized again. My thinking and decision making was certainly colored by this knowledge. The father's psychiatrist had no information of sexual abuse by his patient. Susan had assured me that the sexual and physical abuse had stopped before she began seeing me. In addition I felt protective of Susan's confidentiality and her right to privacy.

I brought up the idea of confronting her father. My reason for wanting to confront the father was complex. I was concerned that perhaps Susan was trying to tell me that the sexual abuse had not stopped or that she was fearful that it would reoccur. I also found it extremely difficult to continue the family sessions. It felt like an elephant was in the room. In addition the dyadic work was arrested. We were treading water and little if any therapeutic work was being accomplished. I felt that as long as Susan and I held onto the secret nothing could be accomplished in healing their relationship. Susan was adamant in her refusal to confront her father or allow me to speak with him about the sexual abuse. She still needed to be able to make it all go away as if it had happened to another little girl or had never happened at all.

The night before Susan was to take her driver's test, her father beat her. She called my office machine as she was choked, punched in the face, pushed to the floor, and kicked. He told her that she should have died last summer when she overdosed and that she was a worthless piece of shit that her mother died for. When the beating ended, he sat on the stairs and asked her for a cigarette and calmly spoke of this as their last night together, begging her not to leave. She called a friend and left the house. I called the child welfare department and Susan was officially removed from the home.

[Months later, Susan and I came to understand this physical attack as her father's inability to allow her to grow-up and separate. It is not an accident that he forced my hand to remove her from his home on the eve of her symbolic independence. He had already bought her a BMW that was waiting for her in the driveway.]

At this point I became exceedingly confused and apprehensive in connection with the legal and ethical dilemmas that I faced. The written report that I was required to submit to the child welfare agency asked for all prior knowledge of abuse. I hired a lawyer who informed me on the legalities of the situation and advised me to hold the emotional (and physical) well-being of my patient as paramount in all decision making. These weeks were stressful as I often doubted myself, worried that I could ultimately lose my license, and of course agonized over what was best for Susan.

As stated above, Susan moved in with her friend but was told she could stay there only until the school term ended. Susan was crestfallen by this news. We were now confronted with the very real prospect of the welfare system returning her to her father. We spoke of confronting her father. The following week Susan and I met with her father and his psychiatrist. Her father denied everything, leaving Susan to feel like she was losing her mind. With Susan's permission, I placed a call to the child welfare worker to disclose all knowledge of prior abuse.

From the day when Susan first confided her deepest darkest secret, that took her almost a year to tell me, we labored together to figure out what was the best action to take. Sessions were often grueling and intense and certainly challenging as Susan struggled to speak about her fears and needs. I reported the sexual abuse hesitantly as I continued to feel ambivalent about the correct course of action. I am still unsure as to how much of my decision was based on a need to alleviate my own anxiety about disobeying the law and how much was in the best interest of my patient. At the time of the report I felt reasonably certain that Susan wanted and needed me to make the phone call.

When Susan first spoke of her incestuous relationship with her father, should I have picked up the phone and made a child abuse report? At that time was Susan strong enough to bear the disclosure? Was our therapeutic relationship solid enough? Was I wrong to wait? Should I have made the call at all? Was it necessary for her safety? Did Susan get the message that I am just like all the others in her life? Was I caught up in an enactment to join hands with her as her abuser? Did I become a harborer of her terrible secret? Was it a test that I failed? Did I disregard the moral value of psychoanalysis of truthfulness? Could there be an analysis if I reported? Could there be an analysis if I did not report?

Moral, ethical, and clinical issues became entwined with a legal dilemma. My own personal morals and values were challenged. Susan was no longer living with her abusive father . . . perhaps there was no need to report . . .

perhaps the truth and fact of her incestuous relationship with her father should have remained in the treatment room. In addition, Children and Youth forgot about Susan. They never followed through to see if her living arrangements were safe or if she was continuing treatment. Once again she became invisible.

Working with Severe Trauma

The following clinical vignettes, from the third year of Susan's analysis, demonstrate how we worked with her severe trauma. At this point Susan was seventeen years old and a senior in high school.

Over the weekend Susan had a terrible experience with her lover, a girl her own age. They had been together for six months as a couple. The girlfriend had attempted to touch Susan's vagina as they made-out and Susan became hysterical, physically throwing her friend across the room. As she sat in my office and sobbed I could hardly make out her words. She spoke in incomplete sentences: "the steps creaking, the doorknob turning, the sound of the door opening." She said she was unable to say the words. It was too terrifying. It was a difficult session.

The next day she looked terrible and was unable to look at me.

> *A: You can't look at me today* (silence). *Maybe it is not that you can't look at me but instead you don't want me to look at you.*

She looks at me and quickly averts her eyes, there is a very long pause and she shakes her head in agreement. I ask her if she can tell me what the feeling is and she asks for pen and paper.

She writes:

> *What shame feels like.*
> *It feels like something is eating me, destroying me from inside out, and I am completely exposed to all who know and that's all that can be seen. It's like it takes over, and there is nothing else left for anyone to see but the horrible tainted ugly side of me. It makes me want to disappear and never have anyone see me again. I am scared of judgment. I hate the shame but I always let it win.*

I read her writing out loud and she tells me that she feels like a monster and that this is what everyone sees, an ugly monster. She tells me that she must have done something to make it happen. We sit in silence, both feeling her great shame.

> A: *Yesterday you said that if you say the words out loud you are terrified of what you will feel. What are you worried will happen?*

She asks for the pen and paper again and begins to write but it is a struggle. Her hand shakes and her tears stain the paper as she attempts to speak through her writing. She writes:

> *I remember the footsteps across my carpet. I remember the feeling of fear that would cause me to tremble as I would lay there silent as possible waiting . . . he would usually stand over my bed for a few minutes or perhaps it was only seconds, I really don't know. I would feel his body . . .*

She couldn't write anymore; her whole body was shaking.

> S: *Last night I wrote about it and burned it. I needed to burn it all up.*

It is imperative to note that while some of Susan's sessions were extremely regressed she was functioning at a high level out in the world. She was once again doing well in school, had applied to colleges in the area so that she would be able to continue her analysis, was working twenty hours a week at a job where she was respected and given extra responsibilities, and socially had developed a wonderful group of friends with whom she had good relationships.

The following session was almost completely nonverbal but one of our most powerful and moving experiences.

I could see from the moment she entered my office that she was not feeling well. The sparkle that had recently entered her eyes was gone, and in its place was what seemed like a pool of endless sadness. After perhaps ten minutes of silence she said she felt sad but did not know why. We sat together for a very long time in silence engulfed in her sadness. She began to try to speak but it was difficult for her to form the words. Finally she asked if she could sit on my floor, but was concerned that I would be angry with her for doing so. She asked several times if it is really all right to leave her chair. She curled up in a fetal position against the radiator behind her chair and began to sob. I asked her if I should also sit on the floor. She nodded her head and I left my chair and joined her on the floor. I remained the same distance from her that we maintain when sitting in our respective chairs. I did this because she needed to know I was with her in her space within her boundaries; not too close and not too far, maintaining optimal distance as with a young child in analysis. This physical arrangement also helped us to maintain eye contact. If I had remained silent in my chair I would have been reenacting all those before me who refused to see her pain, those who could not join her on the floor. Through her tears she related how she used to go into her closet and sit on the floor against the wall; it made her feel better. She was able to tell me that she felt close to me.

Susan yearned for closeness to me and from me, and for love. However, her rage was just around the corner waiting to pounce.

Susan's Rage

Shortly after Susan left her father's home never to return, I had a family emergency and had to cancel her session at the last minute. I left a message on her cell phone, not remembering in my own haste and anxiety that her phone was not functioning. She came to her session and found my office locked. The next day she told me what had happened. There had been some snow the previous night and the roads were icy, so she did not go to school and drove on icy highways over an hour to get to her appointment to find my office locked and uninviting. That night as she drove back to her foster home she thought: *I finally found someone who could be the perfect mother and now I really know it can never happen.*

In the spring I left town to attend my son's college graduation. Upon my return Susan confessed that she had used her computer skills to find out personal details about my family. She related how she now knew where my children went to school, where they were born, among many other details. She felt ashamed that she had also hacked into my graduate school records and found out details about my former career. I felt intruded upon by her aggression. In this action she became my abuser and I her helpless victim, as she aggressively penetrated my private life. She sobbed as she described her frustration about not being able to really be my child. She told me that she had been searching for a mother for so long and now that she finally found the person she thought could fill that void, it was almost intolerable to not be able to have me in this real sense.

Susan and I spent many months in this angry place where she reenacted her abuse and I became her victim. As I interpreted this transference in its many forms she was finally, after many many months, able to express anger toward her mother for not protecting her from her father and not providing a safe caretaker for her after her death.

Before ending Susan's story I want to share one other small part of our work, her sexual identity.

Susan's Sexual Identity

In her sophomore year of college Susan began to question her attraction to women, although she was not sure she was attracted to men either. In this particular session she had just come from the hair salon and her usually pulled-back hair was loose, falling softly around her face. She was wearing a pretty form-fitting colorful top and form fitting jeans with new shoes. She joked about letting her breasts out of hiding and feeling confident about her newfound femininity. She liked the way she felt and she liked the way she looked.

> *S: I tried so hard to look like a boy and feel like a boy. I feel that finally I can just let me be me.*

She told me how her former girlfriend gets very upset when she dresses in "girl" clothes and that she could only be attracted to Susan if she looked like a boy. She added,

> *S: It's competition if I look this way. She worries that I'm thinner and prettier.*

I wondered aloud if she was fearful that boys might find her attractive; she blushed and said she actually likes it that boys are interested, but confided that so far she has not met anyone in whom she has any romantic interest. The session continued and she was very chatty, telling me all about the good grades she had received, her reputation of being the smart girl on campus that everyone comes to for help, and that she had decided to run for student government. The session ended and we both stood up. She froze, terror seizing her as she became mute. She could only flap her arms as if in agony and gesture toward the chair. There on the seat was a quarter size spot of blood; she had gotten her period. The next day, she arrived late, her hair once again pulled back, wearing her old baggy clothes that she bought in the men's department. I did most of the talking as she cried and did her best to contain the overwhelming humiliation and shame that this event had stirred up. She told me she had a memory about blood, her blood, but could not speak the words. At the end of the session she told me she would add it to a journal she was keeping of all the things she cannot say out loud.

Susan experienced excessive shame from what she perceived as her uncontrollable bleeding, and her memories of being sexually damaged by her father came to the forefront. When she got her period in my office (as she spoke excitedly about feeling good about herself and appearing very pretty), she experienced overwhelming fear and humiliation.

Over the next several months Susan began to wear her hair like mine, and dress like me. This attempt to identify with me drew her into a heterosexual relationship with a boy she had known for a couple of years. He asked her to be his girlfriend, she accepted and they had sexual intercourse. Susan stated that this was an impulsive decision: "I just wanted to get it over with and see if I could do it." She was deeply disturbed in her session the next morning, curling up behind her chair against the wall on the floor. She told me she dissociated as she had to do when her father raped her. What caused her to sob uncontrollably was realizing that her body moved on its own, and that she made vocal sounds during sex. However, she felt nothing, neither pleasure nor pain. This relationship ended quickly, as Susan retreated once again into the relative safety of oversized sweatshirts, baggie pants, and hiking boots. We came to understand her flight into heterosexuality as an identification with me. Susan's fantasy was that I did not want her to be gay, but wished she was more like me. Once this was spoken, Susan was able to settle into, and accept herself as a lesbian woman. In her senior year of college Susan fell in love with a woman, whom years later, she eventually married.

Epilogue

Susan remained in her analysis throughout college. Over the years since we parted she has written to me to let me know that she was doing well. She had found love and married, was in a profession where she excelled, and six months ago, became a parent to a beautiful baby girl.

Discussion

Susan learned that anger was a dangerous emotion in her home. In fact displaying any emotion around her father was often met with an abusive reaction. Susan never knew what to expect from her environment, which had an extremely detrimental effect on her psychic development. It was almost impossible for her to navigate her way through the phases and stages of normal development. As an abused child she felt unlovable and worthless and had developed a "bad" self-image and identity. Her whole world denied that Susan was being abused, which reinforced her need to deny what was occurring. Susan denied the abuse but she also denied her rage. "In order to maintain a sense of a protecting other, all anger, disappointment, and frustration need to be directed away. The child cannot blame the parent. [S]he needs him, or the image, too much to allow this to happen. It is her only source of comfort, security, and protection. Herein lies the explanation for the secretiveness, the absence of memory, the resistance to recall, the hypnoid states, the somatic memory, and the apparent absence of anger: it is the inability to resolve the ambivalence with the resultant need to maintain the image of the split-off good parent" (Fischer 1991, p. 53). Her parents and extended family and close friends needed Susan to be invisible, and so she was, but she was not invisible to me and while this was desirable to Susan, at times it was also intolerable. Susan had many stories to tell and they all intertwined as the puzzle of her sexual development and feminine identity revealed itself.

CONCLUSION

Susan grew up in an environment where there was no protection and no escape. There was no adult she could turn to for relief or soothing. Susan must have experienced terrifying flooding affects that threatened her psychological survival. Her sense of self was destabilized as her mind was unable to process her overwhelming chaotic affects, and dissociation became Susan's primary defense. Dissociation is "designed to afford its protection automatically and without self-reflection, which is why it is so hard to work psychoanalytically" (Bromberg 2012, p. 274). Susan's trauma was severe and I imagine she was constantly fighting a tendency toward fragmentation. Susan's father blamed her for her mother's illness and subsequent death and was extremely abusive in every sense. Her mother's passivity and her father's hostile aggression became the foundation of her representational world. Susan's abusive and emotionally impoverished childhood left her with an anaclitic neediness that resulted in substance abuse (Mills 2004).

In the first few years of Susan's analysis, where silence pervaded and Susan often dissociated, I fought to preserve myself as an experienced thinking person. Our analytic goal in the early years of treatment was to create a space that permitted me to witness Susan as nonthinking, while simultaneously preventing her dissociated state from assaulting my ability to think. Susan's analysis was truly "life-saving." Her treatment provided a safe space where she and I could be together in "the shadow of what has been dissociated, including the dread of potential destabilization felt by both analyst and patient when they each face not-me parts of themselves that have been enlisted to prevent awakening" (Bromberg 2012, p. 277). Together, Susan and I created an environment where formally dissociated feelings and thoughts were played-out between us as a narrative. . . . Susan's story gradually took form and was shared. In this way Susan began to heal.

REFERENCES

Amir, D. (2012). The inner witness. *The International Journal of Psychoanalysis*, 93, 879–896.

Bacon, H. and Richardson, S. (2001). Attachment theory and child abuse: An overview of the literature for practitioners. *Child Abuse Review*, 10, 377–397.

Beebe, B. (1985). Interpersonal timing: The application of an adult dialogue model to mother-infant vocal and kinesic interactions. In T. Field and N. A. Fox (Eds.). *Social Perceptions in Infants*, Norwood, NJ: Ablex Pub. Corp.

———. (2000). Co-constructing mother-infant distress. *Psychoanalytic Inquiry*, 20, 421–440.

Beebe, B., Rustin, J., Sorter, D., and Knoblauch, S., (2003). Symposium on intersubjectivity in infant research and its implications for adult treatment. III. An expanded view of forms of intersubjectivity in infancy and its application to psychoanalysis. *Psychoanalytic Dialogues*, 13 (6), 805–841.

Beebe, B. and Sloate, P. (1982). Assessment and treatment of difficulties in mother-infant attunement in the first three years of life: A case history. *Psychoanalytic Inquiry*, 1(4), 601–623.

Brazelton, T. and Tronick, E. (1980). Preverbal communication between mothers and in infants. In D. R. Olson (Ed.). *The Social Foundations of Language and Thought* (pp. 299–315). New York: Norton.

Bromberg, P. M. (2012). Credo. *Psychoanalytic Dialogues*, 22, 273–278.

Cohler, J. (1987). Sex, love, and incest. *Contemporary Psychoanalysis*, 23, 604–620.

Cooper, A. L. (2012). When the lullaby is missing: Healing from an infancy in foster care. *Journal of Infant, Child, and Adolescent Psychotherapy*, 11, 356–367.
Eagle, M. (1995). The developmental perspectives of attachment and psychoanalytic theory. In S. Goldberg, R. Muir, and J. Kerr (Eds.), *Attachment Theory: Social, Developmental, and Clinical Perspectives*. Hillsdale: The Analytic Press.
Ferenczi, S., Abraham, K., Simmel, E., and Jones, E. (1921). *Psychoanalysis of the War Neurosis*. London: International Psychoanalytical Press.
Fischer, R. (1991). The unresolved rapprochement crisis: An important constituant of the incest experience. In S. Kramer and S. Akhtar. (2012) *The Trauma of Incest* (pp. 39–56). New Jersey: Jason Aronson Inc.
Fonagy, P. and Target, M. (1997). Attachment and reflective function: Their role in self-organization. *Development and Psychopathology*, 9, 679–700.
Fonagy, P., Gergely, G., Jurist, E., and Target, M. (2002). *Affect Regulation, Mentalization, and the Development of the Self.* New York: Other Books.
Fonagy, P., Steele, M., Steele, H., Leigh, T., Kennedy, R., Mattoon, G., and Target, M. (1995). Attachment, the reflective self, and borderline states: The predictive specificity of the adult attachment interview and pathological emotional development. In S. Goldberg, R. Muir, and J. Kerr (Eds.). *Attachment Theory: Social, Developmental and Clinical Perspectives*. (pp. 223–279). Hillsdale, NJ: Analytic Press.
Fonagy, P., Target, M., Gergely, G., Allen, J. G., and Bateman, A. W. (2003). The developmental roots of borderline personality disorder in early attachment relationships. *Psychoanalytic Inquiry*, 23 (3), 412–459.
Fraiberg, S. (1982). Pathological defenses in infancy. *Psychoanalytic Quarterly*, 51, 612–635.
Hardy, L. T. (2007). Attachment theory and reactive attachment disorder: Theoretical perspectives and treatment implications. *Journal of Child and Adolescent Psychiatric Nursing*, 20(1), 27–39.
Jaffe, J., Beebe, B., Feldstein, S., Crown, C. L. and Jasnow, M. D. (2001). Rhythms of dialogue in infancy. *Monographs on Social Research in Child Development*, 66(2).
Karen, R. (1998). *Becoming Attached: First Relationships and How They Shape Our Capacity to Love.* New York: Warner Books.
Khan, M. R. (1964). Ego distortion, cumulative trauma, and the role of reconstruction in the analytic situation. *International Journal of Psychoanalysis*, 45, 272–299.
Kramer, S. and Akhtar, S. (Eds). (1991). *The Trauma of Transgression.* New Jersey: Jason Aronson.
Kris, A. O. (1956). The recovery of childhood memories in psychoanalysis. *The Psychoanalytic Study of the Child*, 11, 54–88.
Krystal, H. (1978). Trauma and affects. *Psychoanalytic Study of the Child*, 33, 81–116.
Lieberman, A. F. (1997). Toddlers' internalizations of maternal attributions as a factor in quality of attachment. In K. Zucker and L. Atkinson (Eds.). *Attachment and Psychopathology*. (pp. 277–290), New York: Guilford Press.
Main, M. (1996). Introduction to the special section on attachment and psychopathology: 2. Overview of the field of attachment. *Journal of Consulting and Clinical Psychology*, 64, 237–243.
Meltzoff, A. N. and Moore, M. K. (1977). Imitation of facial and manual gestures by human neonates. *Science*, 198, 75–78.
———. (1989). Imitation in newborn infants: Exploring the range of gestures imitated and the underlying mechanisms. *Developmental Psychology*, 25, 954–962.
———. (1998). Object representation, identity, and the paradox of early permanence: Steps toward a new framework. *Infant Behavior and Development*, 21(2), 201–235.
Mills, J. (2004). Structuralization, trauma, and attachment. *Psychoanalytic Psychology*, 21, 154–160.
Morton, J. and Johnson, M. H. (1991). Conspec and Conlearn: A two-process theory of infant face recognition. *Psychoanalytic Review*, 98, 164–181.
Nachmani, G. (1995). Trauma and ignorance. *Contemporary Psychoanalysis*, 31, 423.
Schore, A. N. (2002). Clinical implications of a psychoneurobiological model of projective identification. In S. Alhanti (Ed.), *Primitive Mental States, Volume II: Psychobiological and*

Psychoanalytic Perspectives on Early Trauma and Personality Development (pp. 1–66). New York: Karnac.

Shengold, L. (1999). *Soul Murder Revisited: Thoughts about Therapy, Hate, Love, and Memory*. New Haven, CT: Yale University Press.

Slade, A. (1998). Representation, symbolization, and affect regulation in the concomitant treatment of a mother and child: Attachment theory and child psychotherapy. *Psychoanalytic Dialogues*, 8, 797–830.

Slade, A., Sadler, L., De Dios-Kenn, C., Webb, D., Currier-Ezepchick, J., and Mayes, L. (2006). Minding the baby: A reflective parenting program. *The Psychoanalytic Study of the Child,* 60, 74–100.

Stern, D. (1985). *The Interpersonal World of the Infant*. New York: Basic Books.

Teicher, M. H., Anderon, S. L., Polcari, A., Anderson, C. M., Navalta, C. P., and Kim, D. M. (2003). The neurobiological consequences of early stress and childhood maltreatment. *Neuroscience and Biobehavioral Reviews,* 27, 33–44.

Trevarthen, C. (1979). Communication and cooperation in early infancy: A description of primary intersubjectivity. In M. Bullowa (Ed.), *Before Speech: The Beginning of Interpersonal Communication.* Cambridge: Cambridge University Press.

Tronick, E. Z. (1989). Emotions and emotional communication in infants. *American Psychologist*, 44, 112–119.

Van der Kolk, B., McFarlane, A., and Weisaeth, L. (1996). *Traumatic Stress: The Effects of Overwhelming Experience on the Mind, Body, and Society.* New York: The Guilford Press.

Winnicott, D. W. (1953). Transitional objects and transitional phenomena: A study of the first not-me possession. *International Journal of Psychoanalysis*, 34, 89–97.

———. (1974). Fear of breakdown. *International Journal of Psychoanalysis*, 1, 103–107.

Chapter Eight

Depression

A Psychoanalytic Perspective

Corinne Masur

Psychoanalytic theory and practice have been much maligned in recent years as irrelevant, insufficiently evidence based, and outmoded. However, much of Sigmund Freud's basic theoretical conceptualization has provided the foundation for contemporary formulations of personality development and organization and for the understanding of psychopathology in adults, especially personality disorders and depression. Psychoanalytic and psychodynamic treatments continue to be viable options for work with patients of many diagnostic categories, including both major depression and briefer depressive episodes. Additionally, there is a growing body of research demonstrating the efficacy of psychodynamic treatment of depression in comparison with newly popular Cognitive Behavioral Therapy (CBT) and Dialectical Behavior Therapy (DBT), which are often considered the more "evidence-based" treatments due to the relative ease with which research can be performed using these treatment modalities.

In regard to depressive syndromes in particular, psychoanalysts can be given credit in the modern era for having developed the original models to explain the etiology and existence of this type of symptomatology. Karl Abraham (1911, 1924), Sigmund Freud (1917), and Sandor Rado (1928) were among the first psychoanalytic theorists to describe depression and to attribute its origins to the loss of a loved one, the loss of love, conflicted anger, developmental trauma, and/or narcissistic vulnerability. Karl Abraham (1911, 1924) provided the initial psychoanalytic framework, remembered today as: depression = anger turned inward.

Sigmund Freud's models of depression included theoretical formulations as to etiology, biological variables, and temperamental vulnerabilities. The experience of loss or abandonment and the quality of early attachment and experience, especially those accompanied by affects such as shame, unpleasure, feelings of loneliness, abandonment, helplessness, and guilt, were considered particularly salient. Such early experiences and affects were posited by early psychoanalytic theoreticians to create vulnerability to depression (Busch, Rudden, and Shapiro 2004).

Abraham was the first of the early psychoanalysts to write about melancholia, saying in 1911 that melancholia is a reaction to the loss of love or to the actual loss through death of a beloved person. In 1924 he described the period of depression following loss and stated that once the mourner can identify with and introject a part of the lost loved one, he can sometimes recover, using the unconscious belief, "My loved object is not gone for now I carry it within myself and can never lose it" (Abraham 1924, p. 437). He also suggested that those who develop a more prolonged depression following the loss of love or the loss of a loved one were predisposed to the development of this psychopathology due to early trauma, e.g., having experienced severe injury to their healthy sense of narcissism (self-esteem) in infancy and/or early childhood due to disappointment in their mother's attention or ministrations. According to Abraham, disappointment in adulthood often provides the trigger for the recrudescence of these earlier feelings in the form of a depressive episode.

In "Mourning and Melancholia," Sigmund Freud worked to "throw some light on the nature of melancholia by comparing it with the normal affect of mourning" (Freud 1917, p. 244). In this chapter he explored the connections between loss, mourning, and depression, which he referred to as melancholia. He described mourning quite clearly: "Mourning is regularly the reaction to the loss of a loved person, or to the loss of some abstraction which has taken the place of one, such as one's country, liberty, an ideal, and so on" (ibid., p. 234). He went on to distinguish this from melancholia: "In some people the same influences produce melancholia (depression) instead of mourning and we consequently suspect them of a pathological disposition," referring here to temperamental predisposition and/or to Abraham's idea of early developmental trauma. According to Freud, "the distinguishing mental features of melancholia are a profoundly painful dejection, cessation of interest in the outside world, loss of the capacity to love, inhibition of all activity, and a lowering of the self-regarding feelings to a degree that finds utterance in self-reproaches and self-revilings, and culminates in a delusional expectation of punishment" (ibid., p. 244). We can scarcely come up with a better description of depression today, even if we look to the *Diagnostic and Statistical Manual of Mental Disorders* (DSM) (as we will do later). Freud went on to say that ". . . the same traits are met with in mourning," however, "the disturbance of self-regard is absent in mourning" (ibid., p. 243). In other words, the individual's sense of self is diminished when depressed, whereas in mourning, it is the outer world which is diminished by the absence of the person who has died.

Freud's description of the psychodynamics of depression can also hardly be improved upon, especially if we substitute the term "depressive" each time he uses the word, "melancholic":

> In mourning we found that the inhibition and loss of interest are fully accounted for by the work of mourning in which the ego is absorbed. In melancholia, (an unexplained or unknown) loss will result in a similar internal work and will therefore be responsible for the melancholic inhibition. The difference is that the inhibition of the melancholic seems puzzling to us because we cannot see what it is that is absorbing him so entirely. The melancholic displays something else besides which is lacking in mourning—an extraordinary diminution in his self-regard, an impoverishment of his ego on a grand scale. . . . The patient represents his ego to us as worthless, incapable of any achievement and morally despicable; he reproaches himself, vilifies himself and expects to be cast out and punished (ibid., p. 245).

In 1924 Karl Abraham produced a second work on melancholia, confirming Freud's conclusions and making some of his own. Abraham wrote that melancholics could not truly love due to their ambivalence toward the love object. The origin of these difficulties, he said, lay once again in early developmental trauma, in their "double disappointment" with both mother and father at the height of the oedipal conflict. Furthermore, he described the melancholic as giving up interest not only in the loved one (thus experiencing loss through a loss of love rather than a loss through death) but also in ever-widening circles of people and interests until he has finally lost interest in everything. Yet at the same time, noted Abraham, the melancholic also holds an attitude of superiority toward himself which will often alternate with an exaggerated attitude of humility. He criticized the idea of his contemporaries (see below) that melancholics have delusions of inferiority. He stated that melancholics "present a picture in which there stands in immediate juxtaposition yet absolutely opposed to one another self love and self hatred" (Abraham 1924, p. 456).

Sandor Rado (1928) expanded on the theories of Abraham and Freud. He wrote that the most striking feature of the depressive individual is the fall in self-esteem and self-satisfaction which the individual experiences. He made a distinction between the depressive neurotic who tries to hide these feelings and the melancholic who suffers openly from "the delusion of moral inferiority," taking offense easily and often behaving as if he were being treated badly. The melancholic, he said, feels a loss of self-esteem when he feels disappointed or offended and he relies on others for attention and praise to reclaim and maintain self-esteem. Rado suggested that those with early narcissistic injury often experience an especially strong desire for attention and praise from others and a particular intolerance for criticism or rejection. He suggested that such patients see the self and others as either all good or all bad (similar to more contemporary theory regarding Narcissistic and Borderline Personality Disorders). In so doing the melancholic individual incorporates both good and bad qualities of loved ones, consciously adopting the good qualities into the ego ideal (who the patient would *like* to be) and unconsciously adopting the bad qualities into the ego, thus setting off an internal war between the ego, the ego ideal, and the superego, with the superego criticizing and punishing the individual for not living up to the standards of the ego ideal.

In regard to neurotic depression, Rado said,

> observation shows that the depressive process . . . is carried out in exact accordance with the mechanism of true melancholia. That is to say that neurotic depression also has as its basis a narcissistic turning-away from reality, the external object being replaced by psychic institutions and an endeavour being made to solve the conflicts on the intrapsychic plane instead of in the outside world, and by means of a regressively activated oral technique. But there is this difference: these processes almost wholly consume the ego of the melancholic and destroy those functions in him which relate to reality, while in a transference-neurosis they are as it were merely superimposed upon an ego which is, indeed, neurotic but is more or less intact. In the depressive neurotic the object and, with it, the relation to reality, are preserved: it is only that the patient's hold on them is loosened and the weak ego has begun to give up the struggle with the world—a struggle which it feels to be unbearable—to turn inwards in a narcissistic fashion and to take refuge in the oral-narcissistic reparation-mechanism. Thus, neurotic depression is a kind of partial melancholia of the (neurotic) ego (Rado 1928, p. 436).

Melanie Klein, in her own metapsychological idiom, introduced the concept of the "depressive position," involving the early perception of the maternal object as a whole, and including a guilty thrust toward reparation (Klein 1935). It should be noted that Klein emphasized the importance of the basic function of consistently dependable good mothering in the infant's mastery of the turbulent intrapersonal and interpersonal dynamics she described (in Stone 1986).

Later, Edward Bibring (1953) suggested that depression arises less from conflict between the ego ideal and the superego and more from difficulty in the regulation of self-esteem arising from early experiences of helplessness. He suggested that early frustrations of a child's dependent needs can lead to a sense of failure and a diminishment in self-esteem (Busch, Rudden, & Shapiro 2004).

Edith Jacobson (1954, 1971, 1975) posited the existence of a "depressive personality" and examined the differences between the oedipal development of the so-called normal individual versus this depressive "personality," concluding that a variety of factors including early trauma could interfere with the child's establishing normal relationships with the parents. She theorized that an actual lack of parental acceptance and/or emotional understanding could negatively affect a child's self-esteem leading to aggressive feelings toward the parents and subsequent guilt. The aggression toward the parent could also be turned against the self as a defensive strategy to protect the loved one and to prevent the self from enacting hostile impulses against the parent in reality (Busch et al.). Jacobson also felt that in reaction to the aggressive feelings toward the parent, the child might develop an excessively perfectionistic ego ideal and unrealistically high standards resulting, of course, in repeated disappointments in the self.

The early psychoanalytic theorists differentiated between a depression focused primarily on interpersonal issues such as dependency, helplessness, and feelings of loss and abandonment, and a depression derived from a harsh, punitive superego—a depression focused primarily on self-criticism, concerns about self-worth, and feelings of failure and guilt.

John Bowlby (1980, 1988), while initially rejected in psychoanalytic circles, was later heralded for bringing biological models to the study of attachment and loss. Bowlby described attachment as an inborn strategy designed to protect the individual as well as the species. He described disruption of attachment in the form of loss or neglect in a three-volume series in which he wrote about the responses characteristic to individuals who have experienced such events. He suggested a sequence of reactions to loss by the infant or young child as including shock, denial, protest, yearning and searching, and ultimately withdrawal and detachment. Bowlby, writing from the object relations and ethological perspectives, briefly discussed the predisposition to depression in anxiously attached and compulsively self-reliant individuals. He noted that anxiously attached individuals seek interpersonal contact and are excessively dependent on others. Compulsively self-reliant individuals are excessively autonomous and avoid close, intimate, interpersonal relationships. According to Bowlby, both of these preoccupations create a vulnerability to depression (Blatt 1990).

Bowlby also distinguished carefully among sadness, mourning, and depression, just as his psychoanalytic predecessors had done. Bowlby stated that sadness is a normal, healthy response to any misfortune; most intense episodes of sadness are elicited by loss whether of a beloved person or a familiar place or social role. The sad person may turn to a trusted other for help, but his own sense of competence and self-worth remains intact and he does not lose hope. Bowlby believed that as long as there is active interaction between the sad individual and the outer world, either in thought or action, the subjective experience of depression is not present. It is when interaction stops that depression sets in, continuing until new patterns of interaction have been adapted and organized toward a new person or goal (Bowlby 1980).

Arieti and Bemporad worked within the interpersonal framework in psychoanalysis and theorized that there are two types of depression, a dominant other type and a dominant goal type. According to Arieti and Bemporad (1978), when the dominant other is lost or the dominant goal is not achieved, depression can result. They discussed two intense and basic wishes in depression: "to be passively gratified by the dominant other" and "to be reassured of one's own worth, and to be free of the burden of guilt" (Arieti & Bemporad 1978, p. 167). In the dominant other type of depression, the individual desires to be passively gratified by developing a relationship that is clinging, demanding, dependent, and infantile. In the dominant goal type, the individual seeks to be reassured of his or her worth and to be free of guilt by directing every effort toward a goal that has become an end in itself.

Sydney Blatt (Blatt 1974; Blatt, D'Afflitti, and Quinlan 1976; Blatt, Quinlan, and Chevron 1990; Blatt et al. 1982) is a contemporary psychoanalytic theorist of depression. He writes from the object-relational, ego psychoanalytic, and cognitive developmental perspectives, and theorizes that a differentiation can be made between an "anaclitic" (dependent) and an "introjective" (self-critical) depression. He discusses the developmental origins, predisposing personality characteristics, clinical manifestations, and unconscious conflicts of these two types. He characterizes anaclitic or dependent depression as containing feelings of loneliness, helplessness, and weakness; he notes that these individuals have intense and chronic fears of being abandoned and left unprotected and uncared for, and states that they have deep longings to be loved, nurtured, and protected. According to Blatt, because there has been little internalization of the experiences of gratification or of the qualities of the individuals who provided satisfaction, others are valued primarily for the immediate care, comfort, and satisfaction they provide. According to Blatt, separation from others and object loss create considerable fear in the depressive (Blatt 1974).

Introjective or self-critical depression, by contrast, is characterized by Blatt and his colleagues as concerned with feelings of unworthiness, inferiority, failure, and guilt. These individuals engage in persistent, harsh self-scrutiny and evaluation, and have a chronic fear of criticism and of losing the approval of significant others. They strive for excessive achievement and perfection, are often highly competitive and work hard, make many demands on themselves, and often achieve a great deal, but with little lasting satisfaction. Because of their intense competitiveness, they can also be critical and attacking toward others in projective process. Through overcompensation they strive to achieve and maintain approval and recognition (Blatt 1974). Basing his discussion on the parallel between these two types of depression (anaclitic and introjective) and the two strands of narcissism discussed by Kohut (idealized parental imago and grandiose self) (Kohut 1971), Blatt et al. (1982) noted that frequent use of narcissism serves as a defense against depression.

Stone (1986) clarified some of what was left less clear by earlier theorists. First, he expanded upon the definition of object loss as a predisposing factor in depressive illness:

> While the idea of "object loss" finds its typical expression in loss of a love object by death, the clinical phenomenology of depressive illness—indeed, at times, of mourning—may be precipitated by an endless spectrum of associatively or symbolically allied phenomena as alternatives—failure in a love affair; departure of a child from home, physically (or psychologically); failure of promotion in a job; loss of money; failure to win a prestigious award to which the individual feels entitled or, in some instances, simply covets, and so on through all of the elements in man's "symbolic universes" . . . Narcissistic injury occasioning loss in the sphere of the individual's "self-love," compounded by degradation of an early idealized object image, is indeed a frequent precipitant of depression (Stone 1986).

Stone also brilliantly and exhaustively summarized and evaluated the existing psychoanalytic clinical literature on depression, finally coming to the following conclusions based on his retrospective scrutiny of twenty-three cases seen over extended periods (fourteen in classical psychoanalytic situations) and his integration of both the old and the new literature on the subject: he states that the considerations of pathologic narcissism, aggression toward the primary object, oral ambivalent regression, and "identification" with the disappointing object, are in varying degree and internal mutual relatedness, important in most if not all cases of true depressive illness, and should be taken into account in evaluating their pathology. He states that while each of these factors is a dynamic entity in its own right, they operate synergistically in the complex of depressive illness. This synergistic relation may derive in part from the common origin of these dynamic elements in disturbances of early infantile experience. The ego state of helplessness, emphasized by Bibring (1953), can be seen as pervasive in this complex. Stone stated that he does not believe that depression is to be viewed as a circumscribed primary affect occurring in a variety of etiological situations, which need only to be analyzed in their own immediate right. He said that the infantile elements in the origin of depressive affect remain important, and should be dealt with to the degree possible. They often cannot be recalled but can be reconstructed with difficulty. They usually have left traces, i.e., in their character derivatives, sometimes warded off until a time of crisis or hidden in countercharacterological formations. Analysis of these last phenomena, while usually difficult, ultimately contributes significantly to the reduction of the substrate of depressive illness.

Charles Brenner (1975, 1979) diverged from the etiological conceptualization of depression as caused by loss, perceived or real, stating instead that depression is often caused by a symbolic castration or disempowerment or as a punishment for sexual, competitive, or aggressive wishes (Busch et al. 2004). Brenner also felt that in some patients success can precipitate depression due to the aforementioned conflict over aggressive and sexual wishes, with the depression serving as the means to diminish the aggression inherent in the achievement of success.

On the other hand Heinz Kohut (1971) saw depressive affect in narcissistically vulnerable individuals as related to chronic feelings of emptiness in response to traumatically unempathic parenting, not unlike Jacobson before him (Jacobson 1954, 1971, 1975).

DEVELOPMENTAL THEORY

As mentioned above, many of the early psychoanalytic theorists who studied depression considered experiences such as early loss or loss of love to be involved in the development of later depression. Research performed by Rene Spitz in the 1940s through the 1960s found that the danger of early trauma and loss lies not just in the predisposition to later depression but also in the impact on the infant or child at the time of the loss. He found that babies in foundling homes who had been abandoned, even though provided with adequate nutrition and hygiene, often developed "failure to thrive" in the second half of the first year of life, leading to marasmus and death if a reunion with their parents was not accomplished. Later it was found that substitute nurturing could be provided for such infants to prevent full blown failure to thrive or marasmus, but that an anaclitic depression of varying lengths and severity often resulted from such separations (Spitz 1965; Robertson and Robertson 1971; Bowlby 1980; Furman 1974).

Between twelve months and three years, the infant or young child who loses his/her mother or is removed from her care and placed with strangers will protest and make urgent efforts to recover her. Such children will eventually give up their protest, withdraw, and sink into despair which can become suffused with anger and hostility (Bowlby 1980). The work of Spitz (1965), Bowlby (1980), the Robertsons (1971), the Furmans (1974), and others demonstrated that infants and children are not only prone to later depression (as discussed above) but may also experience depression in infancy and childhood, a concept which had been rejected for the entire first half of the nineteenth century.

The developmental point of view in psychoanalytic theory refers to just this—the understanding that early experience profoundly affects the individual and his or her intrapsychic life. That depression should develop in childhood or adolescence in an individual who has experienced loss, loss of love, and/or early neglect or abuse has been noted by psychoanalysts in clinical practice and by psychoanalytic theorists (see citations above). Research in the last several decades is just catching up with and affirming this understanding.

Studies derived from Bowlby's work have suggested that loss of one parent in childhood (Brown and Harris, 1978 in Hill 2009) or impaired "bonding" (Perer, Brown and Harris in Hill 2009) is associated with vulnerability to adult depression. Parental "indifference," emotional neglect, and physical neglect have been found to correlate highly with adult depression (Harris, Bown, and Bifulco, in Hill 2009) and a variety of studies have also revealed a high correlation between childhood sexual abuse and adult depression (Fergusson, Horwood, & Lynskey 1996; Hill 2009; Kendler et al.; Mullen, Martin, Anderson, Romans, & Herbison; Nelson et al.; Fergusson and Mullen in Hill 2009).

The etiology of depression has also been looked at from the neurochemical and genetic points of view. It is beyond the scope of this chapter to describe the multiplicity of recent findings in this area. It should be mentioned, however, that evidence is mounting that the early substrate of depression involves the interplay between genetic and environmental influences. For example, Caspi et al.'s (2003) work on the alleles of the 5-HTT gene points to the way in which variations in genes involved in the regulation of relevant neurotransmitters can modify responsiveness to environmental influences such as life events. The study of genetic influences on susceptibility to adverse environments offers a promising way forward in understanding this interplay between genetic and environmental influences in the development of depressive symptomatology (Hill 2009). Moreover, the study of environmental influences on genetics—or epigenetics—is also sure to spread further light on the development of depression in many individuals.

DEFINITIONAL ISSUES IN DEPRESSION

Within general psychiatry and psychology there is no unitary concept of depression. Depressed mood as a symptom may be present in any mental disorder, or be part of the normal range of affect. Psychiatric disorders in which there may be significant depressive symptoms or episodes include bipolar affective disorder (episodes of mania or hypomania and depression), mixed anxiety and depressive disorder, dysthymia, postschizophrenic depression, and adjustment disorders. Substance misuse, brain injuries or diseases, physical diseases, malnutrition, and some medications may also cause depressed mood. Moreover, there is debate about the relative contributions of external stress, biological dysfunction, abnormal personality, genetic factors, and early environmental influence as well as about rates and degrees of recovery and relapse and responsiveness to various treatments (Cole, McGuffin, & Farmer 2008; Farmer & McGuffin 2003; Jacobson 1975; Kendell, in McQueen 2009).

Given an absence of consensus about how best to classify depression, some have recommended that classifications should be based on "unambiguous operational criteria" (Kendall 2000). The DSM of the American Psychiatric Association, and the International Classification of Diseases (ICD) of the World Health Organization, are examples of compendiums using such classification systems. Others, particularly psychoanalytically informed therapists and theorists, have found such classifications artificial and problematic. Within the psychoanalytic framework, depression can better be seen as symptomatic of underlying, often unconscious dynamics including a recrudescence of early affects and/or present-day conflict between the ego, id, and superego, disturbances in interpersonal relationships and the like.

In response to the criticism that the DSM and ICD focus too heavily on externally observable behaviors and too little on internal affects and individual dynamics, the DSMs have become increasingly detailed in the description of psychopathology while also continuing to list symptoms which can be objectively verified. Specific details concerning persistence of symptomatology, cognition, and neurovegetative function (e.g., appetite, sleep disorder, fatigue, or energy loss) are given to assist in making the diagnosis.

The psychoanalytic and psychodynamic points of view assume that every human fact always implies emotion and meaning. The psychoanalytic framework requires that the emotional depth and underlying dynamics be included in describing psychopathology. In 2006, the Psychodynamic Diagnostic Manual was created by the PDM Task Force, a committee of psychoanalytic thinkers from various institutes and orientations in order to classify and describe the spectrum of mental disorders in a way that was both descriptive and attentive to underlying dynamics.

The PDM provides a description of depressive disorders as well as an explanation of the internal experience of depression and a detailed clinical example. The PDM relies heavily on Blatt's conceptualization of anaclitic versus introjective depression when describing the subjective experience of depression, while also including cognitive patterns, fantasies, and preoccupations typical of the depressive. Somatic states and relational patterns are also described.

PREVALENCE AND EPIDEMIOLOGY

According to the World Health Organization, depressive illness is the leading cause of disability in the world in terms of sheer number of people affected

(Bardwaj and Goodyer 2009). Prevalence figures depend on the definition of depression used and the population sampled. Using ICD-10 criteria for depression (excluding adjustment disorders and dysthymia), the Office of National Statistics' (Singleton, Bumpstead, O'Brien, Lee, & Meltzer, in McQueen 2009) survey of psychiatric morbidity for the UK gives the number affected at any one time as 26/1,000 (23/1,000 males and 28/1,000 females), the peak being between the ages of thirty-five and fifty-four years. Adults with depression are more likely to be divorced or separated, living alone or as a lone parent, have no educational qualifications, have a predicted IQ below 90, be unemployed and to have moved three or more times in the last two years. When the less severe concept of mixed depression and anxiety is used the prevalence approaches 10 percent of the population (88/1,000; 68/1,000 males and 108/1,000 females).

CLINICAL COURSE

There is a continuum of distress between normality and depression. In clinically significant depression the natural course of the condition is often prolonged, relapsing, or recurrent. Greater severity of depression is associated with greater risk of relapse. After a depressive episode approximately two-thirds of individuals relapse within 7–12 years (O'Leary & Lee 1996; Surtees & Barkley, in McQueen 2009). Ten years after hospitalization for severe depression, only half the follow-up months are spent at an asymptomatic level; 18 percent of patients never become asymptomatic (Kennedy, Abbott, & Paykel, in McQueen 2009). Death rates are doubled for natural causes of death in depressed individuals, mainly cardiovascular and respiratory diseases (O'Leary & Lee 1996; Surtees & Barkley, in McQueen 2009). A meta-analysis found the risk of suicide in depression to be twenty-one times higher, and in dysthymia, eleven times higher than the population rate (Harris & Barraclough, in McQueen 2009).

DYNAMICS

Psychoanalytic theorists have emphasized the role of narcissistic vulnerability in triggering depression. The basis for this vulnerability varies from theorist to theorist, and includes, as mentioned above, early loss, loss of love, poor parental provision of love and empathy, disappointment in early relationships, fragile self-esteem (based on early experiences of helplessness or a perception of being unloved) and/or fantasies of castration or disempowerment (Busch et al. 2004). This narcissistic vulnerability can lead to sensitivity to disappointment and rejection in later life with these feelings then leading to anger with those who have disappointed. This anger and aggression is often experienced as bad, resulting in conscious or unconscious guilt which contributes to the individual's feelings of low self-esteem and the tendency toward self-denigration and the turning of anger toward the self.

Rudden et al. (in Busch 2004) proposed a core dynamic formulation for depression. They stated that the modulation of self-esteem is often disturbed in depressed individuals with a tendency toward idealizing others and devaluing the self. Disappointment in the idealized other or loss of the idealized other are hypothesized as common triggers in depression. Rudden et al. described the common defenses used by the depressed individual (in an attempt to diminish painful feelings) as denial, projection, passive aggressive mechanisms, and reaction formation. However, they noted that the use of these defenses often leads to an exacerbation of depression.

PSYCHOANALYTIC AND PSYCHODYNAMIC TREATMENT OF DEPRESSION

Psychoanalytic treatment of depression is as old as psychoanalysis itself. As mentioned, Karl Abraham and Sigmund Freud treated depressed patients and wrote about this treatment in some of their earliest papers. In the intervening years, traditional psychoanalysis, long-term psychoanalytic psychotherapy and short-term models of psychoanalytic treatment have been used to treat depressed patients.

The psychoanalyst and the psychoanalytic or psychodynamic psychotherapist see individuals complaining of depressed mood, persistent sadness, frequent crying and/or irritability, anhedonia, and other symptoms of depression perhaps more often than any other type of patient. It has been said that depression is the common cold of mental health. The psychoanalytic model for seeing depressed patients involves providing an open ended, insight oriented treatment situation in which the therapeutic relationship assumes importance. In this relationship, the therapist presents himself both as a highly attuned listener whose job it is to understand the patient's feelings and thoughts (both conscious and unconscious) and as an object for transference, that is, a person onto whom the patient can project his unconscious feelings and early patterns of object relatedness.

In psychoanalysis, the patient will be seen between three and six times per week by a psychoanalyst. It is the analyst's job to make the patient's unconscious material conscious via interpretation. The patient uses the analyst's interpretations to work toward understanding his own conscious and unconscious fantasies, desires, wishes, and feelings, including those which originally predisposed him to depressive symptomatology. Depending on the psychoanalyst's theoretical orientation and formulation of the case, the analyst may work with the patient to ameliorate a harsh and punitive superego and a perfectionistic ego ideal and/or the patient and analyst may work together to use the patient's transference feelings to clarify the nature of the patient's early feelings about his relationships (generally with his parents and other intimates) and to reconstruct the patient's early experience and object relationships. In so doing, the patient comes to understand the origins of his depression, his misperceptions of current relationships based on perfectionistic standards and/or early perceptions, and resulting distortions regarding the nature of relationships, the triggers for depressive feelings, the nature of his own expectations and evaluations of himself, etc. Psychoanalysis often takes from two to many years to complete.

In long-term psychodynamic psychotherapy the patient may be seen over the course of a year to several years. Generally, the use of the transference is diminished due to the decreased frequency of the sessions and the resulting decrease in the intensity and continuity of the clinical work. However, the therapist may use the transference at times to elucidate the patient's dynamics and to make interpretations especially meaningful. A variable amount of support is given to the patient depending on the severity of the patient's depression, with the more depressed patient needing more support. The amount of support given to the patient in psychotherapy is generally greater than that provided in a psychoanalysis. Psychotherapy may be more appropriate than psychoanalysis for the severely depressed patient due to the lack of energy available to such individuals to carry out the tasks of daily life, let alone those involved in intensive treatment. At the beginning of psychotherapy, greater amounts of help and support may be required from the therapist in order to aid the patient in stabilizing, engaging in the treatment relationship, and becoming familiar with and involved in the work of the treatment.

Over the course of long-term psychodynamic psychotherapy the therapist attempts to help the patient to understand his feelings and their origins. Discussion of current life events will eventually lead to deeper material regarding relationships, new and old, experiences with the family of origin and childhood experiences and affects. As the patient puts his feelings and memories into words there is often a new appreciation for the depth of these feelings and a beginning ability to reflect on their meaning. With the growth of trust in the therapist and with the interpretation of defenses, the patient will be able to express deep feelings more fully and openly and to attain some relief from this expression of often long reserved or repressed affect. Eventually, patterns in relationships may be recognized and understood as repetitions from past object relationships. For example, Jacobson's patient Peggy, who had been in psychodynamic psychotherapy, would have no doubt talked at length about her early experiences in childhood. The therapist would have pointed out, over time, the effect these experiences had on Peggy's perception of others, including of the therapist. Peggy would then have been helped to see that her current circumstances were more favorable than those in which she grew up and that the possibility of new types of relationships—including with the therapist—were now possible.

There are also a variety of short-term models of psychodynamic psychotherapy which have been used for research purposes such as (Luborsky et al. 1975, 1993, 1999a and b, 2001), variations of which are increasingly being adopted for clinical practice. One such short-term model of psychoanalytic treatment of depression is Short Term Supportive Psychoanalytic Psychotherapy (STSP), a face to face, six-month individual psychotherapy. The primary goal of this treatment is to cure depression and the secondary goal is to reduce the vulnerability to depression. The latter is accomplished by shaping or altering the internal relationships of the patient. To achieve this goal, two paths can be followed: the adequate interpretation of needs, called the structural approach, and the adequate gratification of needs (called the developmental approach). The two approaches are not mutually exclusive; on the contrary, they are seen as complementary. However, in depressed patients the developmental approach is seen as more appropriate.

STSP relies on "adequate psychoanalytic support" as its curative factor (DeJonghe 2013). In this form of treatment, old relationships with critical others (e.g., the mother and/or father) are theorized as having been internalized by the patient, whereby the patient becomes critical of himself (a simplified version of Abraham and Bibring's earlier conceptualizations). In this form of treatment, the therapist sets himself up as a benign and benevolent figure, the aim being for the patient to experience dissonance between the reality of the therapist as a person and the transference to the therapist as a critical other. In the relationship with the therapist, the patient receives adequate gratification of unmet infantile needs, internalizes the new (therapeutic) relationship and identifies with it and in so doing, the old template for relationships is either corrected or challenged (DeJonghe 2013).

CASE EXAMPLES

Case 1: Psychoanalysis

Camille was a thirty-seven-year-old woman when she presented for treatment. She said, "I want to get to the root of what's bothering me." Camille suffered from numerous somatic complaints: she had chronic neck and back pain, frequent and severe migraine headaches, and digestive disruptions several times weekly. She also suffered from feelings of sadness, frequent crying, inability to achieve orgasm, and periods of lethargy. She was accident-prone and had numerous experiences of having fallen down, car accidents, and the like.

When Camille began psychoanalysis, she was quite happy but after several months of four times weekly treatment her material indicated that she wanted even more time from the analyst. A fifth session per week was offered and Camille was impressed that the analyst had heard and understood her unspoken wish. She accepted the additional session.

The early part of the analysis was characterized by Camille's difficulty talking about what most bothered her. She wished that the analyst could be able to understand her without her having to put her feelings into words, perhaps encouraged by the analyst's having understood and gratified her early wish for additional sessions without her having specifically asked for this. Her material also indicated that she wanted the analyst to be able to "fix" her without having to do any work herself.

Over the course of the treatment, it emerged through reconstruction that Camille's development had been significantly interrupted at age two and a half when her mother became pregnant with twins. Because of significant health issues which made pregnancy inadvisable (and which mother had known about prior to Camille's birth), mother was on bed rest during her pregnancy with Camille and again during her second pregnancy with twins. While she had enjoyed a close relationship with both parents previously, when mother became pregnant with the twins and had to spend significant amounts of time behind closed doors resting, this relationship with mother was replaced by an experience of loss and abandonment. During the analysis Camille uncovered two early memories, one of standing by her mother's bed, patting her mother while she slept, and another of standing by her mother's closed door, wishing she could enter.

As treatment progressed, Camille's anger toward her mother and twin sisters emerged, replacing earlier feelings of defectiveness and desires for self-harm. Camille later was able to express anger toward the analyst and others in her current life, eventually expanding to include nearly everyone except one or two prized friends at a time, with whom Camille would build a sort of latter day twinship.

Later in the treatment, Camille took to her own bed, in identification with mother, no longer feeling able to work. She wanted nothing more than to stay in bed, to read novels, and to watch television. Eventually, as she understood the origins of her depression and her intense anger toward mother and sisters (which she had previously turned against herself and then the analyst), her depression significantly improved, and she began to take better care of herself, exercising regularly, involving herself again in academic and professional activities, and renewing her interest in her family and social life. Her somatic complaints diminished and she sought medical treatment for those that remained.

Case 2: Psychodynamic Psychotherapy

Linda was a young graduate student who entered psychotherapy due to feelings of sadness and depression. While she felt loved by both parents, she often felt that her mother was critical of her and remembered feeling this way from earliest childhood. As the oldest of four girls, she felt that it was her job to please her mother and to be a role model for the younger children. She loved her father and had always found him to be warm and supportive. He was at work a great deal, however, and she had had less access to him growing up than she would have liked.

Over two years of treatment, Linda recognized her competitive and angry feelings toward her mother, seeing the hurt from mother's criticism as partially realistic and partly due to her own feeling of deserving punishment for her less conscious wish to criticize and hurt her mother. She was jealous of her younger siblings, jealous of the attention they received from her mother, and jealous of her mother's power over her father.

By virtue of the treatment, Linda was able to experience and express anger and sadness, and many sessions included Linda crying throughout. She felt attached to and intermittently dependent on the therapist, and worried that the therapist might become critical of her, like her mother had. As the therapist interpreted this transference, Linda became able to understand how mistrustful she had become of others and how this adversely affected her ability to engage in intimate relationships. Gradually she became less sad, more excited about her graduate work, and more aware of the possibility of being able to become closer to and to trust others. She also began to enjoy time with her family, feeling more supported and less criticized. When she felt ready to end her treatment after two years, she expressed her gratitude and her sadness at losing the opportunity to come to talk with the therapist. Several years later, in a chance encounter, Linda told the therapist she was happily married, was working in her chosen profession, and was planning to start a family.

RESEARCH ON PSYCHOANALYTIC AND PSYCHODYNAMIC TREATMENT OUTCOMES FOR DEPRESSION

There is a growing body of research on the efficacy of psychodynamic and psychoanalytic treatment of depression. Although it has been extremely difficult to design research paradigms for such lengthy and complex treatment, an increasing number of scientists are developing methodologies for studying both psychoanalytic and psychodynamic treatment outcomes and the mechanisms by which various treatment variables can help the depressed patient.

Initially, researchers looking at comparative differences between outcomes in psychodynamic and psychoanalytic treatment had to identify what makes these treatments different from others such as CBT or DBT. In their review of the comparative psychotherapy process literature, Blagys and Hilsenroth (2000) delineated seven interventions that distinguished psychodynamic and interpersonal therapy from CBT: (a) a focus on affect and the expression of patients' emotions; (b) an exploration of patients' attempts to avoid topics or engage in activities that hinder the progress of therapy; (c) the identification of patterns in patients' actions, thoughts, feelings, experiences, and relationships; (d) an emphasis on past experiences; (e) a focus on patients' interpersonal experiences; (f) an emphasis on the therapeutic relationship; and (g) an exploration of patients' wishes, dreams, or fantasies. Their conclusions were based in part on a study conducted by Ablon and Jones (1998, 2005), who asked 11 leading psychoanalytic theoreticians and practitioners to rate the 100 items of the Psychotherapy Process Q-Set (PQS; Jones et al.1988) with respect to how characteristic each item was of the principles and activities ideally found in psychodynamic/psychoanalytic therapies. Thus, they identified the distinctive features of psychodynamic/psychoanalytic techniques from both empirical and conceptual points of view, and laid the groundwork for further research in the differential outcomes of psychoanalytic versus other psychotherapies (Zimmerman et al. 2015).

Among others, Blatt (1990), Bastos (2015), Zimmerman (2015), and DeJonghe (2004, 2013) have studied the efficacy of the psychoanalytic treatment of depression. Bastos found that-long term psychodynamic psychotherapy, pharmacological treatment with fluoxetine, and their combination are effective in reducing symptoms of patients with moderate depression. Furthermore, he found that long-term psychodynamic psychotherapy and combined treatment were more effective compared to fluoxetine alone. These findings have implications for patients with depression who may benefit from long-term psychotherapy or combined treatment, or for depressed patients who do not wish to take medications such as fluoxetine.

Zimmerman et al. (2015) are responsible for one of the most significant of the recent studies looking at the efficacy of psychoanalytic treatment and psychodynamic treatment in major depression. They tested whether the long-term effects of psychoanalytic psychotherapy are mediated by the number of sessions and/or by the techniques used in psychoanalytic treatment, performing what they termed a quasi-experimental study comparing psychoanalytic therapy with psychodynamic therapy and CBT for depression. Subjects receiving psychoanalytic therapy reported having fewer interpersonal problems, treated themselves in a more caring fashion directly after treatment, and tended to improve in depressive symptoms and interpersonal problems during a three-year follow-up as compared with patients receiving psychodynamic therapy and/or CBT. Results of statistical analysis suggested that post-treatment differences in interpersonal problems and introject affiliation were mediated by the higher number of sessions, and follow-up differences in depressive symptoms were mediated by the more pronounced application of psychoanalytic techniques.

Specifically and significantly, Zimmerman et al. found that the effect on depressive symptoms and the sustained change following treatment were primarily driven by the therapist's exploration of the patient's fantasy life and discussions of the patient's early memories. In addition, there was some indication for a similar effect on the improvement of introject affiliation during follow-up. Again, significantly, they found that psychoanalytic therapy is effective in helping patients to reduce their interpersonal problems and improve their self-love during treatment. And most importantly, the Zimmerman study provides the first evidence that intensive psychodynamic treatments such as psychoanalytic therapy are effective not only because they are intensive but also because they are psychoanalytic (Zimmerman et al. 2015).

DeJonghe (2004, 2013) studied the efficacy of short-term supportive psychodynamic psychotherapy for depression. The results were aggregated in a mega-analysis and suggest that, in the treatment of outpatients with mild to moderate major depressive disorder, short-term psychodynamic psychotherapy and pharmacotherapy are equally efficacious and that the combination of short-term psychodynamic psychotherapy and pharmacotherapy is more efficacious than pharmacotherapy alone but not more than short-term psychodynamic psychotherapy alone. They therefore considered short-term psychodynamic psychotherapy a valuable extension to the existing options for the treatment of depressed patients (DeJonghe 2013).

Until 2013, the effectiveness of SPSP in ambulatory patients presenting a *DSM-IV* defined, mild to moderate major depressive disorder had been tested in five randomized clinical trials by DeJonghe and colleagues (DeJonghe et al. 2001, 2004; Dekker et al. 2005; Driessen et al. 2008; and Driessen et al., in DeJonghe 2013). A single research group conducted these five trials in similar but different study populations, using an identical research design, with each trial lasting six months. In the first three trials, patients were treated with SPSP, pharmacotherapy, or combined therapy, i.e., the combination of SPSP and pharmacotherapy. De Maat et al. (2007) performed a mega-analysis pooling the original data of three of these studies. The mega-analysis compared SPSP, pharmacotherapy, and combined therapy. Effectiveness was assessed by independent observers. As far as symptom reduction was concerned, the ratings of independent observers did not show differences between SPSP and pharmacotherapy. However, patient and therapist ratings did find differences in favor of SPSP. All three ratings consistently found differences favoring combined therapy over pharmacotherapy. Independent observers and therapists found no differences between combined therapy and SPSP but patients found combined therapy superior. As far as improvements in quality of life were concerned, patients found no differences between SPSP and pharmacotherapy. In several studies by DeJonghe and colleagues

(DeJonghe et al., 2001, 2004; Dekker et al. 2005; Driessen et al., in DeJonghe 2013), patients found combined short-term psychodynamic psychotherapy plus pharmacological intervention superior to pharmacotherapy alone. Kool et al. (in DeJonghe, 2013) demonstrated that the superior effectiveness of combined therapy over pharmacotherapy was found particularly in cases in which depression was combined with personality pathology.

In earlier research, Sydney Blatt looked at introjective versus anaclitic depression, and reported that a number of research procedures (Blatt, D'Afflitti, and Quinlan 1976; Beck et al. 1979; Robins and Ladd 1994; Robins and Luten 1991; Weissman and Beck 1978) had been developed to systematically assess two sets of depressive experiences: (1) a set of depressive feelings that derive from disruptions of interpersonal relations, including feelings of loss, abandonment, helplessness, and loneliness; wanting to be close to, related to, and dependent on others; and being concerned about hurting or offending others for fear of losing the dependent gratification others can provide (which he called anaclytic depression); and (2) another set of depressive experiences that are more internally directed and focused on disruptions of self-definition and self-esteem, and that are expressed in concern about feeling guilty, empty, hopeless, unsatisfied, insecure, self-critical, ambivalent about oneself and others, and lacking in a sense of autonomy and self-worth; about having failed to meet expectations and standards; and about feeling pressured by responsibilities and threatened by change (which he called introjective depression).

The differentiation of these two types of depression led to extensive empirical investigation of the developmental origins, personality characteristics, and aspects of contemporary life situations that characterize these two types of depression in both outpatients and inpatients (for reviews of this research literature, see Blatt and Homann [1992]; Blatt and Zuroff [1992]). Thus, we now understand more fully some of the early and current life experiences that contribute to the development of these two types of depression. We also better understand the functioning of these individuals, both when clinically depressed and in remission, and appreciate more fully the differential vulnerability of each of these two types of depressed individual to various types of stressful life experiences (Blatt and Homann 1992; Blatt and Zuroff 1992]).

The elaboration of a depression associated with themes of loss and abandonment identifies a type of depression overlooked in most studies. These anaclitically depressed individuals often express their depression in somatic complaints, frequently seeking the care and concern of others, including physicians. Depression in these patients is often precipitated by the loss of loved ones, and these individuals may make suicidal gestures by overdosing on prescribed antidepressant medication (Blatt et al. 1982). Research derived from these psychoanalytic observations and formulations illustrate the finding that a self-critical or introjective depression (focused on issues of self-worth, self-esteem, failure, and guilt) is particularly insidious. Individuals who are highly self-critical and feel guilty and worthless are at considerable risk for serious suicide attempts (Beck 1979; Blatt 1974, 1995; Blatt et al. 1982). Powerful needs to succeed, and to avoid public criticism, force some individuals to lives of grinding work in order to achieve. However, according to Blatt, they are always profoundly vulnerable to the criticism of others and to their own self-scrutiny and judgment. In 1995, he said, "[a] harsh punitive superego (Freud 1914, 1923) can be a driving force for achievement, but it can also result in little satisfaction in accomplishments, and through a marked vulnerability to experiences of failure and criticism, in an increased susceptibility to ensuing depression and suicide. Because of the need to maintain a personal and public image of strength and perfection, such individuals are constantly trying to prove themselves, are always on trial, feel vulnerable to any possible implication of failure or criticism, and often are unable to turn to others, even the closest of confidants, for help or to share their anguish" (Blatt 1995, p. 1005). As a result such individuals are vulnerable to intense depression accompanied by suicidal impulses.

GENERAL OUTCOME RESEARCH IN THE TREATMENT OF ADULT DEPRESSION

It is perhaps useful to include a note on outcome research in the treatment of depression in general. In an overview of meta-analysis of outcome research performed over the past four decades, Pim Cuijpers (2008) came up with a variety of interesting findings. First, he said that outcome research in the treatment of depression is problematic. Due to typically small study size and other factors, smaller differences (effect sizes) are hard or impossible to find and interpret due to a lack of statistical power. This brings into question the plethora of recent research preferring one treatment type over another and especially calling certain therapies "evidence based" as compared with other types of psychotherapy.

In his article Cuijpers presented an overview of a series of meta-analyses conducted on the 500 randomized trials that have examined the effects of psychological treatments of adult depression. He saw that several of these interventions have been tested and found to be effective in the treatment of depression. Furthermore, he stated that there are no significant differences between treatments and that effects last for six to twelve months (although it must be noted that generally longer-term outcomes were not measured). He also saw that these therapies are about equally effective as pharmacotherapy in the short-term, and that the combination of psychotherapy and antidepressants is significantly more effective than either of these alone. Therapies are also effective in specific target groups, such as older adults, college students, women with postpartum depression, and patients with general medical disorders. These therapies may be somewhat less effective in chronic depression, and in patients with comorbid substance use disorders. He found that treatments are effective when delivered in individual, group, and guided self-help format. They are less effective when delivered without any kind of human support, i.e., when the intervention is computer based rather than therapist led. He also found that the effects of some psychotherapies have been overestimated due to of the low quality of many trials as well as publication bias.

Moreover, a meta-analysis of outcome research has shown that there is a strong association between the number of sessions per week and the effect size, with a notable improvement being shown in adult patients with depression seen twice per week over once per week. Additionally, evidence was found that while psychotherapy and pharmacotherapy have approximately equal effect size, the positive effects of psychotherapy may last longer than those of pharmacotherapy. Also, individual treatment was shown to be more effective than group treatment and the dropout rate was smaller in individual treatment than in group treatment (Cuijpers 2008).

As a direction for future research, Cuijpers suggested that new psychotherapies for depression are not necessarily more effective than current therapies. He found that now existing therapies appeared to be as effective in the treatment of depression as newly developed treatments. He also suggested that it is not necessary to test treatment formats and therapies in specific populations, because the evidence indicates that all formats with human involvement are effective in all specific target groups. Instead, he recommended that a focus on a reduction of the disease burden of depression should be the starting point for new research. According to Cuijpers, promising areas include research on preventing the onset of depressive disorders, treatments of chronic and treatment-resistant depression, relapse prevention, and scaling up treatments for example by using more guided self-help interventions and training lay counselors in delivering interventions in low-resource settings. Despite the limitations of his study, Cuijpers felt that he could conclude that psychotherapies are essential tools in the treatment of adult depression.

CHILDHOOD AND ADOLESCENT DEPRESSION

Prevalence of Depression in Childhood and Adolescence

Until the 1970s depression was considered uncommon in children, and depression in adolescents was considered a normal developmental phenomenon (Bhardwaj and Goodyer 2009). As mentioned above, it was not until studies were performed in the late 1970s and 1980s that it was shown that adolescents suffer from depression in a similar way to adults (Pearce 1997; Puig-

Antich, in Bhardwaj and Goodyer 2009). Current estimates suggest that one in five adolescents suffer from an episode of depression (Lewisohn, Rohde, and Seeley, in Bhardwaj and Goodyer 2009).

Children who are diagnosed with depression may present somewhat differently than adolescents and adults. Sadness may be replaced by boredom and irritability, separation anxiety, phobias, and somatic concerns. However, it must be noted that sadness may also be present and persistent. Adolescents may also appear more irritable rather than sad, or oppositional and defiant, leading not uncommonly to diagnostic errors, particularly by less well trained professionals such as teachers and school counselors. Adolescents who are depressed may also experience trouble with concentration, anhedonia, and withdrawal from social activities and peers in general. Suicidal thinking is not uncommon and the risk of suicide is heightened by the generally more impulsive nature of adolescents.

Depressive symptoms are prevalent in children and adolescents with 10–15 percent of seven- to seventeen-year-olds reporting clinically significant levels of depression (Bettage et al. 2008, in Weitkamp 2014). Less than 50 percent of children and adolescents experiencing depression are reported to receive any kind of treatment by age eighteen (Kessler, Venevoli, and Merkangal 2001, in Weitkamp 2014).

RESEARCH IN THE PSYCHOANALYTIC TREATMENT OF CHILD AND ADOLESCENT DEPRESSION

The first methodologically sound study on the efficacy of psychoanalytic therapy for young patients with depression compared twenty-five sessions of psychoanalytic psychotherapy with a wait-list control group (Horn et al. 2005, in Weitkamp 2014). Impairment was significantly reduced with a large effect size. Twenty percent of the patients in the intervention group showed a clinically significant change, compared with no patient in the wait-list control group. Although treatment was helpful for some of the depressed patients, the authors concluded that a number of their patients needed longer or more intense treatment. Another randomized controlled trial compared focused psychoanalytic psychotherapy and systems integrative family therapy for childhood depression in nine- to fifteen-year-olds (Trowell et al. 2007, in Weitkamp 2014). The psychoanalytic psychotherapy group received sixteen to thirty sessions plus parent sessions over a nine-month period. At the end of the treatment, 74.3 percent of patients in the psychoanalytic psychotherapy group were no longer clinically depressed. Six months after treatment had ended, 100 percent of cases were no longer clinically depressed compared with 75.7 percent at the end of therapy and 81 percent at six-month follow-up in the systemic family therapy group. This study provided evidence for the efficacy of focused short-term psychoanalytic treatment under controlled conditions.

Weitkamp et al. (2014) conducted a study to further the understanding of the efficacy of psychoanalytic treatment for depression in children and adolescents. In Germany, where the study was conducted, treatment is usually longer in duration, with a maximum of 180 sessions for adolescents and 150 sessions for children reimbursed by the German health insurance companies. The aim of the study was to evaluate psychoanalytic psychotherapies as they are delivered in the naturalistic health care system in Germany, and to extend the findings by Horn et al. and Trowell et al. The results provide evidence that psychoanalytic therapy can significantly reduce target symptoms and increase quality of life for depressed children and adolescents. During the wait-list interval (with minimal treatment), no such significant symptom reduction occurred. The symptom reduction of the intervention group was in the range of moderate to large effect sizes. The patients and the parents in the study both reported a significant improvement. These findings are in contrast to the small to medium effect sizes of CBT and interpersonal therapy for depressive disorders in children and adolescents (Bachmann et al. 2008). The Horn study yielded a clinically significant and reliable change rate of 20 percent for depressed patients treated with twenty-five sessions of psychoanalytic therapy (Horn et al. in Weitkamp 2014). This discrepancy might be due to the longer treatment duration in our sample, with an average duration of twenty-four months (on average ninety-six sessions). In that study, a significant number of patients needed longer treatment than twenty-five sessions. The current data seem to suggest that longer duration of therapy leads to a higher number of significantly improved children and adolescents.

PSYCHODYNAMICS AND TREATMENT OF CHILDHOOD AND ADOLESCENT DEPRESSION

The child with mild to moderate depression is often described by parents as being either low energy, seeming sad and less interested in friends and activities than previously, or as irritable. Parents often report regression in the most recently acquired developmental milestones, difficulty falling asleep and staying asleep, and either an increase or a decrease in appetite and willingness to eat. However, as with all disorders of childhood, individual children present differently and it is up to the clinician to discern whether depression is present based on attaining an extensive developmental history and history of the current problem. Projective psychological testing can be helpful in obtaining a diagnosis of depression in children, even those who do not present with typical symptomatology, when themes of sadness, hopelessness, morbidity and death appear on the Rorschach, Thematic Apperception Test, or House Tree Person Test.

Children presenting with more severe depression may actually look sad, speak about sad topics, and be actively or passively suicidal. Sleep and eating disturbances may be pronounced and the child may or may not be willing to talk with the therapist about their sadness.

For children from the ages of two to twelve or thirteen psychoanalytic play therapy or child analysis is indicated. Through play therapy, a multiplicity of themes may become clear. The child may demonstrate feelings of loss, feelings of being unloved or abandoned, competitive feelings with siblings or parents, feelings of having been replaced by younger siblings, feelings of being less loved or taken care of than siblings, feelings of being unlovable, defective, or bad. The child will often demonstrate these themes and affects using fantasy play with or without including the analyst/therapist. He/she may also illustrate these feelings in artistic productions including drawings, sculptures, Lego productions, etc.

CASE EXAMPLES

Case 1

Bennie was a two-and-a-half-year-old child when he presented for evaluation. His mother was a graduate student who had recently separated from his father. Bennie's mother reported that he was extremely bright, even precocious in some ways, but that he seemed sad and frightened at times. He had watched a Disney video in which a bear showed its teeth and attempted to attack a hunter; this had badly frightened him and he had started to express concerns over leaving the house, meeting dogs on the street, and the like. Mother also wondered what effect her separation from Bennie's father would have on him and she wanted to do her best to help him to develop in a healthy fashion. She went on to say that Bennie was in daycare, spending eight hours a day there five days a week.

Bennie presented as a tentative little toddler, small and inhibited for his age. He looked sad with large dark circles under his eyes and he was noted to glance at his mother frequently, vigilant as to her mood and approval or disapproval of his activities. Initially, he was shy with the analyst, sitting in his mother's lap while she spoke. We talked about Bennie in his presence, mentioning his Daddy and how his Daddy was gone so much now. The analyst talked "for" Bennie, saying how sad this must make him. Mother added that she too was sad sometimes and cried in front of Bennie, saying that she knew this must make him sad too.

After the first session, Bennie began to play in the therapist's office. Interestingly, one of the first things he did was to get out the therapist's collection of play jewelry, to spill it on the floor, running his fingers through it and saying, "I want to be like the other kind of doctor!" Mother and I laughed and wondered if he might be talking about mother's psychoanalyst, whom he had met once or twice and who mother had described as "another kind of doctor, not the kind that examines you and gives you shots."

Bennie was clearly a boy at the beginning of the oedipal period. He longed to be the doctor who got his mother's attention, who mother talked about to him. He imagined this "other kind of doctor" possessing gold and jewels . . . while he was just a tiny little boy. He missed his mother during his long days at daycare and had both the normal developmental need for more time with her alongside his powerful oedipal wishes to have her all to himself.

One of the first interventions made by the analyst was to recommend that mother alter her schedule of classes and teaching so that she could spend more time with Bennie. She did so almost immediately. Secondly, an analysis was recommended. Bennie was a sad, inhibited little boy. Mother had supplied the information that while he cried frequently, Bennie had had very few temper tantrums. He seemed conflicted about his aggression, wanting so much to please mother and to insure that she not leave him that he inhibited his age appropriate anger and desires for omnipotent control and autonomy.

Over the course of two years of four times weekly child analysis, Bennie became outspoken, aggressive and assertive. He went through a period of frequent explosions of rage in the office, expressing his anger with mother, father, and with the analyst, especially around any limitations that were imposed on his play. After one such session he returned the next time singing at top volume, "This little light of mine, I'm going to let it shine. . . ." clearly reveling in his newfound ability to demonstrate his anger.

It became clear that this small boy had indeed inhibited vast amounts of rage. The bear's teeth in the Disney film were *his* teeth, and the bear's attack on the hunter was the attack he wished to make on father for leaving him, on mother for leaving him, on mother's analyst for possessing her (in his mind) and on his analyst for limiting his self-expression (e.g., when he wanted to splash water and soap bubbles all over the office).

After a several-year period, analysis was replaced by psychoanalytic psychotherapy twice weekly and then once weekly, finally ending reluctantly when mother received an academic position in another state. By this time Bennie was a straight A student and a less anxious and more vociferous child.

Case 2

Dana was an eleven-year-old girl who presented at a community mental health center for what her mother termed "a change in behavior." Dana's mother reported that she had been such a good girl up until six months ago, attaining the highest grades in the most difficult classes at her parochial school. Suddenly, according to mother, Dana had started to behave "badly," getting poor grades and refusing to help around the house with the younger children. Dana's father had died some years before and mother reported that Dana had barely reacted to his death.

In the first evaluatory session Dana made a drawing of a house with a rainbow-colored heart over it and a bolt of lightning going through the heart. The drawing Dana made and her associations to it were extremely informative. Dana filled in the detail that her mother had left out. Dana had to move from the house in which she had lived with her father, who had committed suicide there. It seemed to the therapist that the house was a link to the father, and that with its loss Dana's long-delayed mourning began, which then led to a depressive episode. Dana's heart was broken (just as she had described the heart in the drawing); her old house was gone, the place where she had last been with her father, and where, it turns out, he had killed himself, was gone. She had defensively denied sad feelings associated with the loss of her father until the move awakened her deep feelings. Dana's mother had not understood Dana's "change in behavior" or the underlying feelings which had caused the change. Moreover, she has classified her daughter as "bad" for studying less and helping around the house less. The link between the move and the loss of Dana's father had indeed been lost on the mother.

Psychodynamic psychotherapy was recommended for Dana, accompanied by monthly parental sessions to help mother better understand her daughter's feelings. Dana was a very bright girl who was well suited to insight-oriented treatment and able to make use of the therapist's comments. As an eleven-year-old, Dana did not engage in the kind of play that younger children might initiate with the dollhouse or other toys in the office, but she was interested in doing artwork and was capable of talking about her productions. She was able to understand the underlying meaning of her artwork with the therapist's help and over time, to work through her grief, mourning, and depression.

CONCLUSION AND IMPLICATIONS FOR PSYCHOANALYTIC TREATMENT

Childhood adversities including early narcissistic injury, parental neglect, disappointment in parental care, complex dysfunction in the infant-parent relationship and sexual abuse increase both childhood and adult vulnerability to depression. This probably occurs through effects on the concepts of self and other, formation of the ego, id, superego, and ego ideal, the establishment of emotional regulation, object relationships, cognitions, and neurophysiology. The extent, and perhaps the nature, of the effects differ depending on a multiplicity of factors including inborn temperament, environmental circumstances and influences, genetics and their interaction with experience (epigenetics), goodness of fit with parental temperament and practices, and the like. In other words, depression is a disorder that has complex origins and may be arrived along multiple pathways. As such, the highly individualized nature of psychodynamic psychotherapy and psychoanalysis continue to be well suited to the treatment of depressive symptomatology, often in combination with psychopharmacological intervention.

REFERENCES

Ablon, J. S., and Jones, E. E. (1998). How expert clinicians' proto-types of an ideal treatment correlate with outcome in psycho-dynamic and cognitive–behavior therapy. *Psychotherapy Research*, 8, 71–83.

———. (2002). Validity of controlled clinical trials of psychotherapy: Findings from the NIMH Treatment of Depression Collaborative Research Program. *American Journal of Psychiatry*, 159, 775–783.

———. (2005). On analytic process. *Journal of the American Psychoanalytic Association*, 53, 541–568.

Abraham, K. (1911). Notes on the psychoanalytical investigation and treatment of manic-depressive insanity and allied conditions. In *Selected Papers on Psychoanalysis*. London: Hogarth Press.

———. (1924). A short study of the development of the libido, viewed in the light of mental disorders. In *Selected Papers on Psychoanalysis*. London: Hogarth Press.

American Psychiatric Association (2013). *Diagnostic and Statistical Manual of Mental Disorders, Fifth Edition.* Washington, DC, and London: American Psychiatric Publishing.

Arieti, S. and Bemporad, J. R. (1978). *Severe and Mild Depression.* Basic Books: New York.

Bachmann, M., Bachmann, C., Rief, W., and Mattejat, F. (2008). Efficacy of psychiatric and psychotherapeutic interventions in children and adolescents with psychiatric disorders—a systematic evaluation of meta-analyses and reviews. Part I: Anxiety disorders and depressive disorders. *Zeitschrift fur Kinder- und Jugendpsychiatric und Psychotherapyie*, 36, 309–320.

Bhardwaj, A. and Goodyer, I. (2009). Depression and allied illness in children and adolescents: Basic facts. *Psychoanalytic Psychotherapy*, 23(3), 176–184.

Bastos, A. et al. (2015). The efficacy of long-term psychodynamic psychotherapy, fluoxetine and their combination in the outpatient treatment of depression. *Psychotherapy Research*, 25(5), 612–624.

Beck, A. T., Rush, A. J., Shaw B. F., and Emery G. (1979) *Cognitive Theory of Depression.* New York: Guilford Press.

Bibring, E. (1953). The mechanism of depression. In Greenacre, P. (Ed.), *Affective Disorders: Psychoanalytic Contributions to Their Study* (pp. 13–48). New York: International Universities Press.

Bifulco, T. O., Brown, T., and Harris, T. (1987). Childhood loss of parent, lack of adequate parental care and adult depression: A replication. *Journal of Affective Disorders* 12, 115–128.

Blagys, M. D. and Hilsenroth, M. J. (2000). Distinctive feature of short-term psychodynamic–interpersonal psychotherapy: A review of the comparative psychotherapy process literature. *Clinical Psychology: Science and Practice*, 7, 167–188.

Blatt, S. J. (1974). Levels of object representation in anaclitic and introjective depression. *Psychoanalytic Study of the Child*, 29, 107–157.

———. (1990). Interpersonal relatedness and self-definition: Two personality configurations and their implications for psychopathology and psychotherapy. In J. L. Singer (Ed.), *Repression and Dissociation: Implications for Personality Theory, Psychopathology and Health* (1995). (pp. 299–335). Chicago: University of Chicago Press.

———. (1995). The destructiveness of perfectionism: Implications for the treatment of depression. *American Psychologist*, 50(12), 1003–1020.

Blatt, S. J. and Blass, R. B. (1990). Attachment and separateness: A dialectic model of the products and processes of psychological development. *Psychoanalytic Study of the Child*, 45, 107–127.

Blatt, S. J., D'Afflitti, J. P., and Quinlan, D. M. (1976). Experiences of depression in normal young adults. *Journal of Abnormal Psychology*, 85, 383–389.

Blatt, S. J. and Homann, E. (1992). Parent-childinteractioni nthe etiology of dependent and self-critical depression. *Clinical Psychology Review*, 12(1), 47–91.

Blatt, S. J., Quinlan, D. M., and Chevron, E. (1990). Empirical investigations of a psychoanalytic theory of depression. In J. Masling (Ed.), (2017). *Empirical Studies of Psychoanalytic Theories: Volume 3* (pp. 89–147). Hillsdale, NJ: Analytic Press.

Blatt, S. J., Quinlan, D. M., Chevron, E. McDonald, C., and Zuroff, D. (1982). Dependency and self-criticism: Psychological dimensions of depression. *Journal of Consulting and Clinical Psychology*, 50, 113–124.

Blatt, S. J. and Zuroff, D. C. (1992). Interpersonal relatedness and self-definition: Two prototypes for depression. *Clinical Psychology Review*, 12(5), 527–562.

Bowlby, J. (1980). *Attachment and Loss, Vol 3: Loss*. New York: Basic Books.

———. (1988). *A Secure Base: Clinical Applications of Attachment Theory*. London: Routledge & Kegan Paul.

Brenner, C. (1975). Affects and psychic conflict. *Psychoanalytic Quarterly*, 44, 1–28.

———. (1979). Depressive affect, anxiety and psychic conflict in the phallic-oedipal phase. *Psychoanalytic Quarterly*, 48, 177–197.

Brown, T. O. and Harris, T. O. (1978). *Social Origins of Depression: A Study of Psychiatric Disorder in Women.* London: Tavistock.

Brown, C., Harris, C., and Hepworth, C. (1995). Loss, humiliation and entrapment among women developing depression: A patient and non-patient comparison. *Psychological Medicine*, 25, 7–21.

Busch, F., Rudden, M., and Shapiro, T. (2004). *Psychodynamic Treatment of Depression.* Washington and London: American Psychiatric Press.

Caspi, A., Sugden, K., Moffitt, T. E., Taylor, A., Craig, I. W., Harrington, H., McClay, J., Mill, J., Martin, J., Braithwaite, A., and Poulton, R. (2003). Influence of life stress on depression: Moderation by a polymorphism in the 5-HTT gene. *Science*, 301, 386–389.

Cole, J., McGuffin, P., and Farmer, A. E. (2008). Editorial. The classification of depression: Are we still confused? *British Journal of Psychiatry*, 192, 83–85.

Cuijpers, P., van Straten, A., Andersson, G., and van Oppen, P. (2008). Psychotherapy for depression in adults: A meta-analysis of comparative outcome studies. *Journal of Consulting and Clinical Psychology*, 76, 909–922.

DeJonghe, F. et al. (2013). Short term psychoanalytic supportive psychotherapy for depressed patients. *Psychoanalytic Inquiry*, 33, 614–625.

DeJonghe, F., Kool, S., van Aalst, G., Dekker, J., and Peen, J. (2001) Combining psychotherapy and antidepressants in the treatment of depression. *Journal of Affective Disorders*, 64, 217–229.

DeJonghe, F., Hendrickson, M., van Aalst, G., Kool, S., Peen,V., Van, R., van den Eijnden,E., and Dekker, J. (2004). Psychotherapy alone and combined with pharmacotherapy in the treatment of depression. *British Journal of Psychiatry*, 185, 37–45.

Dekker, J., Molenaar, P. J., Kool, S., van Aalst, G., Peen, J., and DeJonghe, F. (2005). Dose–effect relations in time-limited combined psycho-pharmacological treatment for depression. *Psychological Medicine: A Journal of Research in Psychiatry and the Allied Sciences*, 35, 47–58.

de Maat, S., Dekker, J. et al. (2007). Relative efficacy of psychotherapy and combined treatment in the treatment of depression: a meta-analysis. *European Psychiatry*, 22(1), 1–18.

Driessen, E., Cuijpers, P., de Maat, S. C., Abbass, A. A., Jonghe, F. de, and Dekker, J. J. (2010). The efficacy of short-term psychodynamic psychotherapy for depression: A meta-analysis. *Clinical Psychology Review*, 30, 25–36.

Farmer, A. E., and McGuffin, P. (2003). Humiliation, loss and other types of life events and difficulties: A comparison of depressed subjects, healthy controls and their siblings. *Psychological Medicine*, 33(7), 1169-1175.

Fergusson, D. M., Horwood, L. J., and Lynskey, M. T. (1996). Childhood sexual abuse and psychiatric disorder in young adulthood II: Psychiatric outcomes of childhood sexual abuse. *Journal of the American Academy of Child and Adolescent Psychiatry*, 35(10), 1365–1374.

Freud, S. (1917). "Mourning and Melancholia." In Strachey, J. (Ed.), *The Standard Edition of the Complete Psychological Works of Sigmund Freud, Vol. XIV (1914–1916)* (pp. 237–258). London: Hogarth Press and the Institute for Psycho-Analysis.

Furman, E. (1974). *A Child's Parent Dies: Studies in Childhood Bereavement*. New York and London: Yale University Press.

Harris, B. and Barraclough, B. (1998). Excess mortality of mental disorder. *British Journal of Psychiatry*, 173, 11–53.

Harris, T. (2001). Recent developments in understanding the psychosocial aspects of depression. *British Medical Bulletin,* 57, 17–32.

Hill, J. (2009). Developmental perspectives on adult depression. *Psychoanalytic Psychotherapy*, 23(3), 200–212.

Jacobson, E. (1954). Transference problems in the psychoanalytic treatment of severely depressed patients. *Journal of the American Psychoanalytic Association*, 2, 695–705.

———. (1971). *Comparative Studies of Normal, Neurotic and Psychotic Conditions*. New York: International Universities Press.

———. (1975). The psychoanalytic treatment of depressed patients. In Anthony, B., Benedek, T. (Eds.). *Depression and Human Existence*. Boston: Little Brown.

Jones, E. E., Cumming, J. D., and Horowitz, M. J. (1988). Another look at the nonspecific hypothesis of therapeutic effectiveness. *Journal of Consulting and Clinical Psychology*, 56, 48–55.

Kendall, P. A., Sheldrick, R. (2000). Normative data for normative comparisons. *Journal of Consulting and Clinical Psychology*, 68, 767–773.

Kendler, K. S., Kuhn, J. W., Prescott, C. A. (2004). Childhood sexual abuse, stressful life events and risk for major depression in women. *Psychological Medicine*, 34(8), 1475–1482.

Kendell, R. E.(1976). The classificataion of depressions: A review of contemporary confusion. *British Journal of Psychiatry*, 129, 15–28.

Klein, M. (1935). A Contribution to the psychogenesis of manic-depressive states. In *Love, Guilt and Reparation and Other Papers* (pp. 1921–1946). London: Hogarth Press.

Kohut, H. (1971). *The Analysis of the Self.* New York: International Universities Press.

Luborsky, L. (1984). *Principles of Psychoanalytic Psychotherapy: A Manual for Supportive-Expressive (SE) Treatment.* New York: Basic Books.

———. (2000). Psychoanalytic therapies. In A. F. Kazdin (Ed.). *Encyclopedia of Psychology*, Washington, DC: American Psychological Association.

———. (in preparation). A challenge: Empirical psychoanalytic research should be welcomed into the training of more psychoanalysts.

Luborsky, L., Diguer, L., Luborsky, E. and Schmidt, K. A. (1999a). The efficacy of dynamic and other psychotherapies: Is it true that "Everyone has won and all must have prizes"?—An update. In Janowsky, D. (Ed.), *Psychotherapy in the 1990s Indications and Outcomes* (pp. 3–22). Washington, DC: American Psychiatric Press.

Luborsky, L., Diguer, L., Luborsky, E., Singer, B. and Dickter, D. (1993). The efficacy of dynamic psychotherapies: Is it true that "Everyone has won so all shall have prizes"? In N. Miller, L. Luborsky, J. P. Barber, and J. Docherty. (Eds.), *Psychodynamic Treatment Research: A Handbook for Clinical Practice* (pp. 447–514). New York: Basic Books.

Luborsky, L., Diguer, L., Seligman, D. A., Rosenthal, R., Krause, E. D., Johnson, S., Halperin, G., Bishop, M., Berman, J., and Schweizer, E. (1999b). The researcher's own therapy allegiances: A "wild card" in comparisons of treatment efficacy. *Clinical Psychology: Science and Practice*, 6, 95–106.

Luborsky, L., Rosenthal, R., Andrusyna, T., Berman, J., and Shapiro, D. (in preparation). Recommendations for minimizing researchers' allegiance problems in comparisons of psychotherapies.

Luborsky, L., Rosenthal, R., Diguer, L., Andrusyna, T. P., Leavitt, J., Seligman, D. A., Berman, J. S., and Krause, E. D. (2001). The dodo bird verdict is alive and well—mostly. *Clinical Psychology: Science and Practice*, 6, 95–106.

Luborsky, L., Singer, B., and Luborsky, L. (1975). Comparative studies of psychotherapies: Is it true that "Everyone has won and all must have prizes"? *Archives of General Psychiatry*, 32, 995–1008.

Luborsky, L., Stuart, J., Friedman, S., Seligman, D. A., Bucci, W., Pulver, S., Woody, G., Davison, W. S., Krause, E. D., Ermold, J., and Mergenthaler, E. (2001). A collection of complete and tape-recorded psychoanalyses as a research resource: The Penn Psychoanalytic Treatment Collection. *Journal of the American Psychoanalytic Association*, 49, 217–234.

McQueen, D. M. (2009). Depression in adults: some basic facts. *Psychoanalytic Psychotherapy*, 23(3), 200–212.

Mullen, P. E., Martin, J. L., Anderson, J. C., Romans, S. E., and Herbison, G. P. (1993). Childhood sexual abuse and mental health in adult life. *British Journal of Psychiatry*, 163, 721–732.

Nelson, E. C., Heath, A. C., Madden, P. A. F. et al (2002). Association between self-reported childhood sexual abuse and adverse psychosocial outcomes: Results from a twin study. *Archives of General Psychiatry*, 59(2), 139-145.

PDM Taskforce. (2006). *Psychodynamic Diagnostic Manual.* Silver Spring, MD: Alliance of Psychoanalytic Organizations.

Pearce, J. B. (1977) Depressive disorder in childhood. *The Journal of Child Psychology and Psychiatry*, 18, 79–82.

Rado, Sandor (1928). The problem of melancholia. *International Journal of Psychoanalysis*, 9, 420–438.

Robertson, J. and Robertson, J. (1971). Young children in brief separations: A fresh look. *Psychoanalytic Study of the Child*, 26, 264–315.

Robins, C. J., Ladd, J., Welkowitz, J., Blaney, P. H., Diaz, R., and Kutcher, G. (1994) The personal style inventory: Preliminary validation studies of new measures of sociotropy and autonomy. *Journal of Psychopathology and Behavioral Assessment*, 16(4), 277–300.

Robins, C. J., and Luten, A. G. (1991). Sociotropy and autonomy: Differential patterns of clinical presentation in unipolar depression. *Journal of Abnormal Psychology*, I, 100(1), 74–7.

Rudden, M., Busch, F., Milrod, B. et al. (2003). Panic disorder and depression: a psychodynamic exploration of comorbidity. *International Journal of Psychoanalysis*, 84, 997–1015.

Seligman, M. E. P. (1975). *Helplessness: On Depression, Development and Death.* San Francisco: Witt, Freeman.

Short, A. K., Fennell, K. A., Perreau, V. M., Fox, A., O'Bryan, M. K., Kim, J. H., Bredy, T. W., Pang, T. Y., and Hannan, A. J. (2016). Elevated paternal glucocorticoid exposure alters the small noncoding RNA profile in sperm and modifies anxiety and depressive phenotypes in the offspring. *Translational Psychiatry*, 6(6), e837. PMC 4031607.

Spitz, R. A. (1965). *The First Year of Life*. New York: International Universities Press.

Stone, L. (1986). Psychoanalytic observations on the pathology of depressive illness: selected spheres of ambiguity and disagreement. *Journal of the American Psychoanalytic Association*, 34, 329–362.

Weitkamp, K., Daniels, J. K., Hofmann, H., Timmermann, H., Romer, G., and Wiegand-Grefe, S. (2014). Psychoanalytic Psychotherapy for children and adolescents with severe depressive psychopathology: Preliminary results of an effectiveness trial. *Psychotherapy*, 51(1), 138–147.

Zimmermann, J., et al. (2015). Is it all about the higher dose? Why psychoanalytic therapy is an effective treatment for major depression. *Clinical Psychology and Psychotherapy*, 22(6), 469–487.

Chapter Nine

The Dissociative Disorders

Richard P. Kluft

Clinical encounters with the complex array of psychological and somatoform dissociative symptoms presented by distressed individuals, especially those suffering Dissociative Identity Disorder (DID), afford the analyst of today an unparalleled opportunity to walk in the shoes of Sigmund Freud, Josef Breuer, Jean-Martin Charcot, and Pierre Janet. The phenomena that informed and inspired the *Studies on Hysteria* (Breuer & Freud 1893–1895), the foundation of what would become psychoanalysis, come alive in the consulting room, as puzzling and challenging to contemporary clinicians as they were to our fin de siècle counterparts.

It is often said that psychoanalysis began with the study of Anna O. In the *Studies on Hysteria* (Breuer & Freud 1893–1985) Freud speculated that a larval form of DID might be found in every hysteric. Years later, members of Freud's circle would refer to Anna O as Freud's "Miss Beauchamps," drawing analogies between Anna O and the famous DID patient treated by Morton Prince (Jones 1953).

Freud repudiated hypnosis and denied dissociation a central role in his developing formulations. Descriptive/organic psychiatry rose in prominence. Behaviorism came upon the scene. As these approaches attracted adherents, in slightly more than a generation both the grand hysterias and the hypnotic approaches used to treat them became marginalized and displaced from the mainstream. Conflict and repression made no room for dissociation, organic/descriptive psychiatry subsumed DID under the rubric of the new diagnosis of schizophrenia (Rosenbaum 1980), and behaviorism was dismissive of intrapsychic concerns (see Kluft, in press 2018a, in press 2018b).

Mainstream psychoanalysis generally regards Freud's repudiation of hypnosis and his development of a psychology based on the unconscious, conflict, and the analysis of defense and transference as advances, replacing older approaches and understandings with a superior understanding of the mind and a much more effective approach to therapy. Freud's arguments against hypnosis were compromised by understandable era-related limitations of knowledge and his own competitiveness, both as a person and as an advocate for his ideas. At times he distorted and bent facts to suit his arguments (see Breger 2009; Kluft, in press 2018a, in press 2018b; Makari 2008).

Within psychoanalysis, Freud's attitudes toward dissociation and DID have proven profoundly problematic. Berman (1981), Brenner (2009), and Kluft (in press 2018b) ascribe Freud's aversion to these topics in part to his own dissociative symptomatology. Kluft (in press 2018b) adds that by ascribing dissociative symptoms to a failure to maintain mental strength and cohesion, Janet voiced a theoretical stance that may have struck a defensive cord in Freud, and provoked a hostile response.

Indeed Freud's new paradigm brought new insights and advances, but in a manner that repudiated rather than encompassed preexisting relevant clinical findings and clinical experience. Recent efforts to address the psychoanalysis/hypnosis schism (see Brenner 2001, 2004, 2018; Kluft 1995a, 2000, 2018, in press 2018c; O'Neil 2018) have been mounted by dissociation-savvy psychoanalysts appreciative that work with that phenomenon and those conditions are best approached by reclaiming for psychoanalysis much of what Freud once cast aside.

This review will discuss psychoanalytic perspectives on the dissociative disorder through the lens of DID and related disorders. Dissociative amnesia, derealization, and many forms of depersonalization associated with high hypnotizability are commonly encountered as symptoms, but rarely present as autonomous conditions in the analytic context. In contrast, DID is increasingly identified by psychoanalytic clinicians, and its treatment often presents unanticipated and unfamiliar difficulties. The management of most other dissociative phenomena can be inferred from successful approaches to DID.

CONTEXTUALIZING DID

Conditions in which one or more entities recurrently take control of the mind are anthropological commonplaces (Bourgignon 1991). In the context of rituals and/or ceremonies endemic to a culture, they do not represent mental illnesses. Arising outside of such contexts and causing distress and dysfunction, if the entities involved are understood to be ancestors or supernatural entities accepted within the patient's culture and religion, they are described as possession syndromes. In more secular cultures, the entities may or may not refer to supernatural entities or deceased relatives. More commonly, they represent more or less evident identifications with individuals who have played powerful roles in the patient's life, and iconic or stereotypic exemplars of qualities and attributes. In certain subcultures, and in nations and cultures undergoing major changes, possession syndromes from both indigenous and introduced systems of belief may coexist and/or blend with DID.

Until recently, inaccurate but strongly held beliefs that DID was rare, iatrogenic, or a culture-bound syndrome hampered its objective study. However, increasing cross-cultural sensitivity and examination of objective data led to acknowledging the commonalities of possession syndromes and DID in *DSM-5* (American Psychiatric Association 2013). Brand et al. (2016) summarized available scientific data to refute most long-standing but unfounded myths about the condition.

A Brief Introduction to DID

Psychoanalysis is preeminently the study of the mind in conflict, of unconscious fantasies, and the projection and enactment of those conflicts and fantasies within the transference and the analytic situation. As such, it has an inevitable tendency to lean toward Hermeneutic concerns. That is, it demarcates the "realities" it considers relevant, and may understate or be surprisingly dismissive of the importance of other matters. Consequently, much crucial information about DID has received little attention in the analytic literature.

Phenomenology

Until relatively recently, the classical picture of DID involved the overt manifestations of a relatively small number of self-structures that were significantly different from one another. However, Kluft's 1985 study of the natural history of DID, Putnam, Guroff, Silberman, Barban, and Post's description of a series of 100 modern cases (Putnam et al. 1986), and the objective study of switching by Loewenstein et al., Hamilton, Alagna, Reid, & De Vries (1987) contributed to developing what Kluft (1985, 1991) has termed "the new classic picture of DID."

Kluft (1984b) found that only 6 percent of DID patients consistently manifested overt dissociative phenomenology. For the remainder, the condition became overt in response to psychosocial stressors, presenting certain "windows of diagnosability" before its obvious manifestations receded. DID may remain overt for a prolonged period of time if destabilized, either by ongoing stressors or by exploratory treatment. He recommended it be considered what Gutheil (in Kluft 1985) described as a "psychopathology of hiddenness," and should be understood in terms of its underlying structure and patterns of function rather than its intermittently overt phenomena. The landmark study of Putnam and colleagues (1986) clarified the wide range of symptoms associated with the pathognomonic features of the condition. It established that the average number of alters in contemporary DID cases was approximately 16 in women and 8 in men, which previously had been thought to be extraordinarily high numbers. Loewenstein's team studied a DID patient with a random time sound generator (Loewenstein et al. 1987). She was asked to sign in on behalf of whatever alter was in executive control when the sound was heard. Consistent with Kluft's clinical observations and inferences, they discovered that most switches were not noticed by observers, that switches occurred far more frequently than had been suspected, and that many more alters were present and were intermittently active than had been thought to be the case.

DID generally comes to the attention of the analyst due to increasing general psychiatric knowledge about DID, and by clinical happenstance. Bearing in mind this "new classic picture of DID," the usual presentation of most DID patients leaves their condition undeclared, and is often unknown to the patient as he or she comes to analysis. Unsuspected cases of DID may suddenly become manifest in the course of a previously unremarkable psychoanalysis, may be found in connection with attempts to study stalemates and failed analyses, or may even go undetected throughout the course of an extensive analytic process (Kluft 1987).

Biology

This disorder requires the capacity to redistribute attention in a way that permits the profound absorption in one mental organization and set of experiences, absorption so intense that awareness of other similar structures and processes leave the attentional field and may become inaccessible. Absorption is the crux of hypnotizability and of what is called normal dissociation (Butler 2006). This capacity is genetic (Raz, Fan, & Posner 2006). DID is characterized by higher hypnotizability than any other disorder (Frischholz, Lipman, Braun, & Sachs 1992; Dell 2017). Purely psychological formulations cannot encompass and/or explain disorders associated with this biological capacity.

Spontaneous trance and autohypnotic phenomena are intrinsic to DID. They impact treatment even when clinicians make no effort to induce hypnosis. Therefore, the clinician who wishes to work with such patients will need to become knowledgeable about hypnosis, even if the deliberate use of that modality is not part of the clinician's treatment plan. A clinician may scrupulously avoid the deliberate induction of hypnosis (heterohypnosis) without realizing that the patient's autohypnotic capacities and practices and the occurrence of spontaneous trance in response to triggering feelings, sensations, memories, or relational configurations remain vigorous and active in the relational field of the therapeutic endeavor. Psychoanalytic researcher Lester Luborsky (Luborsky & Auerbach 1969; Luborsky & Mintz 1974) systematically documented how feelings in the transference may instigate brief dissociative amnesias within a psychodynamic psychotherapy, serendipitously creating a roadmap enabling the analyst to approach many (but not all) dissociative issues without hypnosis (Kluft, in press).

Highly hypnotizable individuals, even those without diagnosable mental illness, often demonstrate enhanced emotional reactivity and intensity, rapid mobilization of transference and material often considered primary process in nature, heightened suggestivity, a propensity for rapid regression and manifestations often considered psychotic, and may slide in and out of altered states. When they become focused on one subject to the exclusion of others, they may find themselves cut off from usually accessible knowledge and experience compromising of their Generalized Reality Orientation (Shor 1972). When such individuals have experienced traumatization, flashbacks and revivifications, and misperceptions of the present from the past (including mistaking the therapist for another person, usually an abuser) are not uncommon. These phenomena can lead to confusion and terror on the parts of patient and therapist alike, and suggest the false diagnosis of a major psychotic condition. However, they are generally manageable by therapists who are familiar with hypnosis, dissociation, and the dissociative disorders. Steeped in that knowledge, Sigmund Freud and Josef Breuer were better equipped to address such circumstances than most contemporary analysts.

In addition, trauma may bring about biological problems that impair affective regulation (Perry 2013), memory function (van der Kolk 2015), endocrine responses (Yehuda et al. 2013), and create epigenetic alterations with behavioral consequences (Kluft 2017; Meaney 2001; Yehuda & Bierer 2009; Yehuda et al. 2013). Kluft (2017) has speculated that such alterations may underlie the always-challenging repetition compulsion.

Etiology

The psychoanalytic tradition often draws sweeping inferences from the study of individual patients. However venerable, this practice is profoundly vulnerable to sampling error. Here I will bypass such studies, and draw on my experience of assessing well over 2,000 DID patients over a period of forty-seven years, and of bringing over 200 to stable complete integration.

Although crude and simple, the Four Factor Theory (Kluft 1984a) avoids generalizing from individual cases, focusing instead upon what has been proven universal across my experience. In the face of Factor 1, *overwhelming events early in life* (rarely if ever beginning after age eight), a child with the biological capacity for Factor 2, *high hypnotizability* or *absorption*, 3) may develop alternative structures of self based on Factor 3, *a wide variety of possible substrates* including developmental, environmental, relational, and traumatic factors. The *failure of protection and adequate soothing*, Factor 4, which implies ongoing unfortunate experiences and relational failures, makes it difficult for the overwhelmed child to reintegrate before this dissociative adaptation has become established as an ongoing tool of coping. In the face of recurrent overwhelming trauma and/or relational failures, the mind's use of this capacity to sequester the intolerable and permit the creation of mental structures with differential access to autobiographic memory and/or organized around particular states of mind is reinforced as a successful defense. If not healed prior to the adolescent passage, the press to establish identity, put aside residual trauma, and develop more mature sexuality (Blos 1962) all work to solidify such alternate selves as they develop, confronting the clinician with an increasingly more determined and less malleable psychological configuration.

The nature of the trauma experienced, the age of the child at traumatization, the extent of trauma and the identity and number of the traumatizers may exert powerful influences on developmental processes, attachment, object relations, and the like. The vast majority of the DID literature has discussed childhood maltreatment, physical, sexual, psychological, and neglectful, as traumatic triggers in civilian populations in nations at peace. However, medical trauma, painful childhood disease, and overwhelming experiences such as exposure to death, loss, witnessing the mistreatment/destruction of others (by violence, war, disaster, famine, cultural dislocation, etc.), may prove etiological. Family disruption and the impact of congenital difficulties or abnormalities may lower the threshold for the degree of trauma necessary to trigger a DID adaptation.

The Dissociation Perplex

Psychoanalysis has gradually reclaimed the term, "dissociation," but has done so in a plethora of often-confusing, internally contradictory, and manifestly dysfunctional ways. This perplex is the natural outcome of attempts to circumscribe a complex condition in terms of incomplete models drawn from the study of other quite different and generally less difficult to conceptualize models of mental function. They are rarely, if ever, drawn directly from the study of dissociative patients. Currently, over two dozen contemporary definitions of dissociation can be found in the literature.

In order to make their models more convincing and conclusive, their proponents often have banished from consideration phenomena long considered part of the dissociative realm because they do not mesh well with their models. Often, clinical reality is being sacrificed in the formulation of theories which then will be applied to the treatment of that reality.

No available theory encompasses the full realm of dissociative psychopathology. It becomes important to study the individuality of each individual case in order to assess whether available promoted models can play an imperfect, incomplete, but useful role in that particular instance.

I have added here my own observations of dissociative phenomena in DID patients (Kluft 2009):

1. Alters, known as personalities, identities, personality states, etc.
2. Amnesia
3. Identity Confusion
4. Compartmentalization/Modularity Phenomena
    a. Alters, as above
    b. Segregation of some subsets of information from other subsets of information in a relatively rule-bound manner (Spiegel 1986)
    c. BASK (Braun 1988) Dimensions (ablative expressions)
5. Detachment (as in depersonalization and derealization in the perception of self and/or others and also in concerns over whether memories are real or unreal, also seen in alters' lacking senses of ownership or responsibility for the action of other alters)
6. Absorption
7. Altered states of consciousness (e.g., hypnotic/autohypnotic/spontaneous trance)
8. Failures of compartmentalization such as intrusion phenomena, including both alters, memories, and BASK (Braun 1988) dimensions (intrusive expressions)
9. Simultaneous operation of separate self-aware processes or states of mind, including parallel distributed processing, elsewhere thought known phenomena (Kluft 1995b), unconscious thought (Dijksterhuis, Bos, Nordren, & van Baaren 2006), inner-world activities, and creativity by alters not in apparent executive control
10. Simultaneous executive activity by separate self-aware processes or states of mind (copresence phenomena [Kluft 1984b])
11. Inner world and third reality phenomena (events within that inner world that are accorded historical reality and which sometimes intrude into ongoing experiences, and/or impact ongoing experiences from behind the scenes [Kluft 1999])
12. Switching and shifting
13. Multiple reality disorder (Kluft 1991), for which DID, formerly called Multiple Personality Disorder, is the delivery and maintenance system

Both Brenner (2001, 2004, 20009, 2014) and Shengold (1989) combine classic psychoanalytic conflict theory with an awareness of autohypnotic mechanisms. They address dissociation as a defense, and explore the interface of traditional and autohypnotic defenses to ward off the impact of trauma and turmoil.

Numerous authors have used the rubric of splitting to discuss dissociative phenomena (e.g., Davies & Frawley 1994), but this is a problematic stance and fraught with potential for confusion, as implied in Pruyser's 1975 classic "What Splits in Splitting?" Splitting traditionally has been used to describe rather polarized feelings that are incompatible. A typical usage regards the good object/bad object, good subject/bad subject dichotomy. But with splitting comes the connotation of particular patterns of object relatedness and the concerns raised by borderline and narcissistic personality configurations. While this notion has an initial appeal and readily connects to familiar analytic ideas, it is problematic as an explanatory vehicle.

Splitting usually relates to polarized perceptions and experiences of self, object, or both. This is only one of the patterns represented in the formation of personality systems in DID. It is uncommon for most alters to be based primarily on split representations of self and object along the line of particular affective states (e.g., a subject-affect-object unit such as a good self linked with positive affect to good mother), although this may play some part in alter formation.

It is far more common for alters to be based on roles in crucial relational patterns and/or traumatic scenarios, both the roles experienced by the patient and the roles enacted by others. Attachment issues and the preservation of important relationships and reenactments of mistreatment generate both concordant and complementary alter patterns.

Both my clinical experience and unpublished research applying the Core Conflictual Relationship Theme model of Luborsky (Luborsky & Crits-Cristoph 1990) to the verbatim expressions of individual alters have led me to approach the alters neither from a model of repression nor from splitting, but from an appreciation of the purposes they serve. I found that major alters could be studied to determine what they did, why they did it, and how they understood their own roles in transactions and the responses of others.

Let us consider the hypothetical plight of a young girl with good but emotionally cold parents who is groomed and seduced by her Uncle Ben, a warm but perverse individual (see Kluft 1999).

The formation of an alter who holds in isolation awareness of what has occurred permits another to go on as if life were normal, retaining all attachments. The operative principle in the amnestic alter is "this did not happen." However, the victim's mind searches for reasons, and abusers offer rationales to justify their behavior. A child may come to believe that she is bad, and that what has befallen her is deserved punishment. Creation of a "bad" alter whose misbehavior would provoke well-deserved punishment retains the abuser as a positive presence rather than a hostile and degrading miscreant. If sexual experience is to some degree pleasurable, or the child can be convinced that it is, a "sexual" alter identified with arousal may be created, further encouraged by an abuser who tells his victim that she likes what is happening. The sexualized alter reasons, "I must have wanted it." Again, this protects the valued, if conflicted, relationship. Many victims of ongoing abuse, especially those faced into painful submission, discover that they can exert some control over what they endure by initiating sexual advances, avoiding traumatic coercion and inviting a sexual act that is less painful than another. A sexually aggressive alter prepared to use sex as a weapon of control is not an uncommon outcome (Kluft 2017).

It rapidly occurs to a girl that if she were not female, certain unwanted and painful things could not befall her. The wish to be a boy, immune to such approaches, encourages the formation of a male alter, often a "twin" of an abused female alter. The wish to be powerful enough to defend against the abuser may lead to the formation of a protector alter, usually male. Further, the wish to be strong enough to be able to inflict rather than suffer hurt may lead to an alter that is an "identification with the aggressor."

The wish to be able to feel none of the upsetting pain or overstimulation and be protected from such may lead to the creation of an autohypnotic "anesthetic" personality immune from the perception of pain. One anesthetic variant may undertake counterphobic behaviors, encouraging nasty experiences to demonstrate its power. Another mechanism of the flight from pain is the creation of numerous alters associated with particular traumata, or simply the overflow of trauma too excessive to be encapsulated within the previously available alters. This is the most common reason for the creation of very large alter systems (Kluft 1988). Finally, it is typical for all but the most simple cases to include a nurturing, loving protective presence, usually female and maternal, understood to console and care for the injured younger alters. These patterns may be replicated many times over, leading to startling complexity and a large number of alters.

In most instances, at least some of the alters interact, either intermittently or in an ongoing manner, in an inner world that may be experienced with all the intensity of external reality, and may be understood to be as real, if not more real, than external reality. In this inner "third" reality (Kluft, 1991) representations of powerful abusers may reenact the traumatization of representations of the patient at earlier and more vulnerable moments in her life. The toleration of mutually incompatible perceptions of alternative realities by the patient and the need to address this in treatment requires the alert attention of the analyst, and a tremendous amount of skillful and gentle confrontation and clarification.

The Analyst and the Alters

Analysts struggle with how to deal with the manifestations of different senses or states of self that either take on executive control, intrude into other such elements' attempts to assert executive control, or exert their influence by inner voices, command hallucinations, or other manners of exerting direct and indirect influence. Their struggles generally follow one of three pathways, which are not always mutually exclusive.

One approach takes a dismissive stance toward the alters. The analyst might refuse to talk to any alter other than the one the analyst believes to be "the real patient," correcting the speech of patients who speak in the third person or the first person plural, reframing the manifestations of alters as regression, or in terms of their embodying different aspects of a conflict, and similar efforts. These are often rationalized as nonreinforcement, a distinctly nonpsychoanalytic model. This approach assumes that the alters are simply a distraction from the real business of the treatment. While gratifying to the analyst who does not want to deal with dissociative psychopathology, it bypasses all consideration that the personality of a patient with multiple personalities is to have multiple personalities (Coons 1980).

Abused individuals are accustomed to submitting to tyrannical abusers unwilling to deal with their feelings and the impact of their experiences. If enough aspects of the patient attach to the analyst who proceeds in this manner, other alters may resign themselves to withdrawing and remaining silent to please the analyst, who will not appreciate that this adaptation is a compliant negative transference. I have seen over a dozen DID patients who have terminated ostensibly completed analyses without their dissociative disorder's having been treated, and drew the above observations from my study of their experiences.

A second strategy privileges approaching the alters as manifestations of processes over approaching them as entities with firm senses of their own identities. From that stance, Davies and Frawley (1994) offer a masterful approach to the treatment of posttraumatic dissociative phenomena that adheres more closely to the relational paradigm of psychoanalysis than to the dissociative disorders literature.

The most elegant expressions of this "process over structure" stance are found in the work of relational analyst Philip Bromberg (2001) and relational psychoanalytic psychotherapist Richard Chefetz (2015). To oversimplify, they elect to reframe the alters as different ways of being, expressing the hope of thereby avoiding the reification of the alters. Chefetz speaks to patients in terms of "different ways of being you." Bromberg offers thoughtful theoretical formulations, and Chefetz demonstrates his approach at work and shares his decision-making process in presenting and discussing a series of impressive verbatim transcripts.

Brenner's work (2001, 2004, 2009, 2014) addresses both process and structure issues in connection with his approaches to alters, and demonstrates how an analyst aware of both the nature of hypnosis and trance/dissociative phenomena encountered in the analysis of dissociative patients can work with most of these phenomena within a classic psychoanalytic model.

I take a different stance toward dealing with alters (Kluft 2006). I share Coons's conclusion in 1980 that the personality of a person with multiple personalities is to have multiple personalities. Accordingly, I regard direct work with the various alters as integral to the treatment of DID. Since the 1970s I have argued that the term "self states" describes the nature of alters and the clinical challenges they present more accurately and helpfully than terms like personalities/personality states, ego states, subpersonalities, identities, personae, or other similar terms (see Kluft 1988). Since alters characteristically have their own autobiographic memories and are driven by motives not necessarily shared across all parts, I find Kohut's (1971, 1984) description of the self as a center of initiative and experience both realistic and clinically useful. Ullman and Brothers (1993) have written a useful study of the treatment of trauma from a self psychological perspective. My approach overlaps with theirs in part, but is more indebted to my ongoing interest in the intersection of psychoanalysis with dissociation as understood through the lens of hypnosis (see Brenner 2009; Kluft 2000, 2016, in press 2018a, in press 2018b, in press 2018c; O'Neil 2018).

Accordingly, I endeavor to engage rather than dismiss or reframe the alters and their subjectivities in a manner consistent with self-psychology. I have found that empathic engagement with my DID patients across all alters allows for more effective communication, more effective therapeutic alliances involving the alters as active collaborators, more rapid reductions of the shame felt by parts long withdrawn, and reduced instances of crises and self-injury. But further, engaging the alters in this manner encourages them to take similar stances of empathic understanding toward one another, which reduces long-standing mutual avoidances and clashes when these are prominent. Further, an ongoing pattern of attending to rather than bypassing their concerns encourages them to be more concerned about one another and the treatment, supporting continuous contemporary memory and mutual identification, paving the way toward integration.

The patterns of narcissistic injury described by Kohut and Wolf (1978) are frequently encountered within alters' systems, and generally respond well to attention to selfobject hungers and transferences. Moments of real or perceived empathic failure on my part are common. Simplistically, empathizing with one alter may be seen as being dismissive of another, which threatens the stability of the treatment. The exploration of these situations, at times several per session, combined with response to selfobject concerns such as the need for empathic mirroring and the need for the strong presence of an idealized object, contribute to creating an environment in which traumatic events and relationships can be faced and processed with relative safety.

Further, when treating those who often have suffered abuse and neglect from close family members, and who are suffering ongoing traumatic sequelae, many transferences that will remain central throughout the treatment are quite negative, even those cloaked behind an eagerness to please and a fear of rejection. The analyst who takes a remote or aloof stance is likely to be seen as confirming the patient's worst fears; i.e., that under the guise of kindness, the analyst is untrustworthy and potentially both rejecting and abusive.

THE UNIQUE IMPORTANCE OF ANALYTIC TACT AND PRIVILEGING PATIENTS OVER THEORIES AND MODELS IN CARING FOR THE TRAUMATIZED

In approaching the severely traumatized patient, it is imperative for the analyst to avoid the countertransference trap of privileging familiar practices and theories over attention to the individual patient. In a classic article, Waelder (1962) reminds us that clinical observations and correlations are the true heart of psychoanalysis. Summarizing, he points out that while our preferred philosophies and metapsychologies often dominate our thinking, effective clinical work stems from the study of the patient, not the confirmation of preferred abstractions, which are always undergoing change and evolution.

In the spirit of Waelder's wisdom, I strongly advocate the stance that there are many potential developmental pathways, alternatives to the norm forced upon children by unfortunate circumstances. The concept of "growing up strangely" was used by Armstrong (1994) in describing DID as a unique and complex developmental adaptation. Many DID patients have grown up under difficult circumstances little studied in the mainstream analytic literature. It is most respectful to the dignity of the patient and most supportive to the effectiveness of the treatment to become a student of the unique individuality and subjectivity of the patient (Kluft 2016).

Breaches in the therapeutic alliance, crises, or even decompensation may occur when sexual or hostile behaviors are interpreted in terms that attribute either erotic drives or destructive rage to the patient. The following example is extreme, but clear. In the 1970s, a hospitalized DID patient of mine was being covered by a colleague during my vacation. She rapidly gave signs of finding him attractive. He interpreted what he thought were her erotic feelings, and she decompensated and became self-destructive.

On my return, I found my patient miserable, suicidal, and wailing, "You see, those things happened because I wanted them to. It's all my fault!" My patient and her sister had been molested and prostituted by their parents, who had tried to convince them that they wanted the sex forced upon them. My colleague, a very classical analyst of the 1970s, interpreted her interest in him as mature and erotic. In fact, it was the infantile affiliative behavior of a woman who learned early in life that showing sexual interest in a man was her route to acceptance and freedom from coercion.

Distinguishing appearance from underlying meaning is the ongoing task of the analyst. In dealing with DID, this is achieved best by remembering that fear of mistreatment and rejection and the enactments and reenactments that stem from a traumatic past are more likely determinants of erotic and aggressive behavior than libidinal and aggressive drives. I am comfortable with applying Kohut's description of aggression as a deterioration product of relational failure rather than as a primary drive (Kohut 1971, 1977; Kohut & Wolf 1978), and tend to regard overly driven sexual behavior in a similar manner (Kluft 2017). This allows me to approach even extreme situations empathically.

Other common related traps stem from the assumption that analyst and analysand share a common frame of values and understandings. When dealing with patients whose formative years may not have exposed them to many of the experiences and rules of behavior and making sense of the world that are assumed in much of the analytic literature, it is easy to go astray. Faimberg's concept of listening to the patient's listening (2005) helps me consider and inquire into what meanings have been attributed to my words. For example, my research (Kluft 1989, 1990) demonstrates that many of these patients are prone to orient themselves so that whatever pleases powerful abusers or scant sources of support becomes defined as the true reality, and the true sense of what is good. These initially survival-oriented adaptations may lead to very idiosyncratic notions of truth, reality, and what is good or bad. This often is discovered only after some unsettling incident or misunderstanding, from which the analyst learns that a consensual sense of these matters will be forfeited under certain circumstances or in response to certain actual or perceived stressors. It is easier on the analyst, in terms of countertransference pressures, to anticipate lacunae in superego, ego ideal, and reality testing functions. Ongoing attention to what is actually being understood and misunderstood in the therapeutic dyad is most helpful.

TECHNICAL ISSUES IN THE PSYCHOANALYSIS/ PSYCHOANALYTIC PSYCHOTHERAPY OF DISSOCIATIVE SYMPTOMS AND DID

The integration of identity and memory are central goals of the treatment of DID, along with the alleviation of posttraumatic, relational, and dysregulatory symptoms and their associated behavioral and interpersonal difficulties.

Even improvements that fall short of the complete achievement of these goals are profoundly beneficial to such patients.

The analyst looks to the patient to bring an increasingly empowered observing ego to the work of therapy. When dealing with dispersed and reduplicated centers of self-experience and conation, the analyst begins with working with the mind as it presents itself, most commonly in the form of the personality that has presented for treatment, which may be understood, mistakenly, as the real patient.

The analyst hopes to help the patient develop an increasingly functional and complete observing ego that will override the dissociative dividedness increasingly over the passage of time. My approach involves validating the patient's numerous experiences of self, and working empathically within that framework of meaning so persistently that it becomes unnecessary for the patient to maintain it in a "divided" state (Kluft 1995a, 2000). The failure to do so risks inflicting the subjective experience of neglect and betrayal in parts of the mind that do not experience themselves as acknowledged and included as they are. It is difficult to interpret such experiences as transferential when they are being unwittingly repeated, collateral damage inflicted secondary to the analyst's approach.

It has been my experience that the most effective way to bring the various self states into both the therapeutic alliance and the process of therapy in an ongoing manner is to offer them ongoing invitations. A failure to acknowledge, respect, or validate a person inflicts an injury that is likely to include shaming. Alters often experience themselves just as persons experience themselves, and are shamed when treated without acknowledgment or respect.

In my experience, the most cogent approach to conceptualizing shame in the service of formulating clinical interventions is expressed in Nathanson's concept of the "Compass of Shame" (1992). He describes four cardinal script patterns in responding to shame, which, as an affect, severs interpersonal connectedness. These are withdrawal, denial, attack self, and attack other. That is, in order to avoid the full brunt of shame, individuals may withdraw, deny the shame by plunging into distractions (often substance abuse or dysfunctional enactments), attack the self (identifying with those who cause and/or behold/learn of their shame), or try to protect themselves by trying to shame someone else (often those who cause and/or behold/learn of their shame). Alters who feel shamed are loath to participate in the treatment, a situation that may slow, stalemate, or undo the therapy.

My approach to the resolution of these matters is simple and straightforward. I invite the alters to participate by requesting their input as well as those of the alter sitting in my office in ostensible executive control. For example, after a patient has reported a dream and I have heard the associations offered by the alter out at the moment, I may inquire, "If there are any other thoughts or feelings about this, I'd like to hear them as well. Other parts don't have to take the trouble to come out completely. You can speak inwardly and the one sitting here can pass your reactions along. And, addressing myself to the one sitting here, if you become aware of any ideas, sounds, images, or anything else that's not in words, please pass that along, too."

Establishing this form of communication is often an arduous process. It may take months, and success is not guaranteed. The following dialog occurred after a patient described a traumatic dream, the day's residue of which was a violent scene in a movie she had seen the night before, and after she had offered her associations.

> DR: I wonder if any other parts of the mind have something to contribute to our understanding.
>
> PT: (starts to rock back and forth) No. I don't hear anything.
>
> DR: What comes to mind about the way your body is moving?
>
> PT: I'm getting scared. Something inside is saying, "Tell him!" I don't know what that means, but I'm getting scared and my body is rocking more.
>
> DR: Do you think that there's more to tell about that rocking?
>
> PT: (rocking) No. Because it can't be true!
>
> DR: Can't be true?
>
> PT: (rocking) That voice that's saying "Tell him!" is getting louder. And now there's another voice, younger, saying "Mommy loves me! She never hit me!"
>
> DR: So you are holding back something you say can't be true, while at the same time other parts of your mind are saying this something is true, and others are working hard to say your mother loves you . . .
>
> PT: (rocking) OK. OK. When I was a little girl, I thought I was special because my friends got spankings when they misbehaved, and I didn't. They told me my mother must really love me, and that made me feel good. Oh! What a headache! Now it's "Tell him, already, or I will!" I don't want to say it. Do you know what I mean?

DR: My guess is that if I answer you, the parts urging you to talk may feel disrespected. The conflicts that cause you so many symptoms and battles with one another will just go on unchanged.

PT: (rocking) OK. OK. It's true she never hit me. That's true. But I've been remembering that instead of hitting me, sometimes she shook me until I passed out. (stops rocking) A voice inside said, "It's about time you faced the truth!" Another is saying, "Mommy won't love me anymore. You shouldn't have told!"

Here the conflict being analyzed is not between structural components of the mind per se, in the familiar sense of ego psychology. Instead, it is the recapitulation of a young girl's conflicted and mutually incompatible intrapsychic strategies for dealing with abusive treatment by a mother whose love she sought with both terror and desperation.

By inviting the patient's dissociated structures and processes to express themselves, they become far more accessible to intervention, the genetics of the traumatic and negative transferences more amenable to exploration and resolution, and a foundation is established for genuine emotional insight and meaningful change. This approach, here illustrated in the context of a dream, is equally applicable to all aspects of the analytic endeavor. In the flow of the analytic endeavor, it may prove especially useful for the analysis of resistance, enactments, and the deeper understanding of moments of perceived and genuine empathic failure, both between patient and analyst, and among the components of the patient's alter system (Kluft 2000).

CASE PRESENTATION

Lauren, a psychology graduate student, was referred to a psychoanalytic clinic for a low-fee analysis. Evaluators believed she had a hysterical neurotic character. She had difficulties in forming solid relationships with suitable men, and was troubled by her lack of assertiveness in general, but especially with women in authority. This often left her in undesirable subservient positions. On the verge of beginning her career as a mental health professional, Lauren was eager to understand herself better and to address her problems.

For the first four and a half years of her supervised five times per week control analysis, Lauren struggled to work through her highly conflicted relationship with her superficially warm and loving although dictatorial and invalidating mother. Her dysfunctional submissive and passive-aggressive coping styles became manifest in her resistances and in the transference.

Lauren idealized her weaker father, but she had very few memories about him dating from her childhood years. In contrast, vivid experiences with her controlling mother dominated her recollections. Mother and daughter alike described this controlling quality as love and concern, but Lauren admitted that it made her uncomfortable, and more resentful than she usually could admit.

To all outward appearances, Lauren's analysis was progressing well. As time went on, Lauren worked hard on her relationship to her mother, and developed a strong negative maternal transference in which the analyst was seen as granting only provisional warmth and acceptance, contingent upon complete obedience. However, her father remained an obscure figure. The analyst actually remarked that at times it seemed that Lauren talked as if he were not even in the room, and wondered if that might be reflecting something about her feelings toward her father. Lauren rapidly confirmed that observation.

Lauren was an attractive young woman. Lauren was pursued by many men. Two types prevailed. The first consisted of medical students and medical residents, whom she found boring. The second were political radicals, some associated with rather marginal groups that advocated violence. Lauren found them exciting and desirable. The analyst tried to interpret oedipal conflicts that he thought were prohibiting her from becoming interested in "nice but forbidden men" like her father, and pushing her to involve herself with "bad boys." Lauren repudiated these remarks. She often cast the analyst in the role of a profoundly boring good but sexually inadequate man, along with casting him as an intrusive, demanding, and critical mother who could neither be pleased nor satisfied.

Midway through Lauren's fifth year of analysis, she began to hallucinate colored shapes at the foot of the couch. The analyst linked these colors with various affects. Red represented an unacceptable rage that left her overwhelmed with guilt. She could neither explain this rage nor explore it with free association. After a few weeks of working with these hallucinated colors, Lauren rose from the couch in mid-session. In a very different and angry voice, she proclaimed, "You can analyze her, but I'm leaving!"

Lauren had given no prior indication that she suffered DID, although it is possible in retrospect that she may have been dissociating on the couch, but whatever had occurred was misunderstood as regression in the service of the ego. This newly recognized or newly emerging alter was quite angry. It found fault with the analyst in one way after another, and gradually presented a very different and negative picture of Lauren's father. About a month later, another part emerged, fretful about the expression of anger, and determined to be the best little girl in the world. It apologized for the anger and negativity of the first part that had emerged, and tried to convince the analyst that what the angry part had said should be disregarded because it was not nice, and no one wanted to hear it. In some sessions these two parts emerged one after the other and held vigorous debates right in session. During one of these, both raised their voices, prompting the "super-good" part to protest that if they kept shouting, they would wake "the little one." The analyst learned that a child-like part was usually kept asleep, but occasionally "came out to play." It knew nothing painful and negative. The "super-good" part urged the analyst to get rid of the angry part so that the child within would be safe, and could grow up without pain.

It was in this context that all parts began to fear that "someone bad" would come into the office, or that the analyst would attempt to take advantage of Lauren on the couch. Now, a picture of the analyst emerged in the transference that portrayed him as a barely contained sexual predator. Across her parts, Lauren felt she had to turn to look at the analyst frequently lest he be preparing to attack, disrobing, or masturbating. She had traumatic dreams of a "bad man doing bad things to a girl."

Over time, the following picture emerged. Lauren had blotted out all memory of her father's angry tirades, occasional outrageous punishments, and instances in which he had come home intoxicated. On some such occasions Lauren's mother would lock him out of the room they shared. Sometimes he stumbled into Lauren's room in a drunken state and molested her. When she complained to her mother, her mother would not discuss her father's drinking, and chided her for believing her "bad dreams" were actual events.

Memories of mistreatment by father, and memories of bizarre cleansing rituals enforced by mother, emerged and were abreacted. No attempt was made to verify or challenge her memories. If something bothered Lauren, it was explored and processed until it ceased to distress her.

As the above materials were addressed, the nature of Lauren's dreams gradually changed. They no longer involved some vague entity. They now included explicit images of her father doing sexual things to her. As this work was processed, Lauren's negative transferences diminished in intensity. She struggled to make sense of the picture of her childhood and family that had emerged. She came to understand that she dated abusive men both because they were like her father, and because the "super-good" part based on her mother whitewashed the transgressions of the nasty men, while criticizing the nice men who wanted to date her. She came to understand that not only had her mother lied to defend her father and justify her idiosyncratic beliefs about food and cleanliness, but that she was jealous of the better life she thought Lauren might enjoy with a good and successful man. It was as if she was driven to separate Lauren from any decent boyfriend. "She didn't have the courage to face the truth and do something about Dad. She stayed, and I think unconsciously she didn't want me to show her up by escaping." Lauren did not distance herself from her parents, but she set firm boundaries and no longer fell into subservient patterns of behavior in her dealings with them.

By the seventh year of the analysis the angry part, which had endured much of the abuse by both parents, had faded into a vague entity. The "super-good" part, repudiating its identification with mother and abreacting its own traumatic memories, felt it had nothing left to do. Believing it should "really" support Lauren, it merged with her. At this point, the young child part spontaneously experienced itself maturing, several years per month. As it did so, Lauren seemed more content and at peace. She developed a stable relationship with a successful young attorney, and became engaged.

Midway through the eighth year of her analysis, the once youngest part merged with Lauren. Upon this, the angry part, which had born the majority of the abuse by father and mother, and had felt obliged to submit to mistreatment by the undesirable boyfriends and women in authority, came out a final time to offer thanks for the help it had received, and merged. The analysis came to a natural termination at the beginning of its ninth year.

While this highly disguised psychoanalysis was so simple and straightforward that it is not representative of the challenges encountered in the psychotherapy or psychoanalysis of most patients with DID, it has the advantage of illustrating how a patient with DID was treated to the point of stable integration in a classic supervised psychoanalysis.

I was the young candidate analyst who treated her, under the helpful supervision of the late Steven Hammerman, M.D. Although a neophyte analyst, I was already well trained in hypnosis and knowledgeable about DID. This served me well because my process notes on every session were reviewed. As a candidate working with a brilliant but very conservative supervisor, I did not dare to deviate from classic technique.

Lauren had unusually high ego strength, and suffered a very mild case of DID. Most DID patients cannot tolerate a relatively classical analysis because they require more structure and support, or may suffer comorbidities that make it unrealistic to consider them for analysis. Vignettes in the work of Brenner (2001, 2004, 2009, 2014) are more representative of work with more demanding DID patients.

CONCLUSION

While most DID patients are not suitable candidates for psychoanalysis, and many venerable and valued psychoanalytic concepts either are not applicable to work with this group of patients, and may even prove unhelpful if brought to bear, bringing a psychoanalytic awareness to the treatment of DID patients is profoundly useful (Kluft 1995a, 2000). The basic processes of analytic inquiry and exploration offer deep and rich insights that enhance whatever other modalities are brought into play in their treatments (Brenner 2018). Since such patients are recognized with increasing frequency, and may make abrupt and unanticipated appearances in the course of analytic work, it is useful to become knowledgeable about their phenomenology and treatment.

Further, most patients with severe dissociative symptoms can be understood readily through the lens of DID. Dissociative amnesia, dissociative fugue, other less defined dissociative disorders, and some cases of depersonalization disorder share its connection to high hypnotizability and traumatic antecedents.

REFERENCES

American Psychiatric Association. (2013). *Diagnostic and Statistical Manual of Mental Disorders, 5th edition. DSM-5*. Washington, DC: American Psychiatric Press.

Armstrong, J. (1994). Reflections on multiple personality disorder as a developmentally complex adaptation. *Psychoanalytic Study of the Child*, 49, 349–364.

Berman, E. (1981). Multiple personality: Psychoanalytic perspectives. *International Journal of Psycho-Analysis*, 62, 283–300.

Blos, P. (1962). *On Adolescence*. New York: The Free Press.

Bourgignon, E. (1991). *Possession*. San Francisco: Chandler & Sharp.

Brand, B., Sar, V., Stavropoulos, P., Krüger, C., Korzekwa, M., Martínez-Taboas, A., and Middleton, W. (2016). Separating fact from fiction: An empirical examination of six myths about Dissociative Identity Disorder. *Harvard Review of Psychiatry*, 24, 257–270.

Braun, B. G. (1988). The BASK model of dissociation. *Dissociation*, 1(1), 4–23.

Breger, L. (2009). *A Dream of Undying Fame: How Freud Betrayed His Mentor and Invented Psychoanalysis*. New York: Basic Books.

Brenner, I. (2001). *Dissociation of Trauma: Theory, Phenomenology and Technique*. Madison, CT: International Universities Press.

———. (2004). *Psychic Trauma: Dynamics, Symptoms, and Treatment*. Lanham, MD: Aronson.

———. (2009). A new view from the Acropolis: Dissociative Identity Disorder. *Psychoanalytic Quarterly*, 78, 57–105.

———. (2014). *Dark Matters: Exploring the Realm of Psychic Devastation*. London, UK: Karnac.

———. (2018). Catching a wave: The hypnosis-sensitive transference-based treatment of Dissociative Identity Disorder (DID). *American Journal of Clinical Hypnosis*, 60, 279–295.

Breuer J. and Freud, S. (1955). Studies on hysteria. *Standard Edition of the Complete Psychological Works of Sigmund Freud, Vol. 2*. London, UK: Hogarth. (Original works published 1893–1895).

Bromberg, P. (2001). *Standing in the Spaces: Essays on Clinical Process, Trauma, and Dissociation*. New York: Routledge.

Butler, L. (2006). Normative dissociation. *Psychiatric Clinics of North America*, 29, 45–62.

Chefetz, R. (2015). *Intensive Psychotherapy for Persistent Dissociative Processes: The Fear of Feeling Real*. New York: Norton.

Coons, P. M. (1980). Multiple personality: diagnostic considerations. *Journal of Clinical Psychiatry*, 4, 330–336.

Davies, J. M. and Frawley, M. G. (1994). *Treating the Adult Survivor of Childhood Sexual Abuse: A Psychoanalytic Perspective*. New York: Basic Books.

Dell, P. (2017). Is high hypnotizability a necessary diathesis for pathological dissociation? *Journal of Trauma and Dissociation*, 18, 56–87.

Dijksterhuis, A., Bos, M., Nordren, L., and van Baaren, R. (2006). On making the right choice: The deliberation-without-attention effect. *Science*, 311, 1005–1007.

Faimberg, H. (2005). *The Telescoping of the Generations: Listening to the Narcissistic Links between Generations*. New York: Routledge.

Frischholz, E., Lipman, L., Braun, B., and Sachs, R. (1992). Psychopathology, hypnotizability, and dissociation. *American Journal of Psychiatry*, 149, 1521–1525.

Jones, E. (1953). *The Life and Work of Sigmund Freud, three-volume set*. New York: Basic Books.

Kluft, R. P. (1984a). Treatment of multiple personality. *Psychiatric Clinics of North America*, 7, 9–29.

———. (1984b). An introduction to multiple personality disorder. *Psychiatric Annals*, 14, 19–24.

———. (1985). The natural history of multiple personality disorder. In R. P. Kluft (Ed.), *Childhood Antecedents of Multiple Personality* (pp. 197–238). Washington, DC: American Psychiatric Press.

———. (1986). Personality unification in multiple personality disorder. In B. Braun (Ed.), *Treatment of Multiple Personality Disorder* (pp. 29–60). Washington, DC: American Psychiatric Press.

———. (1987). Unsuspected multiple personality disorder: An uncommon source of protracted resistance, interruption, and failure in psychoanalysis. *Hillside Journal of Clinical Psychiatry*, 9, 104–115.

———. (1988). The phenomenology and treatment of extremely complex multiple personality disorder. *Dissociation*, 1(4), 47–58.

———. (1989). Treating the patient who has been sexually exploited by a previous psychotherapist.. *Psychiatric Clinics of North America*, 12, 483–500.

———. (1990). Incest and subsequent revictimization: The case of therapist-patient sexual exploitation, with a description of the sitting duck syndrome. In R. P. Kluft (Ed.), *Incest-Related Syndromes of Adult Psychopathology* (pp. 263–287). Washington, DC: American Psychiatric Press.

———. (1991). Multiple personality disorder. In A. Tasman & S. Goldfinger (Eds.), *Annual Review of Psychiatry, Vol. 10* (pp. 161–188). Washington, DC: American Psychiatric Press.

———. (1995a). Treatment of dissociative disorders. In J. Barber & P. Crits-Cristoph (Eds.), *Dynamic Therapies for Psychiatric Disorders (Axis I)* (pp. 332–385). New York: Basic Books.

———. (1995b). The confirmation and discontinuation of memories of abuse in dissociative identity disorder patients: A naturalistic clinical study. *Dissociation*, 8, 253–258.

———. (1999). Current issues in dissociative identity disorder. *Journal of Practical Psychiatry and Behavioral Health*, 5, 3–19.

———. (2000). The psychoanalytic psychotherapy of dissociative identity disorder in the context of trauma therapy. *Psychoanalytic Inquiry*, 20, 259–286.

———. (2006). Dealing with alters: A pragmatic clinical perspective. *Psychiatric Clinics of North America*, 29, 291–304.

———. (2009). A clinician's understanding of dissociation: Fragments of an acquaintance. In P. Dell & J. O'Neill (Eds.), *Dissociation and the Dissociative Disorders: DSM-V and Beyond* (pp. 599–623). New York: Taylor & Francis.

———. (2016). You have to be carefully taught: Dignity considerations in clinical practice, scholarship, and trauma treatment. In S. Levine (Ed.), *Dignity Matters: Psychoanalytic and Psychosocial Perspectives* (pp. 141–158). London, UK: Karnac Books.

———. (2017). Weaponized sex: Defensive pseudoerotic aggression in the service of safety. *Journal of Trauma and Dissociation*, 18, 259–283.

———. (2018). Reconsidering hypnosis and psychoanalysis: Toward creating a context for understanding. *American Journal of Clinical Hypnosis*, 60, 201–215.

———. (2018a). Freud's rejection of hypnosis: Part I—The genesis of a rift. *American Journal of Clinical Hypnosis*, 60, 307–323.

———. (2018b). Freud's rejection of hypnosis: Part II—The perpetuation of a rift. *American Journal of Clinical Hypnosis*, 60, 324–347.

———. (in press). Freud's rejection of hypnosis: Part III—Toward healing the rift. *American Journal of Clinical Hypnosis*.

Kohut, H. (1971). *The Analysis of the Self.* Chicago, IL: The University of Chicago Press.

———. (1977). *The Restoration of the Self.* Chicago, IL: The University of Chicago Press.

Kohut, H. and Goldberg, A. (1984) *How Does Analysis Cure?* Chicago: University of Chicago Press.

Kohut, H. and Wolf, E. (1978). The disorders of the self and their treatment: An outline. *International Journal of Psychoanalysis*, 59, 413–425.

Loewenstein, R. J., Hamilton, J., Alagna, S., Reid, N., and DeVries, M. (1987). Experiential sampling in the study of multiple personality disorder. *American Journal of Psychiatry*, 144(1), 19–24.

Luborsky, L., & Auerbach, A. (1969). The symptom-context method—quantitative studies of symptom formation in psychotherapy. *Journal of the American Psychoanalytic Association*, 17, 68–99.

Luborsky, L. and Crits-Cristoph, P. (1990). *Understanding Transference : The Core Conflictual Relationship Theme Method.* New York: Basic Books.

Luborsky, L., & Mintz, J. (1974). What sets off momentary forgetting during a psychoanalysis? Investigation of symptom-onset conditions. *Psychoanalysis and Contemporary Science*, 3, 233–268.

Makari, G. (2008). *Revolution in Mind: The Creation of Psychoanalysis*. New York: Harper.

Meaney, M. (2001). Maternal care, gene expression and the transmission of individual differences in stress reactivity across generations. *Annual Review of Neuroscience*, 24, 1161–1192.

Nathanson, D. (1992). *Shame and Pride.* New York: Norton.

O'Neil, J. (2018). Hypnosis and psychoanalysis: Undoing Freud's primal category mistake. *American Journal of Clinical Hypnosis*, 60, 262–278.

Perry, B. (2013). *Brief: Reflections on Childhood, Trauma, and Society*. Houston, TX: Child Trauma Academy Press.

Pruyser, P. (1975). What splits in splitting? A scrutiny of the concept in psychoanalysis and in psychiatry. *Bulletin of the Menninger Clinic*, 39, 1–46.

Putnam, F., Guroff, J., Silberman, E., Barban, L., and Post, R. (1986). The clinical phenomenology of multiple personality disorder: Review of 100 recent cases. *Journal of Clinical Psychiatry*, 47, 285–293.

Raz, A., Fan, J., and Posner, M. I. (2006). Neuroimaging and genetic association in attentional and hypnotic processes. *Journal of Physiology*, 99, 483–491.

Rosenbaum, M. (1980). The role of the term schizophrenia in the decline of diagnoses of multiple personality. *Archives of General Psychiatry*, 37, 1383–1385.

Shengold, L. (1989). *Soul Murder: The Effects of Childhood Abuse and Deprivation*. New Haven, CT: Yale University Press.

Shor, R. (1972). Hypnosis and the concept of the generalized reality-orientation. In C. T. Tart (Ed.), *Altered States of Consciousness, 2nd edition* (pp. 239–267). New York: Anchor/Doubleday. (reprint of 1959 article)

Spiegel, D. (1986). Dissociating damage. *American Journal of Clinical Hypnosis*, 29, 123–131.

Ullman, R. and Brothers, D. (1993). *The Shattered Self: A Psychoanalytic Study of Trauma.* New York: Routledge.

Van der Kolk, B. (2015). *The Body Keeps the Score: Brain, Mind, and Body in the Healing of Trauma*. New York: Penguin.

Waelder, R. (1962). Psychoanalysis, scientific method, and philosophy. *Journal of the American Psychoanalytic Association*, 10, 617–637.

Yehuda, R. and Bierer, L. (2009). The relevance of epigenetics to PTSD: Implications for *DSM-5*. *Journal of Traumatic Stress*, 22, 427–434.

Yehuda, R., Daskalakis, N., Desarnaud, F., Makotkine, I., Lehrner, A., Koch, E., and Bierer, L. (2013). Epigenetic biomarkers as predictors and correlates of symptom improvement following psychotherapy in combat veterans with PTSD. *Frontiers of Psychiatry*, 4, 118.

Yehuda, R., Daskalakis, N., Lehrner, A., Desarnaud, F., Bader, H., Makotkine, I., and Meaney, M. (2014). Influences of maternal and paternal PTSD on epigenetic regulation of the glucocorticoid receptor gene in Holocaust survivor offspring. *American Journal of Psychiatry*, 171, 872–880.

Chapter Ten

Psychoanalytic Aspects of Psychosomatics

Richard Cruz

The complex relationship between mental and emotional life and bodily health and illness is a perennial subject of inquiry. There is mounting evidence that chronic difficulties with self-regulation, hyperarousal, anxiety, and depression affect somatic illness through psychoneuroimmune mechanisms. In this chapter, psychoanalytic literature is reviewed on somatization and its relation to mentalization, affect regulation, and attachment. Implications for psychotherapy and psychoanalytic technique are discussed. Selected literature is also reviewed on self-states and dissociation in physical/neurological illness in childhood and adulthood and on treatment approaches.

BIOLOGICAL MEDIATORS OF STRESS

Chronic psychological stress renders the hypothalamus-pituitary-adrenal (HPA) axis either overactive or underactive, and is associated with abnormal inflammatory activity involving cytokines (Luyten et al. 2012). Luyten also notes that with increasing levels of stress, patients rely excessively on maladaptive secondary attachment strategies, either avoidant or clinging, and have mentalizing impairments, particularly in embodied mentalizing, difficulty reflecting on one's bodily experiences and sensations, and their relationship to mental and emotional states in self and others (ibid.). Recently appreciated psychoneuroimmune effects include the importance of T cells in memory and learning and the increased risk of depression and cardiac disease posed by elevated cytokines (Arehart-Treichel 2012).

EARLY PSYCHOSOMATIC CONCEPTS

Early in the psychoanalytic literature (Kaplan 1980) there is a broad conceptualization of the dynamics of conversion hysteria applied beyond the symbolic expression of unconscious conflict in organs innervated by the voluntary neuromuscular and sensory-motor nervous system to the proposed expression of specific unconscious fantasies in clearly organic symptoms such as fever and bleeding (Groddeck 1929) and in disturbances in organs innervated by the involuntary/autonomic nervous system, e.g., bleeding in ulcerative colitis (Ferenczi 1926). Alexander later distinguished psychosomatic symptoms as occurring only in organ systems innervated by the autonomic-sympathetic/parasympathetic nervous system and having no specific psychic meaning as in classical conversion hysteria, but being the results of prolonged physiological stress states (1950).

Alexander's concepts drew on research by Canon on physiological aspects of the "fight or flight" response and by Selye on the general adaptation syndrome to stress associated with adrenal cortical hormonal activation. Alexander, French, and Pollock (1968) went on to propose a series of fixed unconscious conflictual constellations in several illnesses including asthma, peptic ulcer, hypertension, rheumatoid arthritis, hyperthyroidism, and ulcerative colitis. Repressed hostility was hypothesized in essential hypertension, and fear of self-destructive impulses was surmised in hyperthyroidism. Fear of separation and dependency conflicts were noted in asthma with asthma attacks being seen as "suppressed cries" for mother. A number of investigators have gone on to propose constellations of maladaptive personality traits in other physical illness. Hard driving "Type A" heart attack prone personalities have been described by Dunbar (1954) and by Friedman and Rosenman (1959, 1970) with physiological characteristics of adrenal cortical activation and elevated serum lipids. Bahnson and Bahnson (1969) describes "cancer prone" personalities who deny and repress conflict, seldom project for defense, and hypothetically somaticize depression over losses as neoplasm. The preceding defense/personality constellation theories have been criticized as not applying to all or even most cases of the same disease. The speculative work on cancer seems not so different from Groddeck's mysterious transformation of id to organic illness in a complicated multifactorial disease (1929).

SOMATIZATION, MENTALIZATION, AND ATTACHMENT THEORY

In the 1960s and early 1970s, psychosomatic researchers in France and the United States described a "psychosomatic personality" (McDougall 1989) style. "La pensee operatoire" or operatory thinking is described as "a pragmatic and affectless way of relating both to oneself and to other people, a form of relationship that appears to be largely delibidinized" (McDougall 1989; Marty & de M'Uzan 1963). Sifneos described "alexithymic" characteristics in psychosomatic patients, including "a relative constriction in emotional functioning, poverty of fantasy life, and inability to find appropriate words to describe their emotions" (Sifneos 1973, p. 1). This deficit in verbal emotional expression has been hypothesized to be a sort of neurological deficit (Hoppe & Boogen 1977; Jessimer & Markham 1997; Lane 1997) that predisposes the patient to experience emotional disturbance as bodily distress in the absence of an adequate verbal outlet. Sifneos (1973) saw "alexithymic" patients as poor candidates for psychoanalytic psychotherapy.

McDougall, by contrast, writes of psychosomatic patients she has worked with intensively in psychoanalytic psychotherapy or analysis, suffering from an apparent "absence of affect":

> The word that seemed most appropriate to describe them was that they were "disaffected." In coining this term I hoped to indicate that such people had in fact experienced overwhelming emotion that threatened to attack their sense of integrity and identity. This hypothesis challenged the theory of neuroanatomical defects, based on observations in psychosomatic centers, as an explanatory hypothesis to account for the phenomenon of alexithymia. I came to the conclusion that my patients, unable to repress the ideas linked to emotional pain and equally unable to project these feelings delusionally onto the representations of other people, simply ejected them from consciousness. They were not suffering from an inability to experience or express emotion, but from an inability to contain and reflect over an excess of affective experience (McDougall 1989, pp. 93–94).

Over subsequent decades, controversy has ensued over questions about the restrictive affect and impaired symbolization noted in psychosomatic patients, more commonly referred to as alexithymia in American and English psychoanalytic and psychosomatic literature. What is the relationship to somatization? What is the etiology? What is the best treatment approach?

Somatization has been defined (Moore & Fine 1990, p. 183) as:

> the tendency to react to stimuli (including drives, defenses, and conflict between them) physically rather than psychically. Also termed (by Flanders Dunbar) the somatic short circuit, somatization describes the shift of psychic energy toward expression in somatic symptoms. Somatization includes both conversion reactions and organ-neurotic (psychophysiological) disorders.

It is hypothesized (Nemiah, Freyberger, & Sifneos 1976; Nemiah 1977; Taylor, Bagby, & Parker 1997; Taylor & Bagby 2013, p. 104) that the alexithymic deficit in the cognitive processing of emotions leads to a focusing on, and amplification of, the somatic sensations accompanying emotional arousal, and/or to physical action as an immediate response to unpleasant arousal. This is thought to explain the proneness to somatization among high alexithymia individuals, as well as their tendency to regulate tension through compulsive behaviors such as smoking, binge eating, and abuse of alcohol or drugs.

Verhaeghe and colleagues (2007) questions whether alexithymia is a causative factor in somatization or an "accompanying side effect in a disordered state." Taylor (1993; Taylor & Bagby 2013) has reviewed studies noting high rates of alexithymia among patients with substance abuse disorders, panic disorder, and posttraumatic stress disorder (PTSD). Alexithymia overlaps with autistic spectrum disorder involving core disturbances in speech and language and social relationships (Frith 2004; Fitzgerald & Bellgrove 2006; Hill, Berth, & Frith 2004). Taylor (2003; Taylor & Bagby 2013) cites studies noting high levels of alexithymia in functional gastrointestinal disorders and essential hypertension but lower levels among patients with Franz Alexander's other so-called classic psychosomatic illnesses (1950). Taylor and Bagby (2013) notes that alexithymia can be associated with trauma and considered secondary to the dissociation (Bucci 1997) among the symbolic—verbal and imaginal—and subsymbolic—sensorimotor and visceral—elements within emotional schemas as a result of psychic trauma. High rates of alexithymia have been noted in Vietnam veterans with PTSD (Shipko, Alvarez, & Noviello 1983) and Holocaust survivors with PTSD (Yehuda et al. 1997).

Though the term somatization may be broadly used to encompass both conversion and other somatic disorders, a distinction can be made between conversion disorders as hysterical psychoneuroses and other somatic disorders including panic disorder, somatization, and somatoform disorder as actual neuroses conceptualized by Freud (McDougall 1980; Lichtman 2010; Taylor 2003; Verhaeghe, Vanheule, & de Rice 2007). Conversion disorders were conceptualized by Freud as involving repression of neurotic conflict with symptom formation related to intact symbolic thinking with:

> emotions represented cognitively as nameable feelings as well as sensations and associated images. Being an expression of conflictual repressed fantasies, the symptoms tell a story and follow psychic laws. In contrast, in patients with somatization symptoms, emotions are not well represented symbolically and there is a lack of underlying fantasy activity. In these patients, the symptoms begin in the body and follow somatic laws. Whereas conversion symptoms involve higher-order neurocognitive functioning, somatization symptoms involve lower level physiological perturbations (Kirmayer and Santhanam 2001; Taylor 2003, p. 503).

Gottlieb (2003) and Lichtman (2010) note that Janet (1889) conceptualized short-circuiting of mind and somatization of pathology without symbolic recognition of conflict.

Taylor and Bagby (2013, p. 118) notes etiological possibilities for alexithymia that include an inherited trait, the impact of trauma in childhood or adulthood, and the result of interaction between a vulnerable temperament and environmental/developmental factors. Taylor and Bagby (2013) and Katz (2010) both comment that McDougall relates alexithymia to deficits in the mental representation of emotions and empathic failure in the early mother-child relationship. McDougall (1989, p. 47) tells us that in "grave psychosomatic illnesses, it has been my experience that certain highly charged emotional thoughts which the mother cannot bear, become totally forbidden or foreclosed thoughts for her child." Katz (2010) remarks that the overwhelmed caregiver may not be able to maintain enough sense of separateness from what the troubled child is feeling to soothe the child and contain and symbolize the feelings. The child may then be left in a state of rageful hyperarousal without words to help contain the experience that will affect the body. Katz further notes that "the achievement of psychological separation . . . is a barrier to severe psychosomatic illness," presumably because the awareness of another's psychic experience as different requires symbolic representation with which emotional experience can be reflected upon and contained.

Fonagy and Target (1997; Fongay et al. 2002; Fongay, Bateman, & Luten 2012) have developed a broad construct of mentalization which incorporates attachment theory and which has implications for understanding alexithymia, in that it involves the caretaker's trying to understand the emotional state and intentions of the child, mirroring the child such that the child feels recognized and affirmed and learns to understand himself as separate from his caretaker, and as able to put his feelings and intentions into words. Embodied mentalizing (Luyten et al. 2012, p. 124) is defined as "the capacity to see the body as the seat of emotions, wishes, and feelings and the capacity to reflect on one's own bodily experiences and sensations and their relationships to intentional mental states in the self and others." Having developed the ability to represent and symbolize internal states, the child is assumed to have a capacity for self-regulation (Pedersen, Poulson, & Lunn 2015). Luyten and colleagues (2012) proposes an interactive relationship between stress regulation, attachment, and mentalization relevant to functional somatic disorders including chronic fatigue syndrome, fibromyalgia, temporomandibular pain syndrome, and chronic pelvic pain. The capacity for mentalization is conceptualized as fostered by secure attachment and good enough mothering in early preoedipal development, and is hypothesized to promote resilience to high levels of stress in later life, reinforcing secure attachment, personal agency, and affect regulation. The capacity to mentalize is "context dependent and cannot be maintained by anyone across all contexts" of interpersonal and physical stress (Pedersen et al. 2015, p. 673). Luyten et al. (2012, p. 125) see insecure attachment and early adverse experience as increasing vulnerability to stress-related disorders including functional somatic disorders in patients with biological, genetic, and neurophysiological predisposition, through dysfunction of the hypothalamic-pituitary-adrenal axis and associated immune reactions.

Luyten (2012, p. 128) questions whether alexithymia is the cause of functional somatic disorders since "empirical research clearly suggests that only a limited subgroup of patients with functional somatic disorders (i.e., those with a history of severe attachment disruptions and/or trauma) show clinically elevated levels of alexithymia and lack of emotional awareness" (Pedrosa Gil et al. 2008). Impairments in embodied mentalizing in functional somatic disorders are often related to specific experiences and physical symptoms rather than to general deficits in emotional awareness, and are the consequence rather than the cause of functional somatic disorders and involve high arousal or stress. "Symptoms can be considered as an 'attack' on the capacity to reflect, particularly on the capacity to see the body as a 'lived body' that one has ownership of and is fundamental in our relatedness to others." (Luyten et al. 2012, 128). Luyten (ibid.) cites the work of Driver (2005), who describes "the 'otherness of the illness' in chronic fatigue syndrome patients which leads to regressive fears and fantasies," and the work of Schattner and colleagues (2008), who describes lupus patients, dreaming of their illness as an "internal object," "some sort of creature," who threatens the individual from within and needs to be calmed.

Luyten (ibid., p. 127) describes a regressive process, in which mentalizing impairments and maladaptive "secondary attachment strategies" may be a consequence of functional somatic disorders. "Attachment deactivating" strategies regulate stress by denying attachment needs, while "attachment hyperactivating" strategies involve demanding, clinging behavior. Such chronic interpersonal stress may further aggravate functional somatic disorders.

Luyten (ibid., p. 131) concludes that although impairments in mentalizing and "alexithymic" features are often the result rather than the cause of functional somatic disorders, interventions aimed at recovery of this capacity can be expected to be effective. Pedersen et al. (2015) question whether an ability to mentalize necessarily entails a capacity to regulate affects. He cites the cases of five women with bulimia nervosa who have a high ability to mentalize on a Reflective Functioning Scale but have difficulty regulating emotions and use the eating disorder to compensate for these difficulties. These women "are relatively skilled at reflecting on their own and others' thoughts and emotions" (Pedersen et al. 2015, p. 671) but leave the "impression of girls who far too early in life were forced to relate more to their parents' emotions than to their own" (Pedersen et al. 2015, pp. 691–92) as a survival skill in chaotic family environments. One suspects that these struggling women have impaired embodied mentalization despite having the capacity to reflect on their own and others' emotions.

TREATMENT CONSIDERATIONS

DeWolf (2014), reporting from the Netherlands, notes that 20 to 50 percent of primary care doctors' patients have unexplained somatic complaints and 16 percent have somatoform disorder. These somatizing patients have a three times higher incidence of anxiety and depression. Of these patients 50 to 75 percent improve over a year and 10 to 30 percent deteriorate. The subsequent risk of real somatic disease is small, for example, 1 percent for patients initially diagnosed with irritable bowel syndrome and 0 to 12 percent for patients initially diagnosed with conversion disorder. He estimates that less than a third of these patients would be psychologically minded and amenable to referral for psychotherapy. He notes that Karen Horney observed as early as the 1940s and 1950s that "psychosomatic patients did poorly in psychoanalytic treatment because of a lack of emotional awareness, paucity of inner experience, minimal interest in dreams, concrete way of thinking and an externalized style of living" (DeWolf 2014, p. 32).

Taylor and Bagby (2013, p. 103) note that:

> psychoanalysts have continued to report that patients with a high degree of alexithymia make little progress in psychoanalysis or psychoanalytic psychotherapy. McDougall (1972, 1984) referred to these patients as anti-analysands and used the word disaffected to describe their affect pathology; she warned of the potential for prolonged periods of "stagnation" if they are taken into analysis. And Krystal (1982–1983, 364) concluded that "alexithymia is possibly the most important single factor diminishing the success of psychoanalysis and psychoanalytic psychotherapy." There was general agreement that the communicative style of alexithymic patients often evokes feelings of dullness, boredom, and frustration in the therapist.

Despite pessimism that psychoanalytic treatment is contraindicated in functional somatic disorders, a meta-analysis of clinical trials of several short-term dynamic psychotherapies suggests efficacy for a range of somatic disorders (Abbass, Kisely, & Kroenke 2009). In considering treatment options for functional somatic disorders a recent short-term dynamic psychotherapy model based on Fonagy and associates, mentalization and attachment theory (Luyten et al. 2012) will be outlined. Case studies of longer-term psychoanalytic psychotherapy by McDougall (1974), Ogden (1999), and Katz (2010) will also be reviewed with a focus on countertransference.

Luyten outlines a sixteen-session course of treatment which focuses on "restoring the capacity for stress regulation by a focus on (a) typical attachment strategies in response to stress and (b) recovery of the capacity for (embodied) mentalizing" (Luyten et al. 2012, p. 131). He sees the first 4 sessions as engagement of the patient and formulation of an interpersonal affective focus for treatment. The therapist works to identify core anxieties mobilized by starting therapy and attachment to the therapist. Initial sessions often focus on past experiences of being misunderstood, which are explored along with the attachment activation or deactivation strategies elicited to manage the anticipated experience of being misunderstood. Shared understanding of what might go wrong may help avert premature ending of therapy or other avoidant behavior. The therapist resists forcing biopsychosocial theory on the patient but tries to use the patient's own experience to demonstrate how psychosocial factors may affect physical symptoms, recognizing limitations to discussing these issues posed by variable impairment in mentalizing associated with exacerbation of physical symptoms. Arriving at the interpersonal affective focus involves "identifying a recurrent cognitive-affective relational or attachment pattern that is associated with onset and perpetuation of symptoms . . . underpinned by a . . . non-conscious representation of self-in-relation-to-another and a defensive function of this constellation" (Luyten et al. 2012, p. 132). For example, a patient with avoidant, attachment deactivating defenses might see himself as autonomous and well intentioned in relation to others who are seen as judgemental and nonunderstanding. Depression, anger, and helplessness may be accompanied by denial of feelings of dependency with frustrated "attempts to gain approval and love of others" (ibid., p. 132). By contrast, a patient with clinging, attachment hyperactivating defenses might see himself as caring and concerned, perhaps a compulsive caregiver, while others are seen as indifferent and uncaring. The interpersonal affective focus is aimed at collaboratively addressing maladaptive, self-defeating defenses that attempt to compensate for feelings of helplessness and hopelessness.

Luyten describes the middle phase of sessions 5 to 12 as working through and consolidation, focusing on "the patient's ability to reflect on the (bodily) self, others and the self-in-relation-to others" (ibid., p. 133). Patients with avoidant, attachment deactivating defenses are often seen as adopting a dualistic "mind is 'the self' and body is the 'other'" view of their subjective experience.

> The focus is on reinvestment of the body with positive affective meanings and linking interpersonal experiences with bodily experiences and vice versa (e.g., recognizing that feeling "tense" may actually mean that one is angry at someone). In patients using hyperactivating strategies, this phase often entails finding words to express feelings and to differentiate between different sensations,

> feelings and experiences. For many patients, this implies changes in terms of a life narrative characterized by incoherence and inconsistence toward a more coherent view of one's own past and present, and the relationship between both. In general, during this phase, a different way of relating to one's bodily self and to others emerges, fostering broaden-and-build cycles associated with more effective regulation of distress. Interventions in this phase include (a) supportive interventions (i.e., reassurance support, empathy), (b) basic mentalizing interventions aimed at affect recognition, differentiation, and amplification as well as more advanced expressive techniques such as interpretation, and addressing the transference relationship when appropriate, and (c) directive techniques (e.g., encouraging the patient to try out new ways of relating) (ibid., p. 133).

The final phase of sessions 13 to 16 in Luyten's program is described as "empowerment." A "goodbye" letter is written by the therapist and shared with the patient, aimed at reviewing work to date, focusing on the final sessions, and providing a reference once therapy is over. Luyten finds such letters can be both supportive and challenging, perhaps provoking strong affects including anxiety and depression over ending. The letter aims to realistically appraise gains, disappointments, and future vulnerabilities and risk of relapse. Directive techniques are described as central in this phase to empower patients, encouraging them to "actively explore and try out new ways of thinking, feeling, and relating to others and themselves" (ibid., p. 134). Luyten cautions that the therapist may overestimate the patient's reflective capacities particularly when stressed over interpersonal issues. "Interventions that strongly rely on insight and reflective capacities are therefore likely to be more harmful than helpful" (ibid., p. 134–35), perhaps in patients with "more significant biological and/or environmental vulnerability and psychiatric comorbidity." Such patients may benefit in addition from longer-term psychotherapy, pain management, physical therapy, psychiatric medication, family interventions, and social casework.

Longer-term psychoanalytic psychotherapies and psychoanalyses involving psychosomatic patients or psychosomatic countertransference reactions have been reported by highly experienced clinicians including McDougall (1974, 1980, 1989), Ogden (1999), and Katz (2010). Such treatments are often described as very difficult for patient and analyst alike with the potential for impasses and negative therapeutic reactions. These analysts have often found understanding of countertransference important to their work.

McDougall (1974, pp. 458–59) notes:

> Much of the success or failure of the analysis of the psychosomatic dimensions of the personality depend on the extent to which the transference is able to bear the coming alive of archaic instinctual impulses, and consequent ego perturbation. Perhaps the limits of the analytic process in these cases are the limits of the analyst. One does not always "survive" as an inner object for one's patients

> and then the mother-nursling failure is repeated once more and the psychosomatic defences hold firm. On the other hand the analytic process can produce overwhelming change even though to do this may lead the rock to feel great pain and the island to cry for many years to come (a reference to Simon and Garfunkel's folksong "I Am a Rock").

In 1980 McDougall (pp. 457–459) commented that,

> everybody possesses a certain "psychosomatic potentiality personality" which reveals itself under conditions of psychic stress . . . so-called normal neurotics (which we could suppose includes the majority of psychoanalysts) with today's longer analyses invariably come to reveal the sectors of their personality structure where there too, somatic symptoms, narcissistic problems, addictive behavior, second-hand ideas and discharge in action have taken the place of psychic work—of thinking and feeling, . . . a burden . . . frequently painful and humiliating.

McDougall (1989, p. 13) recalls her own childhood reaction of a recurrent rash precipitated by visits with her strong-willed grandmother. After working with an alcohol-addicted parent of a psychotic child, McDougall (2001, p. 7) resolved to quit smoking, and became more aware of painful affects that prompted her to smoke, as if to get rid of her feelings. McDougall (1980, p. 457) contrasts normal neurotics with psychosomatic patients who are "more exposed to serious psychosomatic organization than those who have constructed neurotic barriers—or even psychotic ones—against psychic conflict and stressful circumstances." She reflects that she came to question her earlier view of psychosomatic patients as "devoid of repressed fantasy content capable of being verbalized . . . with no direct symbolic meaning such as we find in the unconscious structure behind neuroses . . . and radical elimination of any representation of intense affect" when she found that some patients revealed in analysis what she termed "archaic hysteria," "back and forth movement between somatization and massive anxiety state . . . concerned to ward off fears of imminent death, bodily disintegration and loss of identity feeling—psychotic rather than neurotic symptoms" (McDougall 1980, pp. 457–58).

In *Theaters of the Body* (1989, pp. 55–67) McDougall gives a vignette from the analysis of a psychiatrist who struggles with depression and irritable bowel syndrome after the suicide of a woman patient, to:

> illustrate a certain type of mental functioning which in my opinion increases psychosomatic vulnerability (among other possible symptomatic outcomes). Such mental structures appear to become organized in early childhood, when the mother-child relationship has failed to give rise to an internal representation with caretaking functions (with which the child needs eventually to identify if he is to acquire the capacity for both physical and mental self-care). On

> the one hand, there is an idealized, inaccessible, and omnipotent mother-image, potentially able to take away all suffering and satisfy every wish; however, this plays a persecutory role in that the child can neither deserve nor attain this grandiose ideal. On the other hand, there is a rejecting and death-bearing image of mother with whom the child, once he has become an adult, will identify, consequently behaving in similar manner to his own child-self. When, in addition, the father appears to have played a rather muted role in the child's life, being therefore represented in his inner world as someone indifferent to his child's well-being, such patients act as shockingly careless parents towards themselves. They tend to look either to the world of others or to addictive substances to repair their sense of damage. These combined factors contribute to a disturbed sense of subjective identity with a concomitant lack of distinction between self and object. This favors the persistence of unrecognized psychotic anxieties regarding one's bodily and psychic integrity and eventually facilitates psychosomatic expressions (McDougall 1989, p. 58).

McDougall's patient suffers a bout of irritable bowel syndrome during the analyst's vacation break. Upon McDougall's return the patient's associations to his bowel symptoms include his frustration with his wife for wanting a third child and a horrible nightmare of roasting and cannibalizing a child. His further associations include recalling a similar dream reported by his psychotic patient who reported a dream of boiling her youngest (the third) child before suiciding by setting herself on fire. He complains "I can't bear to think I made this dream. The very thought makes me ill . . . I'm as psychotic as my patient. I understand now why she committed suicide. I feel such hatred for myself. I can't tolerate this dream" (McDougall 1989, p. 62–63). The patient explores with McDougall his sense of guilt as a "baby killer," not wanting his wife to have a third child as he didn't want his emotionally unavailable mother and physically injured, depressed father to have another child. He elaborates on his guilt over his patient's suicide, calling himself "an incapable murderous mother" to his patient. McDougall hypothesizes that during her absence, primitive archaic fantasies were mobilized for her patient and that his body "reacted as though it had been poisoned because he was deprived of the knowledge of wordless fears and the primitive fantasies that were just becoming capable of verbalization" as if there was a "breakdown in dream functioning . . . no adequate discharge of tension through hallucinatory dream formation, nor does the psychic structure lead to psychotic manifestations." She continues that perhaps her patient "felt the need to be back in the analytic relationship before allowing himself to make this frightening nightmare. Through my absence on vacation, I too no doubt joined the cohort of 'killer-mothers' in his internal world." She hypothesizes that the patient's mother "failed to ensure the basic maternal function of shielding against overwhelming stimuli both from within and from without" leading to the "creation of a 'false self' and . . . later of character defenses against psychotic anxieties . . . which mask a persecutory representation of his mother." She reports that colitis resolved as

> he became progressively more tolerant of his wild ("baby-killer") child-self and better able to parent his distressed child, he ceased identifying with the rejecting internal mother. He also began to allow the creation of dreams that more adequately fulfilled their function, so that the severity of his insomnia decreased. Little by little he ceased to react like "burned baby," became less lost in his everyday life, and actually began to look forward to creating a third baby with his wife, since he no longer needed this place for himself" (McDougall 1989, pp. 64–67).

In a panel discussion of psychosomatic case presentations by Joyce McDougall and Stanley Coen (2000), questions are raised about the difference between metaphoric attribution of meaning to somatic phenomena and the establishment of causality. McDougall (1989) hypothesizes that early trauma that cannot be encoded symbolically or be expressed verbally is expressed bodily. Charles Hanly (2011) similarly talks of "somatization . . . and 'desomatizing' retrieval of . . . repressed affects in the transference" (McDougall and Coen 2000), the mechanism of which is unclear. While analysis of some hysterical somatic symptoms such as pseudocyesis may reveal guilt over well-symbolized fantasies and wishes to be impregnated by an oedipal father, other psychosomatic patients present with more vague hypochondriacal symptoms without clear symbolic meaning. Coen (1992) advocates that "rather than conceiving of most somatic symptoms as themselves expressing conflicted wishes, it seems more appropriate to consider patients' affect tolerance and need for hypochondriacal elaboration with regressive, pathological modes of relatedness."

> Perhaps we do better to eschew causal mechanisms, as this panel's clinical material would seem to indicate, instead to examine a given patient's need to defend against and express conflict through an intense focus on bodily experience. We did not have access to clinical material demonstrative of McDougall's proposal that early unverbalised affects may be expressed somatically. As this panel illustrated, most patients shift their focus from bodily concern to psychic conflict, as they become able, with appropriate analytic help to tolerate previously unbearable feelings, wishes, and needs" (McDougall and Coen 2000, 160–61).

Related to the difficulties with maternal empathy, mirroring, and mentalization is Andre Green's concept of the Dead Mother (Kohon 1999). The concept of the "dead mother" describes a clinical phenomena in which "the mother remains alive, but she has psychically 'died' for the child. This produces a depression in the child, who carries these feelings within him or her into adult life, as the experience of the loss of mother's love is followed by the loss of meaning in life" (Kohon 1999, preface). Ogden (1999) describes his work with a woman civic leader with "diffuse anxiety" and the belief "that something was seriously wrong in her life." He describes struggling with at times overwhelming somatic countertransference feelings which:

> felt equivalent to losing the use of my mind. I experienced a form of claustrophobia during the hours and on occasion defended against this anxiety by obsessionally counting the minutes until the hour would be over. At other times I fantasied ending the hour prematurely by telling the patient that I was ill and needed to end the session. I would sometimes "pass the time" by counting the beats per minute of my radial pulse (Ogden 1999, p. 131).

Though Ogden does not describe the patient as having psychosomatic symptoms, he notes that the "patient's sense of deadness could not initially be symbolized and instead was enacted (entombed) in the lifelessness of the analytic experience itself" (Ogden 1999, p. 130). Ogden views his experience as part of the "intersubjective analytic third . . . understood as created by the unconscious interplay of analyst and analysand . . . an evolving experience that is continually in a state of flux as the intersubjectivity of the analytic process is transformed by the understanding generated by the analytic pair."(Ogden 1999, p. 131).

Ogden reflected on his fantasy that he "was being made ill by prolonged exposure to the lifelessness of the analysis" and "began to develop a sense of the meaning of the patient's diffuse anxiety and her sense that she was caught in something awful she could not identify." Ogden told her that he felt:

> she had given up on being able to create a life for herself. Instead she felt she was giving me the forms with which she had filled her time in hopes that I could create a life for her from these pieces. The patient responded by describing the way in which her life . . . consisted . . . of never actually making anything herself . . . but used other people's lives and the things that they made (the lives of her employees, her husband, her au pair, and her two children) as a substitute for her own ability to create something that felt like a life of her own (Ogden 1999, p. 132).

In subsequent months the patient recalled the death of a friend's child and went on to express that she felt she had "not been able to love and be with her children in the way that she wished she could have been." Ogden discerned the

> beginnings of a process in which the patient's experience of deadness (both in her imagined inability to grieve and in her identification with her friend's dead child) was being transformed from an unthinkable thing-in-itself (a fact experienced by both the patient and myself as a non-verbally symbolized sense of deadness of the analysis) into a living, verbally symbolized experience of the

> patient's (and my own) deadness in the analysis. An intersubjective analytic space had begun to be generated in which the deadness could be felt, viewed, experienced, and spoken about by the two of us. Deadness had become a feeling as opposed to a fact (Ogden 1999, p. 133).

Katz (2010) describes the analytic treatment of two women with multiple somatic problems and a history of severe trauma beginning when they were toddlers. She summarizes:

> although both were gifted verbally, some of the deepest and most authentic experiences in our work were derived from noting and then reflecting upon physical sensations or experiences they had in the room with me. The body became a vehicle into which unprocessed feelings were emptied. The words to say it, contain it, and reflect upon it came much later in the course of treatment" (Katz 2010, p. 430).

She describes patients who as young children suffered from their parent's empathic failures. Later difficulties with separation were associated with unstable self and object representations, and impaired self-soothing and mentalizing abilities. She describes her patients' conflicted relationships, depending on others as self-objects and attachment figures for self-regulation as well as meeting overdetermined needs for an outlet for aggression, self-punishment, and dependency needs. One of Katz's patients, a teacher, suffered multiple traumas including loss of a live-in nanny at age two and a half, sexual abuse by her father, a depressed Holocaust survivor, and later sexual molestation by an older cousin. As described by Katz, she

> used speech as a bodily way of processing thought, rather than as a technique for containing and reflecting upon her experience. Words, hers and mine, were at times objects of love and at times objects of hatred, and she used her mouth to incorporate or evacuate them. She accomplished the same kind of evacuation of chaotic or disturbing experience with other parts of her body as well—with her skin, her breathing, her sleep patterns—and in so doing established the "illnesses" that brought her to therapy (Katz 2010, p. 432).

Katz goes on to describe the patient's father as not helping her

> to modulate or contain the fears and passions that he kindled. On the contrary, when she woke up scared one night at the age of seven and came to him for solace, he dismissed her fears, telling her that she had to "learn to live with these things." Unable as yet to handle terror alone, (she) had her first asthma attack—a bodily expression of her longing for her mother (who was also an asthmatic, and who was not home that night) and her anger at her father for abandoning her to the fears that he himself had evoked (ibid., p. 433).

Katz notes that the patient idealized her early in the analysis, but

> her loving admiration shattered at the slightest disappointment or limit, and the eating and drinking would soon be followed by a dismissive spitting out. "I'm not into that psychoanalytic stuff . . . You don't know what you're talking about" . . . for a long time she was emotionally detached from her crucial memories and there was a disconnect between her verbal discourse and her nonverbal communications (ibid., p. 434).

The patient tentatively began to respond to Katz's line of interpretation that she was angry with the analyst for not helping her enough. The patient recalled a family story about her returning from camp when she was three and by her parents' report saying to a toy doll, "Don't worry. You don't need a mommy. I will take care of you." When Katz responded suggesting "that she was giving up on me as she had given up on her mother—hating me for not taking better care of her, she moaned and heaved a sigh. This had happened before, but this time (she) recognized a link between what was going on in her mind and what happened in her body and commented, 'Something is happening when I begin to moan.'" Katz continues that her patient's

> memories were so dissociated from affect that for a long time, the only access we had to her affective experience was through mine. When I found myself tearful, or angry, or afraid in response to a memory that (she) recalled only in a detached way, I would communicate these feelings to her so that she could locate them in herself–she experienced them physically, in a heaviness in her chest, say, or in moaning sounds. When she could feel them, she could believe that they belonged to her. This helped her gradually integrate them into her own mind and experience. We concentrated on the messages her body conveyed and slowly began to marry her bodily experience with her memories, and open them up to reflection and words, the tools of mindfulness . . . (her) body which had been for a long time the dumping ground of a disempowered psyche, became our best source of psychological insight. When she felt understood by me, (she) might experience a twinge in her stomach or her vagina. Through these bodily changes, as opposed to the facile but soon discarded intellectualized verbal insights of our early work, she became, for the first time aware, and mindful of her own emotional experience. We paid close attention to the way (she) dealt with psychological discomfort by expelling it from awareness and to how those attempted expulsions were reflected in physical symptoms. When she tried to keep from voicing her irritation at a student who reminded her of things she hated in herself, her throat would start to itch. We came to understand that she was stifling her own voice, the voice that was itching to express her anger. Itches like that, (she) told me, were always an asthma precursor, and asthma was an old symptom associated with being alone and uncared for (ibid., p. 434–50).

In Katz's view (ibid., p. 430), separation and independence are a threat to her psychosomatic patients—associated with punishment or abandonment. Dependence, either in a loving relationship or in illness, is also a threat risking invasion and shame. This is seen as due to a lack of emotional object constancy and mentalizing and self-soothing abilities from early parental failures in empathy, mirroring, and emotional containment. She sees her nonmentalizing, poorly verbalizing, patients as having "few ways of expressing power except through their bodies" and sees treatment as providing the containment through embodied mentalizing that "parents had failed to offer while she was young."

ALIEN SELF-STATES AND SELF-REGULATION IN PHYSICAL HANDICAPS

Much of the previously reviewed psychosomatic literature has focused on what might be conceptualized as dissociated psychosomatic self-states often associated with a history of abuse, neglect, and/or early parental failures in empathy, mentalizing, and emotional containment. Dissociated self-states may also be seen in physical and neurological handicaps both developmentally in childhood and in adults who have severe illnesses. These patients might be seen as struggling with traumatic internal overstimulation associated with their illnesses. Relationships with caretakers and attachment figures also play a critical role. Adaptation to physical illness in childhood or adulthood can be seen as an interaction between coping abilities shaped by early object relations and ability to mentalize, the vicissitudes and severity of the patient's illness, and the patient's relationship with significant others including attachment figures who may serve as self-objects, assisting with self-regulation. Disturbances in mentalizing process may reflect the effect of trauma as well as the effect of nonadequate mirroring (DeWolf 2014). An experience reported in physical illnesses is the sense of an "Alien Self" (DeWolf 2014), "one's body starts feeling like an 'alien self-part,' a machine that is out of control" (Luyten et al. 2012), or a "'little man,' 'the dwarf,' 'the imp' or the like within themselves" (Niederland 1965). It is of interest how specific illnesses result in traumatic overstimulation and impair ego functioning and mentalizing abilities.

The sense of self and treatment approaches are outlined in several psychotherapy case vignettes of neurological disorders including a child with Tourette's disorder, an adult with spasmodic torticollis, an adult with chronic fatigue syndrome and encephalomyelitis, and adults suffering catastrophic cerebrovascular insults.

Tourette's syndrome is a disorder of the basal ganglia with chronic motor and vocal tics, which begins in early grade school or even preschool years, progresses in severity in adolescence, and may diminish in adulthood. Cohen (1991) sees Tourette's patients as having the ego deficit of a defective stimulus barrier which renders them vulnerable to traumatic sensory-motor tics.

Tics may be associated with a psychotic–like blurring of ego boundaries. For example, a depressed eight-year-old boy sees "a face melting in and out of the wall" as he experiences a repetitive facial tic (Cruz 2002). The boy also lies on the floor in the office and repeatedly shrugs his shoulders and quacks. He talks about peers in school mocking him and calling him the "Penguin," referring to a villain in Batman superhero comics. In fantasy play he elaborates on the story of the "Penguin" being abandoned, flushed down the sewer, by his parents who can't bear to look at his defective out of control body. He plays out the "Penguin" taking revenge on the citizens of Gotham City. Another ominous squawking bird "Pipsqueak" appears and foretells that the "Penguin" is coming to "shake up" the city. The boy proceeds to play out stories about another aggressive villain/superhero, the doomsday robot "Terminator" in Arnold Schwarzenegger films. He appears to play out fantasies of what might be wrong with him, having Tourette's syndrome, and what might be done to fix him. Can the "Terminator's" brain chip be replaced or reprogrammed to permanently change him from a dangerous predator to a strong protector of the weak? If he cannot be fixed, the only solution is to leave him to self-destruct by exploding or melting into a cauldron of liquid metal. Therapy is aimed at helping the boy with his disorganizing rage over feeling unwanted and unloved by his parents and peers due to his neurological defect. The handicapped child's angry sense of being unloved and unwanted as he is has been noted by Freud (1915), Jacobson (1959), and Winnicott (1917). DeWolf (2014, p. 59) hypothesizes that "when a child cannot develop a representation of his own experience (the self) through adequate parental mirroring, he internalizes the image of the rejecting caregiver as part of his self-representation, a discontinuity within the self, an 'alien self.'"

The treatment approach to a child with Tourette's includes psychoeducation of child, parents, and school staff, aimed at understanding and acceptance of embarrassing tics which the child has little control over. Individual psychoanalytic psychotherapy often also focuses on the child's fear of losing control, heightened by his tics, and questioning superstitious magical thinking which inhibits the child in socializing and productive activity. Superstitious thinking may be seen as "omen formation" (Terr 1984), when a child searches for predictive omens and distorts time sequences, struggling to deal with unbearable helplessness associated with psychic trauma. Terr's observations on the formation of omens and retrospective significances in victims of psychic trauma may contribute to the understanding of the development of sensorimotor premonitory experiences in patients with Tourette's syndrome. Leckman (1992) notes that such premonitory experiences are reported three to five years after the initial onset of tics. In this boy's case the ominous little bird "Pipsqueak" heralding the "Penguin" wreaking havoc, likely reflects his attempt to explain the traumatic ego-alien experiences of Tourette's syndrome including premonitory sensations prior to the discharge of tics. Terr (1984, p. 650) notes that "a traumatized child or adult sifts through the past repeatedly until he discovers the 'reason' he suffers. This reason or 'omen' becomes a permanently grafted appendage to the psychic trauma."

Taylor (1993) reports the case of an angry avoidant thirty-one year old man suffering from acute onset of spasmodic torticollis, a disorder of the basal ganglia with involuntary spasms of his neck muscles that resulted in a sustained torsion of his head. He has symptoms of depersonalization and complains that his torticollis is "killing him." He is troubled by angry dreams in which he "deliberately smashed a glass sculpture of a woman or some other glass object" (Taylor 1993, p. 586). The patient's subsequent dreams and associations about cold, distant, rejecting women led Taylor to conceptualize:

> the failure of (his) mother to establish a close bond of understanding and enjoyment of her child . . . left (him) deprived of a maternal introject with soothing and protective functions. Instead, the maternal image was split into a cold and persecutory representation that threatened psychic or even physical death, along with an idealized part-object that offered comfort and love (Taylor 1993, p. 585).

Taylor reports that "acknowledging his awareness of the patient's psychic pain and linking it to the deficiencies in family relationships . . . restored a stabilizing positive transference and helped activate memories of pleasant childhood experiences with an aunt" (Taylor 1993, p. 586) as a sort of idealized adoptive mother. Taylor's treatment narrative moves back and forth between periods of disorganizing rage and chaotic violent fantasies (the patient verbalizing fears that he could be a murderer, rapist, or child molester) often precipitated by the analyst's empathic failures and periods of consolidation in which the patient reflects on his rage being excessive and hurtful and restrains himself from verbally attacking his girlfriend and the analyst, wishing to repair the relationships, feeling that these are caring relationships to be valued. Taylor reports that torticollis remitted about three years into a six-year course of weekly psychoanalytic psychotherapy. He summarizes that:

> throughout the analytic treatment, attention was given to repairing deficits in the patient's self-organization, and to elevating chaotic impulses and inchoate emotions from a primitive sensorimotor level of experience to a mature representational level where they could be valued for their signal function and modulated through imaginal activity and communication with others. Analysis of the patient's pathologic internal object relations modified his self-organization, and enabled him to establish regulatory interpersonal relationships that complemented his enhanced self-regulatory capacities (Taylor 1993, p. 592).

Driver (2005) reports the case of a twenty-six-year-old woman with chronic fatigue syndrome and myalgic encephalomyelitis who is depressed and unable to work. The patient suffered from chronic migraine headaches in sessions and the analyst also found herself experiencing headaches in the sessions. The analyst interpreted "Perhaps you are wanting me to know what the headaches feel like so I will be able to unravel what causes them." The analyst took the patient's response, "No, you don't mean you've got the headaches, do you?" (Driver 2005, p. 159) as evidence that the patient feared that the analyst experienced the headaches as an "unconscious aggressive attack" from the patient. Driver's countertransference feeling was that the patient "could not/would not use (the analyst) as a maternal object," reminding the analyst of Andre Green's concept of the Dead Mother.

> It was impossible at this stage for (her) to think about her headaches as a part of herself or reflect on the experience of the headaches in terms of what they might be communicating . . . the headaches were experienced as persecutory objects and unconscious attacks that were "killing her off" and there was a parallel anxiety and "belief" that they killed off anything that could process them. . . . Within my countertransference I felt that she was communicating her desperation and anger towards an unresponsive, helpless mother. The attack . . . expressed through headaches remained . . . split off . . . unavailable to conscious thought . . . (ibid., pp. 159–60).

The analyst describes the patient's swings between exhausting overactivity and passive underactivity and "her ignoring of her needs (that) seemed to reflect the 'absent' or dead mother who was too lost or internally preoccupied to reflect on and process experience" (ibid., p. 160). She goes on to remark that:

> The pressure to be active, either by the patient or countertransferentially within the analyst, is immense . . . over activity defends against the fear of "nothingness," . . . the deathlike sense of underactivity, . . . (and the) lack of an internal maternal reflective function . . . my interpretations from my counter-transference were partly organized around trying to connect thought to experience and partly to reflect on the symbolic and transference dynamics in relation to Jane's internal world and her internal objects (ibid., pp. 164–67).

The analyst remarks that the analytic process helped "to develop the capacity of her ego to relate to her body-self and her psyche-self so that needs, issues, and conflicts could be struggled with, made more conscious and not collapse into symmetry (poles of 'just' the physiological or 'just' the psychological) and confusion" (ibid., p. 170).

Salas (2012) describes the cases of several patients who experience catastrophic reactions with an altered sense of self, a "disorganized inner state," after acute brain injury. He proposes that catastrophic reactions activate

> attachment mechanisms by default, mobilizing the patient to look for a significant other to regulate him/herself from outside . . . high levels of arousal, triggered by a catastrophic reaction during interpersonal conflict, impact on mentalizing, which is a self-regulatory function that generates representations of our own and other's mental states . . . lesions to different brain areas might impair specific self-regulatory and other self-other regulatory components, requiring adaptation of psychotherapeutic technique to these particular profiles (Salas 2012, p. 77).

He describes the case of a seventy-year-old professor with a dominant hemisphere stroke and expressive language difficulties. He is near panic at times when he struggles to express himself but is calmed by the presence of his family. Conversations among several people are particularly frustrating with interruptions, topic changes, and changes in tense. He manages to communicate more comfortably one on one, "especially . . . when he feels calm and knows people will wait until his ideas emerge." He prepares for conversation and his orderly presentation is a way of "preserving the words that may allow him to describe how he feels . . . protecting his valued but scarce thoughts" (ibid., p. 79).

Salas (ibid., 78) notes that "in more tragic circumstance, brain damage may also impair the capacity to use others as a source of external regulation—for example by compromising the ability to emotionally connect to others." A married man develops acute paranoid jealousy of his wife after a traumatic brain injury to his right frontal and parietal regions, associated with deficits in memory and emotional object constancy. His therapist notes: "To him I existed only when I presented myself concretely in front of him" (ibid., p. 84). The patient has profound difficulty with self-regulation and using others as a source of self-regulation, since potentially self-soothing, mentalizing ability, understanding his emotions and intentions and his wife's, is impaired along with his memory difficulties. The wife becomes increasingly frustrated with her husband and has increasing difficulty with mentalizing while with him. The therapist clarifies his deficits for her and, given his difficulty with retaining any more complex verbal encounter, focuses on his wife communicating her emotional reaction of feeling hurt when he criticizes her. Though such encounters are emotionally draining for the wife, the strategy seems to have some immediate though short-lived calming effect for the husband (ibid., p. 87).

SUMMARY

Though somatization is broadly used to refer to both classic hysterical conversion disorders and psychophysiological disorders, most of this review has focused on the latter. The hypothalamic-pituitary-adrenal (HPA) axis and the immune system mediate the impact of emotional distress on bodily function. The significance of the clinical finding of difficulty with symbolization, mentalization, and affect regulation in psychosomatic patients noted by investigators including Marty, Sifneos, McDougall, and Fonagy is less clear. Though mentalization/symbolization difficulties may be associated with increased somatization, it is uncertain whether these difficulties are causative of psychosomatic disorder. Mentalization/symbolization difficulties may be aggravated by physical illness, pain and psychic trauma and may also be associated with limitations of ego functioning in autistic spectrum disorders. McDougall (1980) and Fonagy and colleagues (2002) point to the interaction between early childhood temperament, parent-child attachment patterns, and parental empathic difficulties as major determinants of the capacity for mentalization and self-regulation. Reflective functioning appears to promote self-regulation and decrease somatization. However in some eating disorder patients, Pedersen, Poulsen, and Lunn (2015) notes that high reflective functioning, perceiving the emotional state of self and others, may not extend to embodied mentalization and self-regulation. In such cases, high reflective functioning may represent a survival skill in conflicted interpersonal relationships beginning in the family, while eating disorder symptoms may serve a less than ideal self-regulatory function.

Perhaps a third of primary care doctors' patients present with unexplained somatic complaints and perhaps a third of these are psychologically minded and amenable to referral for psychotherapy. In this context, much supportive work and medication treatment of associated anxiety and depression is done by nurses and physicians who may benefit from psychological and psychiatric consultation.

Short-term supportive psychoanalytically informed therapy can be helpful for psychosomatic disorders by encouraging mentalization and verbalization of somatic distress and interpersonal tensions with some limited sense of mastery while discouraging regression to impasses or negative therapeutic reactions more likely in long-term psychodynamic psychotherapy or psychoanalysis.

In longer-term psychotherapy and psychoanalytic cases reported by McDougall (1972, 1974, 1984), Ogden (1999), Taylor et al. (1997), and Katz (2010), the analyst's reflection on difficult sometimes somatic countertransference, e.g., malaise, panic, headaches, appears to have been critical to negotiating impasses and helping patients understand and verbalize previously unbearable affect. Coen (1992) suggests that while it is difficult to validate working analytic paradigms in treating psychosomatic cases (e.g., split idealized and devalued maternal introjects, an emotionally "dead" and unempathic mother, or disordered attachment patterns), there is clinical improvement and a decrease in somatic symptoms when the analyst is able to help patients bear previously intolerable wishes, feelings, and needs.

When more specific neuropsychological deficits and handicaps can be identified in some somatic disorders, e.g., fear of loss of control, loss of ego boundaries, and magical thinking in basal ganglia disorders; fluctuations in energy and mood in chronic fatigue syndrome; and fear over expressive language deficits or loss of emotional object constancy in brain injury; difficulties may be focused on therapeutically.

REFERENCES

Abbass, A., Kisely, S., and Kroenke, K. (2009). Short-term psychodynamic psychotherapy for somatic disorders: systematic review and meta-analysis of clinical trials. *Psychotherapy and Psychosomatics*, 78(5), 265–74.
Alexander, F. (1950). *Psychosomatic Medicine: Its Principles and Application*. New York: Norton.
Alexander, F., French, T., and Pollock, G. (1968). *Psychosomatic Specificity. Vol 1: Experimental Study and Results*. Chicago: University of Chicago Press.
Arehart-Treichel, J. (2012, August 3). Burgeoning field of study could impact psychiatry. *Psychiatric News*. Retrieved from http.//psychnews.psychiatryonline.org/doi/full/10.1176/pn.47.15
Bahnson, M. and Bahnson, C. (1969). Ego defenses in cancer patients. *Annals of the New York Academy of Sciences*, 164, 546–57.
Bucci, W. (1997). Symptoms and symbols: A multiple code theory of somatization. *Psychoanalytic Inquiry*, 17(2), 151–72.
Coen, S. (1992). Psychosomatic avoidance of conflict. In S. Coen, (Ed.). *The Misuse of Persons: Analyzing Pathological Dependency* (pp. 156–72). Hillside, NJ and London: Analytic Press.
Cohen, D. (1991). Tourette's syndrome: A model for integrating psychoanalysis and biological perspectives. *International Review of Psychoanalysis,* 18, 195–209.
Cruz, R. (2002). The handicapped super-hero: The traumatic sense of self in a Touretter. Unpublished manuscript, honorable mention for Rieger Psychodynamic Psychotherapy Award, American Academy of Child and Adolescent Psychiatry.
DeWolf, M. (2014). Psychoanalysis and psychosomatic disorders, from soma to psyche: Related to DSM, attachment, mentalization and affect regulation. Unpublished lectures to Lithuanian Society for Psychoanalysis and University of Vilnius. Retrieved from http://thijsdewolf.nl/aangenaam
Driver, C. (2005). An under-active or over-active internal world? An exploration of parallel dynamics within psyche and soma, and the difficulty of internal regulation, in patients with chronic fatigue syndrome and myalgic encephalomyelitis. *Journal of Analytical Psychology,* 50(2), 155–73.
Dunbar, F. (1954). *Emotions and Bodily Changes*. New York: Columbia University Press.
Ferenczi, S. (1926). *Further Contributions to the Theory and Technique of Psychoanalysis*. London: Hogarth Press.
Fitzgerald, M. and Bellgrove, M. (2006). The overlap between alexithymia and Asperger's Syndrome. *Journal of Autism and Developmental Disorder,* 36(4), 573–76.
Fonagy, P., Bateman, A., and Luyten, P. (2012). Introduction and overview. In A. W. Bateman, and P. Fonagy (Eds.). *Handbook of Mentalizing in Mental Health Practice.* (p. 312) Washington, DC: American Psychiatric Publishing.
Fonagy, P., Gergely, G., Jurist, E., and Target, M. (2002). *Affect Regulation, Mentalization and the Development of the Self.* New York: Other Press.
Fonagy, P. and Target, M. (1997). Attachment and reflective function: Their role in self-organization. *Developmental Psychopathology,* 9, 679–700.
Freud, S. (1915). Some character-types met with in psycho-analytic work. In J. Strachey (Ed.). *Standard Edition of the Complete Psychological Works of Sigmund Freud, Vol. XIV*

(1914–1916: On the History of the Psycho-Analytic Movement, Papers on Metapsychology and Other) (pp. 311–15). London: Hogarth Press and the Institute for Psycho-Analysis.
Friedman, M. and Rosenman, R. (1959). Association of specific overt behavior pattern with blood and cardiovascular findings: Blood cholesterol level, blood clotting time, incidence of arcus senilis and clinical coronary artery disease. *Journal of the American Medical Association*, 169, 1286.
Friedman, M., Byers, S., and Rosenman, R. (1970). Coronary-prone individuals (type A behavior pattern): Some biochemical characteristics. *Journal of the American Medical Association*, 212, 1030.
Frith, U. (2004). Emanuel Miller Lecture: Confusion and controversies about Asperger syndrome. *Journal of Child Psychology and Psychiatry and Allied Disciplines*, 45(4), 672–86.
Gottlieb, R. (2003). Psychosomatic medicine: The divergent legacies of Freud and Janet. *Journal of the American Psychoanalytic Association*, 51, 857–81.
Groddeck, G. (1929). *The Book of the It.* New York: Nervous and Disease Publishing.
Hanly, C. (2011). Narcissism, hypochondria and the problem of alternative theories. *International Journal of Psychoanalysis*, 92(3), 593–608.
Hill, E., Berth, S., and Frith, U. (2004). Brief report: Cognitive processing of own emotions in individuals with autistic spectrum disorder and in their relatives. *Journal of Autism and Developmental Disorders*, 34(2), 229–35.
Hoppe, K. and Bogen, J. (1977). Alexithymia in twelve commissurotomized patients. *Psychotherapy and Psychosomatics*, 28(1–4), 148–55.
Jacobson, E. (1959). The "Exceptions," an elaboration of Freud's character study. *Psychoanalytic Study of the Child,* 14, 135–54.
Janet, P. (1889). *L'automatisme Psychologique*. Paris: Alcan.
Jessimer, M. and Markham, R. (1997). Alexithymia: a right hemisphere dysfunction specific to recognition of certain facial expressions? *Brain and Cognition,* 34(2), 246–58.
Kaplan, H. (1980). History of psychosomatic medicine. In H. Kaplan, A. Freedman, and B. Sadock (Eds.). *Comprehensive Textbook of Psychiatry/III, Vol. 2, 3rd edition* (pp. 1849–51). Baltimore/London: Williams &Wilkins.
Katz, A. (2010). Healing the split between body and mind: Structural and developmental aspects of psychosomatic illness. *Psychoanalytic Inquiry*, 30(5), 430–44.
Kirmayer, L. and Santhanam, R. (2001). The anthropology of hysteria. In P. Halligan, C. Bass, and J. Marshall (Eds.). *Contemporary Approaches to Hysteria* (pp. 251–70). Oxford: Oxford University Press.
Kohon, G. (1999). *The Dead Mother: The Work of Andre Green.* London/Philadelphia: Brunner-Routledge.
Krystal, H. (1982–1983). Alexithymia and the effectiveness of psychoanalytic treatment. *International Journal of Psychoanalytic Psychotherapy,* 9, 353–88.
Lane, R. (1997). Is alexithymia the emotional equivalent of blindsight? *Biological Psychiatry,* 42(9), 834–44.
Leckman, J. (1992, October 22). Clinical case conference: Tourette's syndrome and associated disorders. Unpublished discussion, presented at American Academy of Child and Adolescent Psychiatry Annual Meeting, Washington, D.C.
Lichtman, C. (2010). Psychosomatic medicine: A psychoanalyst's journey through a somatic world. *Psychoanalytic Inquiry,* 30(5), 380–89.
Luyten, P., van Houdenhove, B., Lemma, A., Target, M., and Fonagy, P. (2012). A mentalization-based approach to the understanding and treatment of functional somatic disorders. *Psychoanalytic Psychotherapy*, 26(2), 121–40.
Marty, P. and de M'Uzan, M. (1963). *La pensee operatoire. Revue Francaise de Psychanalyse*, 27, 1345–56.
McDougall, J. (1972). The anti-analysand in analysis. In S. Lebovici and D. Widlocher (Eds.). (1980). *Ten Years of Psychoanalysis in France* (pp. 333–54). New York: International Universities Press.
———. (1974). The psychosoma and the psychoanalytic process. *International Review of Psycho-Analysis*, 1, 437–59.

———. (1980). A child is being eaten. I: Psychosomatic states, anxiety neurosis and hysteria-a theoretical approach. II: The abysmal mother and the cork child—a clinical illustration. *Contemporary Psychoanalysis,* 16, 417–59.
———. (1984). The "disaffected" patient: Reflections of affect pathology. *Psychoanalytic Quarterly*, 53, 386–09.
———. (1989). *Theaters of the Body: A Psychoanalytic Approach to Psychosomatic Illness.* New York: Norton.
———. (2001). The psychic economy of addiction. In J. Petrucelli and C. Stuart (Eds.). *Hunger and Compulsions: The Dynamic Treatment of Eating Disorders and Addictions* (pp. 4–26). Northvale, NJ and London: Jason Aronson.
McDougall, J. and Coen, S. (2000). Affect, somatisation, and symbolisation. *International Journal of Psycho-Analysis,* 81(1), 159–61.
Moore, B. and Fine, B. (1990). *Psychoanalytic Terms & Concepts.* New Haven: Yale University Press.
Nemiah, J. (1977). Alexithymia: Theoretical considerations. *Psychotherapy and Psychosomatics*, 28, 199–206.
Nemiah, J., Freyberger, H., and Sifneos, P. (1976). Alexithymia: A view of the psychosomatic process. In Hill, O. (Ed.). *Modern Trends in Psychosomatic Medicine* (pp. 430–39). London: Butterworths.
Niederland, W. (1965). Narcissistic ego impairment in patients with early physical malformations. *Psychoanalytic Study of the Child,* 20, 518–34.
Ogden, T. (1999). Analysing forms of aliveness and deadness of the transference-countertransference. In G. Kohon (Ed.). *The Dead Mother: The Work of Andre Green* (pp. 128–48). London/Philadelphia: Brunner-Routledge.
Pedersen, S., Poulsen, S., and Lunn, S. (2015). Eating disorders and mentalization: High reflective functioning in patients with bulimia nervosa. *Journal of the American Psychoanalytic Association,* 63(4), 671–94.
Pedrosa Gil, F., Scheidt, C. E., Hoeger, D., and Nickel, M. (2008). Relationship between attachment style, parental bonding and alexithymia in adults with somatoform disorders. *Journal of Psychiatry in Medicine*, 38(4), 437–51.
Pedrosa Gil, F., Weigl, M., Wessels, T., Irnich, D., Baumuller, E., and Winkelmann, A. (2008). Parental bonding and alexithymia in adults with fibromyalgia. *Psychosomatics*, 49(2), 115–22.
Salas, C. (2012). Surviving catastrophic reaction after brain injury: The use of self-regulation and self-other regulation. *Neuropsychoanalysis*, 14(1), 77–92.
Schattner, E., Shahar, G., and Abu-Shakra, M. (2008). "I used to dream of Lupus as some sort of creature": Chronic illness as an internal object. *American Journal of Orthopsychiatry*, 78(4), 466–72.
Shipko, S., Alvarez, W., and Noviello, N. (1983). Towards a teleological model of alexithymia: Alexithymia and post-traumatic stress disorder. *Psychotherapy and Psychosomatics*, 39(2), 122–26.
Sifneos, P. (1973). The prevalence of "alexithymic" characteristics in psychosomatic patients. *Psychotherapy and Psychosomatics*, 22, 255–62.
Taylor, G. (1993). Clinical application of a dysregulation model of illness and disease: A case of spasmodic torticollis. *International Journal of Psychoanalysis,* 74, 581–94.
Taylor, G. (2003). Somatization and conversion: Distinct or overlapping constructs? *Journal of the American Academy of Psychoanalytic and Dynamic Psychiatry,* 31(3), 487–508.
Taylor, G., Bagby, M., and Parker, J. (1997). *Disorders of Affect Regulation: Alexithymia in Medical and Psychiatric Illness.* Cambridge: Cambridge University Press.
Taylor, G. and Bagby, M. (2013). Psychoanalysis and empirical research: The example of alexithymia. *Journal of the American Psychoanalytic Association,* 61(1), 99–133.
Terr, L. (1984). Time and trauma. *Psychoanalytic Study of the Child,* 39, 633–65.
Verhaeghe, P., Vanheule, S., and de Rice, A. (2007). Actual neurosis as the underlying psychic structure of panic disorder, somatization, and somatoform disorder: An integration of Freudian and attachment perspectives. *Psychoanalytic Quarterly*, 76, 1317–50.

Winnicott, D. (1971). Case I "Iiro" *aet* 9 years 9 months. In *Therapeutic Consultations in Child Psychiatry*. New York: Basic Books.

Yehuda, R., Steiner, A., Kahana, B., Binder-Brynes, K., Southwick, S. M., Zemelman, S., and Giller, E. (1997). Alexithymia in holocaust survivors with and without PTSD. *Journal of Traumatic Stress,* 10, 93–100.

Chapter Eleven

Back to Freud's Beginning

Looking at Neuroscience through a Contemporary Psychoanalytic Lens

Susan P. Sherkow and Kate Lieberman

"Psychoanalysis" is commonly understood to be a process directed at understanding a person's inner world. Only recently has psychoanalysis come under the scrutiny of a neuroscientific lens. Ironically, from the beginning, Freud's clinical experience as a neurologist triggered his curiosity about the impact of mental activity and emotions on the body, which led to his formulating models of the *psyche,* formulations that he considered to be related to activity of the *brain.* We can only marvel at Freud's creating a corpus of psychoanalytic knowledge in the context of what was as yet uncharted neuroscientific terrain.

Over time, Freud progressively revised his sense of the relationship between *mind* and *brain* by framing them in schematic constructs, for example the "topographic" or "structural" models. We have no doubt that, had he been able to weigh in on any disagreement about whether the Mind, or Consciousness, or Sense of Self exist outside of neuronal pathways, Freud would have come down firmly on the side of "everything is wired!"

It is impossible in the space of a chapter to do justice to the relationship between observable behaviors and brain function, whether we are looking at Freud's complex contributions or at our current body of knowledge. At the very least, we know that any change in psychological function implicitly references *a simultaneous change in the neurobiological patterns inside the brain* (Edelman 2012; Kandel 2007). In other words, our work in psychoanalysis not only addresses manifest and latent emotions and conflicts, but also simultaneously alters connectivity along neuronal pathways. Thus, it behooves us *now,* as we believe it did Freud, to think of analysis as a tool to change patterns of established neurophysiological connections that are continuously affected by, and that in turn affect, our behavior and our relationships: patterns in the brain that appear to us as actions, feelings, thoughts, and intentions.

Tracing the evolution in neuroscience from Freud's time until the present requires narrowing both the scope of Freud's enormous contribution to psychoanalysis and the scope of current exploration of the connections between psyche and soma. Thus, in this chapter, we limit the lens with which we will examine "neuroscience" to specific aspects of "neurodevelopment." Furthermore, in attempting to bridge the gap between Freud's efforts to find physiologic correspondence to "the psyche" and our own current psychoanalytic theories of neurodevelopment, we have searched for a useful common denominator. We have found a springboard from Freud into contemporary neuroscience in the concept of a *Mental Representation.*

From the psychological point of view, the term "mental representation" is used to describe a conscious or unconscious structure that is organized by, and in turn organizes, intentions, interactions, and stimulations of all kinds that have emanated from both external experience and internal experience. Mental representations do not occur in a vacuum, but are connected to other representations, some conscious, others not. In this chapter, we will address those aspects of early development that pertain to the concept of mental representations, with the understanding that the neurodevelopmental process is one in which experience is registered through connectivity within the neurocircuitry of the brain. Given the limitations of space, we have chosen to further narrow that focus to how mental representations derive from the earliest internalizations of the maternal object, using a case of a five-and-a-half-year-old boy to illustrate this process.

THE HISTORY OF THE CONCEPT OF "MENTAL REPRESENTATION"

If we truly start at Freud's beginning, we observe that Freud's aim was to explain "psychic" or "mental" activity: *how* the "mind" represents an impulse or emotion; the nature of the *behavior* of the *impulse/emotion;* the *movement* of the impulse/emotion; and, then, its *object.* To accomplish this aim, Freud needed to be able to "locate" this mental activity in the brain, *without yet having a map of where psychological events exist.* Nor did he have a commonly accepted name for either the "*events*" or the "*structure*" of this mental activity.

In 1905, in the '"Three Essays on Sexuality," Freud first coined the word "mental representation" to stand in for the impulse/emotion, which he called, temporarily, an "ego-libido," giving a location from which the libidinal forces can move to or away from the object, and calling this process a "cathexis." In pointing to the *movement* of sexual excitations and hypothesizing that these cathexes can move *toward* an object, or *retreat,* he added that they can be perceived consciously or be repressed (Freud 1905, p. 217; Freud 1919, p. 200). He importantly further deduced that mental representations can be of a real object or of a fantasy (Freud 1907, p. 46).

Freud then introduced the concept of *internalizing the cathexis of the object* (Freud 1917), clearly identifying a mental representation as within the neurobiological apparatus of the brain. Importantly, perceiving the complex process of emotional engagement as emanating from a neurobiological structure became useful in describing the functions of mental representations, and how they might help us understand essential aspects of development.

By 1919, Freud had "located" the schema of a "mental representation" within the topography of conscious, unconscious, and preconscious, and, in describing the element of *movement of a mental representation from one neuroanatomical structure to another,* postulated that mental representations *can be repressed,* thus framing the role of mental representations in psychodynamic formulations (Freud 1919, p. 200).

Grasping that mental activity can be traced in terms of movements between *registrations* of "excitations," and furthermore that the *connections* between the excitations and the object toward whom these excitations are directed, can be very complex and multidimensional, was seminal. Freud was working toward understanding that these excitations are *moving along a neural pathway,* accessing parts of the brain that are connected to each other and fire simultaneously, and are mediated by mental representations of all of the various aspects of the excitations. It is not hard to see how close Freud came to understanding that registrations of past and present, of wishes, fantasies, actions, intentions, guilt, conflict, and all aspects of theories of mind were neurophysiologically connected.

In summary, Freud's work in trying to operationalize "registration" or "cathexis" of external and internal experiences and their emotional attributes (i.e., "affect") in the mind/brain/mental apparatus, laid the foundation for the dialogue over the next century of how we come to know the object world. In other words, through mental representations, we come to imbue the object world with registrations of emotions, which gradually connect to cognitive processes, cumulatively creating "the mind/brain apparatus" that is collectively our thoughts, feelings, ideas, intentions, and condition.

Beyond Freud, students of development continued to try to map psychic events and relationships within the mental apparatus, i.e., the brain. Historically, reinforcement of the usefulness of the schema of "mental representations" emerged through exploration of a *developmental* model of the mind. One such moment occurred in 1968, during a panel discussion of object constancy between Arlow, A. Freud, Lampl-de Groot, and Beres. In discussing the problem of object constancy, Lampl-de Groot pointed out that "without the development of the child to the point where it has the *capacity* to form a mental representation of the object *which remains* in the psychic apparatus . . . "object constancy" in Miss Freud's sense would not be something of which the child would be capable" (Arlow, Freud, Lampl-de Groot, and Beres 1968, p. 507). Furthermore, in 1970, Anna Freud proposed that the processes of developing *symbolic function* derive from the structures created through mental representation (A. Freud 1970, pp. 32–33).

Last but not least, Fonagy extended and broadened the apparent functions of mental representations from where Freud and Anna Freud left off, pursuing an exploration of the biological nature of mental processing in terms of how a baby *internalizes the object world.* Fonagy proposed that "making meaning" begins through creating mental representations of one's own feelings, experiences, thoughts, and intentions, as well as mentally representing what one understands about another person's state of mind, feelings, and experiences (Fonagy and Target 1998; Fonagy, Gergely, Jurist, and Target 2002). "The capacity to mentalize," or Theory of Mind, describes representations of all behavior and experiences that are located within the anatomy of a brain that not only cognates, but registers and uses its cognitive knowledge through interconnectivity to understand oneself and others (Fonagy 1991).

THE LINK TO CONTEMPORARY NEURODEVELOPMENT

Current developmental theory and research confirm what Freud suspected, that everything that a baby experiences from the time of conception, and certainly postconception, has a physiological basis (Edelman 2012; Kandel 2007). Central to our work as psychoanalysts is our understanding that the distortions we encounter in our patient's view of self and other, distortions that ultimately lead to symptom formation and character differences, stem from mental representations of lived experiences that are encoded in the brain (i.e., wired), and thus uniquely individual (Edelman 2012; Kandel 2007; Klin and Jones 2007).

Like Freud, we understand that in the course of development, a child's libidinal forces—his endowment—create stimuli that are processed together with external stimuli—his environment—by virtue of their interconnectivity. Through his unique registration of nature and nurture, a child makes meaning of his emotional world. Indeed, our current thinking about the inextricability of mind and body has rendered the perspective of "nature" and "nurture" to be inseparable perspectives of the same process.

In other words, an infant's experience is formed by bidirectional perceptions of an object, a creative process that is co-constructed between the perceiver and the perceived, where the perception of the object is mediated by complex, interconnected registrations of the *experience* of that object. These capabilities are moderated by nature and nurture in the form of, for example, core information, emotional state, dyadic expectations, and capacity for reciprocity (Fonagy, Gergely, Jurist, and Target 2002; Gergely and Watson 1996; Stern 1974).

A baby's ability to make a representation is also contingent on the extent to which the baby's brain is capable of *registering* internal and external information. For example, a deaf or blind child, unable to register sounds or sights, highlights how an aspect of the internal environment can determine what and how the child processes, and how he makes use of available information. Similarly, the presentation of symptoms in an autistic child represents atypical connectivity that interferes with receiving, sorting, processing, and making use of both internal and external information and experience. (Glezerman 2013; Kanna, Uddin, Kenet, Chugani, and Muller 2014; Klin and Jones 2007; Sherkow 2015).

NEURODEVELOPMENT FROM THE PERSPECTIVE OF THE INFANT

The study of "neurodevelopment" addresses itself to the possible biological substrates of normal and abnormal expressions of four components of experience: emotions, cognition, sociability, and intentionality. First, the simplest substrate to describe is the component of feelings: the instinctive, intuitive ingredients of relating and being attached, what has been called "implicit relational knowing" (Tronick 2007; Lyons-Ruth 1998, 1999; Beebe and Lachmann 1988, 1994). These innate, preverbal, positive or negative emotions become increasingly connected to an object, in all the complexity that emotional connections entail, including sensory responses, emotion-laden memories, stimuli triggers, and what we hypothesize comprises the emotional attachment to mental representations of the object.

While infants in the state of precognition are understood to have "implicit knowledge" by virtue of instinct and intuition, it is a common mistake to use the word "know" in the context of early infancy. Early in development, "implicit knowing" is, by definition, unconscious, precognitive, registration of experience (Klin and Jones 2007; Piaget 1973). Implicit knowing comes to be explicit through formations of synapses that, through experience and myelinization, connect emotional and cognitive circuits, leading to the ability to use logic and to scaffold information (Sherkow 2013; Kandel, Dudai, and Mayford 2014). We use the word "experience" to mean mental, physical, interpersonal, and intentional events of all kinds, understood to be registered in the brain (Fonagy et al. 2002; Baron-Cohen, Leslie, and Frith 1985; Sherkow 2013; Fallon and Sherkow 2013).

Secondly, cognition (or "thinking") is a formal, gradually emerging process driven by physiology: increasing connectivity within the brain gives the growing child the ability to use language to represent experience and feelings, and allows experiences and memories of experiences to be formed, stored, retrieved, and verbalized. The evolving language and cognitive systems are in constant flux, as more and more information, from both inside and outside, is processed and integrated in the brain (Edelman 2012; Klin and Jones 2007; Fallon and Sherkow 2013).

The third component of neurodevelopment can be described as the gradual internalization of interpersonal experiences that underlie the capacity for social ability and independence. Our developmental perspective focuses on the way babies process social information: Winnicott (1958) proposed that a baby learns "who he is" through the gradual development of his experiential state being mirrored in his mother's expression. Thus, the processes of internalizing mother's caretaking, in all of its complexity, are governed by interpersonal, reciprocal mechanisms through the creation of mental representations of self and the mother (Jacobson 1954).

The fourth component, intentionality, is relatively new to psychoanalytic thinking, but hardly to neuroscience. We know that the baby does much of the work of understanding, translating, and using his experience of his mother—this is his "intention" at work (Beebe and Lachmann 1988, 1994; Stern 1974; Tronick 2007; Winnicott 1958). His motor apparatus also registers intentional information from the first time a baby moves a muscle; he registers awareness of his movements, certainly, when he reaches for something, an "awareness" neuroconnection that in turn connects to registrations in his pleasure/reward centers (Klin and Jones 2007; Piaget 1973).

MENTAL REPRESENTATION IN THE INTERNALIZATION PROCESS

The challenge of transposing an analytic model of the development of the mind into neurodevelopmental terms begins with understanding how the creation of patterns, predictability, and reciprocity between mother and child evolve in development, providing a child with the regulatory coping mechanisms and skills that allow him to evolve independently of his parents (Klin and Jones 2007; Qian and Lipkin 2007; Sherkow 2015). One way to address this challenge is to focus on one component of the process of forming mental representations, namely "internalization." Here "internalize" is used as a verb to refer to any aspect of an infant "taking in" any aspect of the mother/mothering relationship, including but not limited to the baby's incorporation, introjection, and identifications of mother/mothering. Importantly, we recognize that the processes of development are contingent both on a child's endowment and on the contributions of mother and mothering.

To elaborate, the infant's experiences of mother's actions, emotions, sensations, and attitudes during the critical first three years of life are processed through his sensory, proto-cognitive, and body-bound capacities. We know that a mother organizes her baby's activities according to her own conscious and unconscious needs, and that her baby, through mutual mirroring, cueing and scanning, incorporates her mother's attributes and expectations (Fonagy et al. 2002; Gergely and Watson 1996). We also know that due to inborn, genetically influenced traits, babies differ in their responses to these ministrations (Mahler, Pine, and Bergman 1975; McDevitt 1975; Pine 1982). The literature is replete with research by Beebe, Trevarthan, Stern, and Tronick, among others, offering proof that a baby's brain does some of the work of development! Another example comes from the literature on learning styles: critical to an infant "reading" his mother's intentions and affects is his ability to categorize what he "reads" (Fonagy et al. 2002; Trevarthan 1979; Stern 1974; Qian and Lipkin 2011).

Integral to this process, from birth, is the child's implicit formation of representations of his mother, himself, and his mother-self pair in action. Neurodevelopmentally, this process can be described as follows: early experiences are continually processed in the infant's brain as rudimentary mental representations, and these representations "wire together" biologically in the form of synaptic connections. Increased brain connectivity allows for the development of ever more complex mental representations, in the form of patterns we recognize as "object relations," "attachment," and the integration of dyadic experiences of being mothered (Sherkow 2015).

A good example is one from the earliest days of infancy. A typically developing infant, napping in his crib, naturally cries or fusses when he is hungry, and an attuned mother responds to the cry by entering the room to feed her baby by bottle or breast. The infant's brain registers this sequence of events, including the physiological sensation of hunger, the crying response, and the subsequent arrival of satiation and soothing, which is wired to the neural reward center. The typically developing infant comes to recognize this pattern in the form of a mental representation (really, a complex of connected mental representations) of the dyadic interaction. Once this mental representation is in place, the typically developing infant stops crying upon mother's arrival at the door; by recognizing mother, he is able to anticipate the satiation and soothing which has historically followed her appearance. In response, mother feels delight at her baby's ability to recognize her, leading to mutual delight in the infant, and the groundwork for positive circular interactions.

To conceptualize this process on a neurobiological level, we can say that the neurocircuitry, which underlies the infant's mental representation, allows him to begin to predict events in the world around him. When mother appears at the door, he is able to wait calmly for her to walk to him and feed him; the temporal space between mother's arrival and the satiation of her bottle or breast represents the infant's ability to delay gratification. This first experience of reality testing leads, with repetition, to the infant's scaffolding and integrating other similar experiences, and thus the ability to tolerate more complex moments of delay of gratification with increasingly varied forms of satisfaction or soothing. Over time, he learns to *categorize* both experiences of satisfaction and occasional dissatisfaction as such.

Furthermore, the ability to make predictions from experience, and to delay gratification, allows the calmly waiting infant to label and therefore symbolize the mental representation of mother. He soon begins to say "Mama" when he sees her at the door, a proto-symbol that in its first incarnation stands for the entire mental representation of the dyadic process of mother arriving to soothe/feed him. Likewise, "Bye-Bye" stands for the sequence of waving at mother as mother and baby separate. These proto-symbols take the form of gestures (e.g., waving) and words (e.g., Mama), and are therefore *intentional* and *actions*; thus, on a biological level, they signal that the brain is making complex associations between 1) representations of objects, physiological sensations, and intentionality, and 2) verbal and gestural activity (the cognitive brain). All of these competencies (i.e., predictability, delay of gratification, and symbolization) form the building blocks of self-regulation and independent functioning, which require a range of flexible coping abilities.

Importantly, the capability to manage transitions through predictability and anticipatory anxiety is a key component of categorical learning, which allows for integration of internal and external messages (Qian and Lipkin 2011). In order for the infant to develop a thoroughly predictable symbolic substitute for the soothing qualities of mother, he must learn to differentiate mother's various behaviors, commands, wishes, and moods; these numerous incarnations of the same mother require increasingly scaffolded (neurobiologically wired) mental representations of her (Sherkow 2013; Sherkow 2015). Subsequently, a neurotypically developing child can use his early experience of being mothered, including the pattern-making in their relationship, to make order out of the chaos of his feelings, perceptions, and, later, his toys, organizing not only his blocks into towers, lining up his cars, but also his feelings into compartments and his impulses into rule-bound discipline.

UNDERSTANDING MOTHERING (OR MENTAL REPRESENTATIONS)

As stated previously, infants present a variety of cues to their mothers to indicate their needs, tensions, and pleasure. The mother's contribution to this neurodevelopmental process is that mothers respond selectively to only certain of these cues. Mothers transmit, intergenerationally, their own developmental processes of the mental representations of internalization and identifications that they have made with their own parent(s). They also bring to the table representations of other aspects of their development, such as their prior experiences of caring for others, their maternal fantasies stemming from consolidation of the oedipal period, and their narcissistic investment in having an infant.

One important aspect of mothering involves mentalizing and sharing joint attention, which organize and help scaffold a baby's experiences, as well as allow him to selectively and appropriately mirror, imitate, and reciprocate in impacting on another's thoughts and feelings. Needless to say, all of these capacities are driven by mental representations. However, when a mother has historically experienced difficulty in her own processes of projection and identification, infant distress and failure to internalize a regulating maternal figure may result. For example, a mother whose internal object representations are weighted heavily toward angry and irrational objects might perceive her infant's normal distress as likewise angry and irrational, causing her to be overwhelmed with anxiety, freeze up, or otherwise defend against her seeming failure by avoiding or overstimulating her infant.

When all goes well in a child's development, issues of "neuroconnectivity" or "neurodevelopment" on the one hand, or "quality of mothering" on the other hand, do not get raised. While we have emphasized, above, the correlation between developing neurocircuitry and the formation of internalization/mental representations of mothering in the infant, we have not commented on the impact on a mother of a child who ultimately receives the diagnosis of autism spectrum disorder, attention-deficit/hyperactivity disorder (ADHD), or learning disorders. What would those children look like in the earliest stages of infancy? How would their wiring, already neurobiologically "programmed," to some extent, impact mothering?

A mother will certainly become anxious or feel inadequate if, for example, she finds that her best efforts to soothe her child and to help him self-regulate, having "predictably" presented him with patterns, flounder upon his neurocircuitry: the child does not—cannot—internalize her best efforts. Sensitive mothers of children on the autism spectrum identify that their infants fail to recognize the patterns of maternal care, such as arriving with milk and the message "help is on the way." One hypothesis is that these children are "wired" such that they cannot recognize or make use of the patterns formed by mental representations, so that each appearance of mother at the door seems novel. It is not known if this difference is a product of a diminished neurophysiologic capacity to recognize patterns, or possibly a diminished capacity of the brain to scaffold information.

What is known, however, is that such moments of distress and failure to regulate can lead to formations of mental representations between mother and baby that are less than optimally attuned. We know from Fonagy et al.'s work that attunement is optimal at somewhere around 80 percent, so it is expected and natural that some percentage of the time both mother and child will be disappointed (Fonagy, Gergely, Jurist, and Target 2004). Problematically, mothers of children who ultimately receive neurodevelopmental diagnoses cannot possibly be aware in the earliest stages of development that their increasing sense of discord or anxiety, when the sense of attunement seems to be far less than 80 percent, is beyond their control.

CLINICAL APPLICATION

Clinically, we are treating children who fall into a diagnostic category we are struggling to define, but nonetheless seem to have much in common. These children follow a pattern best described as "being on the edge of the autism spectrum" and having "uneven development"; children whose combination of innate wiring and environmental difficulties lead to a diminished ability to internalize the process of being mothered.

Perhaps the most striking feature of these children is the way in which they are observed to react aggressively against another person or to erupt into an uncontrollable tantrum seemingly "out of the blue." For instance, one young boy, Peter, was referred to Dr. Sherkow[1] at the age of five-and-a-half years for violent aggressive outbursts at school and in public. (From this point forward, "I" or "me" refers to Dr. Sherkow.) An extremely bright, verbally gifted, adorable, and otherwise sweet-tempered youngster, his outbursts were unusual in that they were seemingly unprovoked, mysterious, and irrational. There was nothing about him or in his history that suggested he was on the spectrum.

Indeed, he did not exhibit any of this symptomatic behavior *with me* until the fourth week of our work together, and it seemed to come, indeed, out of nowhere. He had been playing with a Fisher Price toy vehicle, and suddenly swiped at me with the car, with a guileless grin on his face. Another time, he poked me in my buttocks with a sharp object as I was walking in front of him to the waiting room, smiling again guilelessly. Yet another incident was one in which he segued from nonaggressive baseball batting practice to smacking me with the bat, and when I startled, smacking me again and again. In instances such as these, he moved from 0 to 100 in a split second, with no warning, and with not a hint of expectation on my part of what was to follow: no pattern, no predictability.

What accounts for this type of apparently "out of the blue" aggressive action? Because of their insufficient internalization, such children seem to be unable to access a sense of a regulating maternal figure. They are therefore unable to make sense of their emotions (predominantly fear, anxiety, and anger) or to predict their own reactions. For these children, the internal is externalized, so that their feelings are experienced as coming at them from their environment, and thus environmental stressors, which activate their feelings, are experienced as monstrous, larger-than-life attacks.

As a result, these children tend to react to situations that evoke internal anxiety or anger as if the world is punishing or actively sabotaging them. Negative environmental stimuli (for instance, changes in routine or separations), as well as their internally generated stimuli and responses, are experienced as external forces beyond their control. Without access to "wired" internal representations of mothers who could understand and regulate their own (and their children's) anxiety about changes, they are left to attempt to exercise their intentionality by taking control of and attacking the "external forces" by lashing out.

Clinically, these children have demanded from me a change in my technical approach. Confronted with their sudden concreteness and outbursts of aggression, I learned that before addressing what appears to be conflictual material, I need to address the aspects of their aggressive response to external forces that impeded their accessing neurotypical, neurotically-determined compromise formations. I must help them process emotions that emerge in response to underdeveloped aspects of their early development—those aspects which disrupted their internalization, leading to difficulty with predictability, patterning, and categorizing, and thus subsequent deficient development of strategies to manage transitions and, in some, to function typically at their age level. This therapeutic task is accomplished by addressing the very specific transference manifestations of this atypical wiring, before I can employ the conventional techniques of child analysis to address their dynamic picture.

The case excerpts that follow were selected from the treatment of a young boy, Cameron, whose psychodynamics/neurobiological wiring can be understood best through this lens. At the age of four years, Cameron presented with a significant impairment in his ability to regulate tension, anxiety, and rageful emotions. He came from an intact family in which both parents were highly educated and were functioning successfully in the workplace. His parents were familiar with psychoanalytic therapy, sensitive to their child's need for psychological intervention, and agreed to four-times-weekly treatment. However, his mother struggled with her own developmentally determined difficulties; as a result she had difficulty initiating and maintaining reciprocal interactions with her son, as well as mirroring his experiences in a way that allowed him to register, metabolize, and make sense of his experience.

Cameron appeared cognitively gifted in many ways, particularly in verbal processing. However, he struggled in school because his rageful outbursts could not be contained by authority figures under any circumstances. These included tantrums where kicking, hitting, and biting of classmates occurred at times that often appeared to be unprovoked; one could not see the "trigger" and thus was at a greater than usual loss as to how to address the trigger. Because he was so gifted, his teachers' and parents' expectations that he would apply his superior cognitive skills to manage his emotions inevitably contributed to his feeling more different and defective than the other children. In turn, this conundrum seemed to serve to increase his anxiety and thus seemed to compound an initial outburst by fueling a secondary aggressive response to being called out for the initial outburst. Cameron's mother likewise responded to him with increasing hypervigilance and intrusiveness related to her own fears and anxieties, which also magnified his reactions.

Cameron underwent neuropsychological testing, with inconclusive results. He presented with a picture that fit no diagnosis. While his receptive and expressive verbal skills were noted to be "excellent," his visuoperceptual and motor capacities were significantly compromised; in particular, he was found to have impaired sequencing abilities that compromised his recognition of visuospatial patterns. Further, he was found to lack the "desire for adult approval that motivates many children his age." In short, testing painted a picture of a child with neurological wiring which manifested as "uneven development"; at one time, he might have been diagnosed as pervasive developmental disorder, not otherwise specified, but he was not clearly in the range of autism spectrum disorder, despite sharing some of its features. His testing results were likewise not consistent with diagnoses of oppositional defiant behavior, learning disabilities, ADHD, or psychopathy.

Cameron's difficulty internalizing a soothing, regulating maternal figure can thus be conceptualized as a product of both his neurocircuitry and his experience with a mother who could be confusing and dysregulating. Below, I present excerpts of a session with Cameron, which provide good examples of the clinical manifestations of this insufficient internalization: in other words, how Cameron experienced his environment, as well as his internal emotional states, as an attacking force outside of his control. At the time of the session, Cameron was five and half years old and had already been in analysis for one and a half years. He was beginning to be able to make use of *me*, the analyst, as a substitute regulating maternal figure; his increasing internalization of a regulating "maternal" internal representation was allowing him to experiment with reciprocal play. These gains were consolidated over the course of a two-week Christmas vacation, from which he had just returned:

> *Cameron enters the playroom with his mother and yells "No!" at me when I try to follow them. I wait by the door for a few minutes; when I do enter, I see Cameron and Mom playing catch with beanbags of different colors and shapes. As Cameron tosses each beanbag to mother, he identifies it by color and/or shape.*
>
> Cameron: *Tossing the beanbag:* "Now it's pink, and an oval."
>
> Mother: "I got it! Oh my goodness, this is so incredible." *She catches it.* "Ready, one, two, three!" *She throws it back. He catches it and puts it on the table.* "Well done, Cameron!"
>
> C: *Selects another from the table, and tosses it.* "Now it's a triangle."
>
> M: *The beanbag flies over her shoulder, but she catches it.* "I got it." *She throws it back.*
>
> C: *Picks a red beanbag and throws it to Mom without announcing it. It is tossed too close to her face, but she catches it just as she has the others; she puts it on her nose, as if she didn't catch it, and says:*
>
> M: "That was a funny one. I almost ended up like Rudolph. Mommy's a red-nosed— what? Goofball. Scootch back, my handsome prince. One, two, three hoppapumpkin." *She tosses the beanbag back. Cameron catches, and selects another to throw.*
>
> M: *Whispering:* "I love you Cameron." *He moves toward her; she kisses his head.*

Mother's behavior here is quite confusing. Their play had been reciprocal, tossing and catching. However, her words do not match the actions. She responded as if she had been hit on the nose by a beanbag (though she was not), and responded by calling herself a "goofball" (since she feared she would not catch it)—or was she accusing Cameron of being a goofball (because his aim was off?). Then, she tells Cameron, "I love you," and kisses him on the head. This sequence suggests that she thought he intended to hit her with the beanbag. Her response—denial—would be quite confusing for Cameron.

C: *Speaking in a silly voice,* "Now make a stack!" *Mom joins him in trying to stack the beanbags, like pancakes—clearly an impossible task to throw and catch a stack at a time.*

C: *He throws a stack of beanbags at her,* "Here mommy!"

Here is a concrete demonstration of Cameron's confusion, mirroring his mother's confusing behavior: he throws everything (all the beanbags) at her, as she has thrown all her confused thoughts at him. Had she simply said, "You are being goofy," it would have labeled his behavior (throwing "wildly") in an acceptable way. Furthermore, it would have kept the interaction acceptably ambiguous—the throw would have been "no one's fault." Instead, mom's confusing response lacked clarity and exaggerated the "blame," placing it on Cameron. As a result, Mom and Cameron are not on the same page; their play lacks synchrony, patterning, and regulation. Cameron seems to imitate Mom's lack of predictability, and Mom in turn becomes angry and protests:

M: "I can't catch all those at once; I only have two hands. Even if I were a very good catcher I couldn't catch them all at once."

C: "I just gonna give it to you! Ahh!" *He throws the whole stack at Mom. Most fall around her; two fall on her lap.*

M: "Splat. But the yellow one landed right in my lap, isn't that nice."

C: "Now give the pile to me."

M: "Beanbags. Beanbags for sale, 50 cents a beanbag."

After Mom's confusing play interruption, I decide to step in and attempt to provide some external regulation. I use the technique of inviting displacement to allow Cameron to sort out his feelings. I offer myself, as a more neutral object than mother, on the premise that Cameron actually does have a mental representation of *me* as an alternative regulator of emotions.

Dr. Sherkow: "Do you want me to be a target and you can throw the beanbags at me, Cameron?"

C: "That's not how it works!"

He is right. *We* cannot play reciprocally if he and his mom cannot, and Cameron understands this, so that when I try again to regulate him by offering to play at throwing something else, he responds:

C: *Screaming,* "No no no no no that's not how the rule goes!"

DS: "Oh, ok. I just thought we—"

C: *Interrupting me,* "You're not following the rules."

DS: "Oh, I'm so sorry. I will follow the rules."

Now I've agreed that we can have and will follow the rules of predictable behaviors and reactions in order to handle transitions. He then turns to his mother:

C: "Mommy, you follow the rules."

M: "And what are the rules?"

C: "You only have to throw beanbags. To someone."

DS: *I hand the beanbags back to Mom,* "Here you go."

M: "Shall I, one at a time? So you can catch them."

C: "No, not one at a time, a whole bunch!"

Here, Mom agrees to play by the rules (i.e., to allow the play to be regulated), but shortly thereafter she breaks the rules (i.e., interrupts the play):

M: "A whole bunch! That's awfully tricky. Be careful, ready, one two three!" *She tosses the beanbag pile to him.*

DS: *Watching Cameron catch most of the beanbags,* "Look at that, amazing."

M: *Gathers up all the beanbags in her hands and covers Cameron with them and with kisses.* "There they are! And on every branch there was a monkey, and on every—"

C: *Suddenly throws several bean bags hard past her head.*

M: "Oh, no no no, that was too hard. That could've hurt me."

Here Cameron shows direct aggression at his mom for failing to be reciprocal and play the game according to the rules she had just agreed to, in other words, for failing to help him regulate his feelings of internal confusion, which are compounded by the changes in schedule surrounding our recent vacation. I make an interpretation:

DS: "I think it's awfully scary to have so many changes on a Monday morning after vacation. We haven't seen each other for two weeks.

C: *Pulls out a large toy fire engine and presses its buttons to create a mixture of loud sounds—siren and engine noises.*

This shift, a response to my interpretation, signals the emergence of imaginary play in this session, while nevertheless continuing to overstimulate us with a projection of his feeling of internal "craziness."

DS: "He's calling for help!"

C: "No we can't, we're just playing 'call!'"

DS: "Oh, only 'call,' not 'call for help?' Just 'call?'"

M: "Just 'call.'"

DS: "Ok. Can I make a call?" *In child's voice, pretending to be Cameron,* "Ding-a-ling-a-ling—Ding-a-ling-a-ling."

M: "Hello?"

DS: *Talking in child's voice,* "Hello, I feel so lost"

M: "Oh I'm terribly sorry, is there anything I can do to help?"

DS: *In child's voice,* "Can you help me feel better? Because you're a good mommy."

M: "I'd be happy to."

DS: "Aww, it's so hard—"

C: *Restarts fire engine noises, drowning both of us out.*

M: "It's very difficult the last few days, since vacation, everything's been so crazy, things aren't quite back to normal . . ."

C: "That's not playing! That's too busy." . . . *Blasts fire engine noises. Then, he lies down on the floor, facing away from us, and starts rolling the truck back and forth.*

We can literally witness Cameron's ambivalence about "taking in the object" and "rejecting the object:" as Mother is talking to me about their vacation, he alternates between letting her talk, and using the sounds of the fire truck to "scream" over her. Because he is dysregulated, still overwhelmed with anxiety and anger at his mother, his brain cannot tell the difference between my words, mother's words, and the fire engine noises. He is not ready for words; words are "too busy." I thus interpret:

> DS: "That's so true, Cameron. What you are thinking (in your mind) maybe is the busiest of all. It's easier to not think and just let things roll back and forth." *Gets on floor to join Cameron,* "I think I'll try that, maybe it'll make me feel better, I'll just try rolling. . . ." *Cameron and I both roll our trucks back and forth.*

To sum up, we first see Cameron attempt to assert control over his environment by making rules for play; however, his mother refuses to follow them. Following an escalation, Cameron begins to soothe himself by rolling the truck, controlling *it*, letting me watch him, and internalizing my soothing, controlling, regulatory mental representational world. Now his play becomes more symbolic.

> C: *Picks up the fire truck.* "There's a fire! And this is the fire engine."
>
> DS: "Do you need a truck to help you with the fire?"
>
> C: "Noo, this is perfect."
>
> DS: "Just perfect. . . . I'm so glad you found the perfect solution. Great."
>
> C: *Plays with engine and makes noise over the "fire" he's putting out.* "The fire's out!"
>
> DS: "Wow, that's a really wonderful fire truck. It put the fire out right away."
>
> C: "It has control pipes."

Cameron tells me that the fire truck has "control pipes." This is new. . . . I have never heard of this phenomenon related to the fire engine. He then points out the hoses.

> DS: "Are you in charge of helping him with his control pipes?" *He says it is the truck's job to turn the control pipes on and off, as he keeps playing at putting out the fire.*

C: *Keeps playing at putting out the fire, doesn't answer.*

DS: "That's a very important job, the one that turns pipes on and off."

At this point, Cameron shows a play association by moving to a bin of wood blocks; he begins building a house, creating a roof with a chimney as well as a "cozy cave" inside. He says he needs the cave to be dark, but then expresses a worry: he needs a light to see if an intruder will enter the cave. We put little figures into the house, representing himself and his brother; he states that he is worried that someone is hiding inside and wants the fire engine to protect the house. He has now clearly shifted from nonsymbolic, to semi-symbolic, to symbolic play, expressing conflict emanating from oedipal anxieties, which we address:

C: "The fire engine is staying in the cave because it doesn't want to get bashed and banged."

DS: "I see; so it's safe in there, huh?"

C. "I want to build a wall."

DS: "To make sure he's in there nice and safe."

Cameron's "walls" here symbolize his need/wish for rules and regulation. With walls, rules, and self-regulation, he can see the "enemy" as something that can be controlled, and he can be in charge.

C: "Now they're asleep!"

DS: *Pretending to be asleep, talking in child's voice and snoring:* "I hope I don't have bad dreams! I hope I don't wake up in the dark! It's so hard to sleep in the dark, I can't see anything, but I hear noises . . . I don't know what's out there. . . . I don't even like being alone."

C: "But don't worry, the fire engine is— is—is keeping the eyes closed!"

DS: "Oh, keep the eyes closed, that's the secret. But what if they open in the middle of the night? What if I'm lying there like this, and my eyes open POP, because I had a bad dream, POP, and my eyes open, and my bad dream's going WOOWOOWOOWOO and I can't get rid of it. What do I do?"

C: "He blew it away."

DS: *Starts blowing:* "I'll huff and I'll puff and I'll blow that bad stuff away. I hope this works."—*blows more*—"Oh, I'm going back to sleep."

C: "They are holding their eyes closed."

DS: "Oh, that's good."

C: "They're not dreaming anything."

DS: "Oh, that's good."

C: "And they're stillll plenty asleep."

Two Years Later

As I continued to work with Cameron over the next two years, he has shown great improvement. He has sufficiently internalized me as a regulating figure so that he can more effectively self-regulate; he can now go to school and attend a play group. He has come to internalize a sense of his mother as a chaotic figure, which he has been representing symbolically in the play as "stormy."

The following material at age seven-and-a-half shows in one example, he is playing with kinetic sand (which is sand with an osmotic capacity to stick together when lumped, but behaves like wet sand when raining down from above). He creates a huge storm of sand that rains down on our toy cars as they compete in a race. He calls the storm a "snowstorm." His car can plow through the storm, but my car is stuck in the globs of sand-as-snow. He declares that we need a snow plow to dig my car out.

C: "Let's invent a small little plow."

DS: "Ok! Sure, I can make a little plow."

C: "Move!"

DS: "Oh no! Can we get a plow to clean up the tracks of my car so it can go a little further? Is that plow helping?"

C: "It's stuck!"

DS: "It's stuck! There is a plow but the plow is stuck."

C: "And broken!"

DS: "And broken, so it makes it harder for the car to go . . ."

C: "Ok! Wait! The race is starting!"

DS: "The race is starting!"

C: *The car, made out of kinetic sand, starts to fall apart.* "It's coming apart! Look! I made a. . . . There's a mechanic."

DS: "Look! They called the plow, and the plow is broken, is that what you said?"

C: "They fixed it!"

DS: "Oh, they got a mechanic. . . . Oh!"

C: "They made a new. . . . They made an invention. Here, he made a snow blower."

DS: "A snow blower! Oh my God! Look!" *Begins to blow on the kinetic sand-as-snow.* "Looks like we could be successful now. We can get that ramp back and we can go move ahead. We've got a snow plow that . . ."

C: "Snow blower!"

DS: "I mean that blows the snow away."

Cameron becomes the snow storm and starts throwing kinetic sand on the cars' path.

DS: "Oh, it looks like the stormy mom came back! She was angry one day, upset . . . Her sunny mood is gone, oh no . . ."

C: "I know how to stop it."

DS: "How?"

C: "Just. . . . Actually she was mistaken."

DS: "She was?"

C: "She wanted him to never make it to the end, so she's breaking it apart."

DS: "She never wanted him to make it to the end so she's breaking it apart? Oh, my goodness, that answers the question. She didn't want him to get to the end. She never wanted him to get to the end of the race."

C: "That's why she was dropping all this sand . . ."

DS: "That's why she was dropping all the sand and the snow. She never wanted him to get to the end. Oh, wow . . . !"

Cameron throws more sand in a more aggressive way

DS: "Oh, look, so much anger, and unhappiness. . . . So much unhappiness . . ."

At first, Cameron personifies the storm without naming it; in our play, we put into words that he seems to be suffering from a stormy "Mother" who is impeding his progress; from his perspective, she gets in his way in the play race, as in real life: she is late, she is disorganized, she talks about wanting to have more babies . . . she just talks too much! The storm in this play represents his once entirely externalized conflict, the symbol of his disorganizing, rage-evoking mother, who is obstructing his progress, but against whom he now has developed defenses, like snow blower machines and analysis (while identifying with the analyst as rescuer and interpreter). Further, he can now "discuss" his increasingly oedipal anxieties in therapy in the form of puppet plays about, for instance, unicorns who want to be all powerful, or about dinosaurs, sharks, and caterpillars, all of whom are villains with poisonous venom.

CONCLUSION

Cameron presented as verbally gifted, yet "unevenly" developed, and often aggressive child, whose clinical picture is typical of children whose neurocircuitry leads to a failure to internalize a mental representation of a soothing, predictable, need-satisfying maternal figure. Without this internalization, the developmental tasks of self-regulation, the ability to manage transitions, to predict, to categorize, and to symbolize suffer enormously. Compounding the problem, mothers of these children who have difficulty with internalization often blame themselves; their feelings of guilt and anxiety leave their children feeling inadequate, and a vicious cycle of anxiety and heightened sensitivity to failure results. In Cameron's case, his mother was indeed quite dysregulating.

Most striking in the case of Cameron is the externalization of his inner world, a result of his inability to access a regulating maternal mental representation and subsequent difficulty making sense of, predicting, and regulating his own internal stimuli and reactions. When Cameron was referred to me, he appeared to operate out of a vacuum—his aggressive behavior was erratic and seemed irrational, mysterious, or "out of the blue." Over the course of the analysis, he was, gradually, able to internalize *me* as a substitute soothing, regulating "maternal" figure. These *wired* internal representations allowed him to make sense of his emotions, to put words to his inner and external reality, and to categorize his experiences. The shifts in his play from nonsymbolic to symbolic mirror the evolution of his anxieties, from fear of an overwhelming and seemingly monstrous/attacking environment to Oedipal issues (i.e., anxiety about me replacing his mother). Finally, analysis allowed Cameron to be able to see his mother for who she is—while she is often intrusive and dsyregulating, he can now hold his own ground and weather her "storms."

NOTE

1. Dr. Sherkow also saw the case that followed, Cameron, in psychoanalysis. In addition, Cameron interacted with Dr. Lieberman in two different ways. Dr. Lieberman was often in the Sherkow Center when Cameron had his sessions, and he enlisted her, as well as interns and externs who were at the Center, to participate in his races and ball games. Dr. Lieberman also participated in running the psychotherapeutic social skills group in which Cameron participa ted, starting at age seven. From this point forward, "I" or "me" refers to Dr. Sherkow.

REFERENCES

Arlow, J. A., Freud, A., Lampl-de Groot, J., and Beres, D. (1968). Panel discussion. *International Journal of Psycho-Analysis*, 49, 506–512.

Baron-Cohen, S. (1995). *Mindblindness: An Essay on Autism and Theory of Mind.* Cambridge, MA: MIT Press.

Baron-Cohen, S., Leslie, A. M., and Frith, U. (1985). Does the autistic child have a "theory of mind"? *Cognition*, 21, 37–46.

Beebe, B. and Lachmann, F. (1988). The contribution of mother-infant mutual influence to the origins of self and object representations. *Psychoanalytic Psychology*, 5, 305–337.

———. (1994). Representation and internalization in infancy: Three principles of salience. *Psychoanalytic Psychology*, 15, 1–37.

Edelman, S. (2012). *The Happiness of Pursuit: What Neuroscience Can Teach Us about the Good Life.* New York: Basic Books.

Fallon, T. and Sherkow, S. (2011). *Disordered Thought and Development: Chaos to Organization in the Moment.* Lanham, MD: Jason Aronson.

Fonagy, P. (1991). Thinking about thinking: Some clinical and theoretical considerations in the treatment of a borderline patient. *International Journal of Psycho-Analysis*, 72, 639–656.

Fonagy, P. and Target, M. (1998). Mentalization and the changing aims of child psychoanalysis. *Psychoanalytic Dialogues*, 8, 87–114.

Fonagy, P., Gergely, G., Jurist, E. L., and Target, M. (2002). *Affect Regulation, Mentalization, and the Development of the Self.* London, UK: Karnac.

Freud, A. (1970). The symptomatology of childhood: A preliminary attempt at classification. *Psychoanalytic Study of the Child*, 25, 19–41.

Freud, S. (1905). Three essays on the theory of sexuality. In J. Strachey (Ed.), *The Standard Edition of the Complete Psychological Works of Sigmund Freud, Vol. VII (1901–1905): A Case of Hysteria, Three Essays on Sexuality and Other Works.* London: Hogarth Press and Institute of Psychoanalysis, 1953.

———. (1907). Letter from Sigmund Freud to C. G. Jung, Undated. In W. McGuire (Ed.), *The Freud/Jung letters: The Correspondence between Sigmund Freud and C. G. Jung* (pp. 38–40). Princeton, NJ: Princeton University Press, 1974.

———. (1917). "Mourning and Melancholia." In J. Strachey (Ed.), *The Standard Edition of the Complete Psychological Works of Sigmund Freud, Vol XIV (1914–1916): The History of the Psycho-analytic Movement, Papers on Metapsychology, and Other Works.* London: Hogarth Press and Institute of Psychoanalysis, 1953.

———. (1919). "A child is being beaten": A contribution to the study of the origin of sexual perversions. In J. Strachey (Ed.), *The Standard Edition of the Complete Psychological Works of Sigmund Freud, Vol XVII (1917–1919): An Infantile Neurosis and Other Works.* London: Hogarth Press and Institute of Psychoanalysis, 1955.

Gergely, G. and Watson, J. S. (1996). The social biofeedback theory of parental affect-mirroring: The development of emotional self-awareness and self-control in infancy. *International Journal of Psychoanalysis*, 77(6): 1181–1212.

Glezerman, T. (2013). *Autism and the Brain: Neurophenomenological Interpretation.* New York: Springer.

Harrison, A. M. and Tronick, E. Z. (2007). Contributions to understanding therapeutic change: Now we have a playground. *Journal of the American Psychoanalytic Association*, 55, 853–874.

Jacobson, E. (1954). The self and the object world. *Psychoanalytic Study of the Child*, 9, 75–127.

Kana, R., Uddin, L., Kenet, T., Chugani, D., and Muller, R-A. (2014). Brain connectivity in autism. *Frontiers of Human Neurosocience*, 8, 1–4.

Kandel, E. (2007). *In Search of Memory: The Emergence of a New Science of Mind.* New York: W. W. Norton & Company, Inc.

Kandel, E., Dudai, Y., and Mayford, M. (2014). The molecular and systems biology of memory. *Cell*, 157, 163–186.

Klin, A. and Jones, W.(2007). Altered face scanning and impaired recognition of biological motion in a 15-month-old with autism. *Developmental Science*, 11(1), 40-46. Doi.org/10.1111/1467-7687.2007.00608.x

Lombardo, M. V., Chakrabarti, B., Bullmore, E. T., MRC AIMS Consortium, and Baron-Cohen, S. (2011). Specialization of right temporo-parietal junction for mentalizing and its relation to social impairments in autism. *Neuroimage*, 56,1832–1838.

Lyons-Ruth, K. (1998). Implicit relational knowing: Its role in development and psychoanalytic treatment. *Infant Mental Health Journal*, 19, 282–291.

———. (1999). The two-person unconscious: Intersubjective dialogue, enactive relational representation, and the emergence of new forms of relational organization. *Psychoanalytic Inquiry*, 19, 576–617.

Mahler, M. S., Pine, F., and Bergman, A. (1975). *The Psychological Birth of the Human Infant: Symbiosis and Individuation.* New York: Basic Books.

McDevitt, J. B. (1975). Separation-individuation, and object constancy. *Journal of the American Psychoanalytic Association*, 23, 713–742.

Piaget, J. (1974). *Memory and Intelligence.* NY: Basic Books.

Pine, F. (1982). The experience of the self. *Psychoanalytic Study of the Child*, 37, 143–168.

Qian, N. and Lipkin, R. M. (2011). A learning-style theory for understanding autistic behaviors. *Frontiers in Human Neuroscience*, 5, 51–17.

Sherkow, S. (2011). The dyadic psychoanalytic treatment of a toddler with autism spectrum disorder. *Psychoanalytic Inquiry*, 31, 252–275.

———. (2015, March). *Helping parents and therapists understand and cope with autism spectrum disorder.* TEDx talk presented at the Lycée Francais, New York, NY.

Sherkow, S. P. and Harrison, M. D. (2014). *Autism Spectrum Disorder: Perspectives from Psychoanalysis and Neuroscience.* Lanham, MD: Jason Aronson.

Sherkow, S. and Harrison, A. M. (2013). *Autism Spectrum Disorder: Perspectives from Psychoanalysis and Neuroscience.* Lanham, MD: Jason Aronson.

Sing-Curry, V. and Husain, M. (2009). The functional role of the inferior parietal lobe in the dorsal and ventral stream dichotomy. *Neuropsychoelogia*, 47, 1434–1448.

Stern, D. (1974). Mother and infant at play: The dyadic interaction involving facial, vocal and gaze behaviors. In *The Effect of the Infant on Its Caregiver*, M. Lewis and L. Rosenblum. New York: Wiley, pp. 187–213.

Trevarthen, C. (1979). Descriptive analyses of infant communicative behavior. In H.R. Shaffer (Ed.), *Studies in Mother-Infant Interaction* (227–270). New York: Academic Press.

Tronick, E. (2007). *The Neurobehavioral and Social-Emotional Development of Infants and Children.* New York: W. W. Norton & Company, Inc.

Winnicott, D. W. (1958). The capacity to be alone. *International Journal of Psychoanalysis*, 39, 416–420.

Chapter Twelve

Culture, Socialization, and Creativity in Analytic Practice

Monisha Nayar-Akhtar

INTRODUCTION AND HISTORICAL REVIEW

Psychoanalysis in the United States is in a state of flux in both its clinical practice and in its training. While the exact reasons for this remain unclear, most would agree that the challenges faced from other competing treatment models, which provide more time-contained and less expensive mental health interventions, as well as perhaps the astronomical cost of psychoanalytic training itself, has impeded its growth. Certainly, the caricatured portrayal of psychoanalysis by the film industry and the denouncement by other, sometimes prominent, mental health colleagues has also added to its vanishing image on the national mental health landscape. Ironically, despite this rather dismal picture, there continue to be significant advances in both psychoanalytic technique and theory. These broaden the depth and scope of the discipline, often leading to enhanced ways of working with populations that would otherwise have been unable to avail themselves of this form of intervention, nationally. More importantly, they draw attention in the social contexts in which the individuals reside, creating a culture of transforming psychoanalytic ideas and reaching across geographical boundaries and casting a wider net of appeal. This has in more recent years led to a growing excitement about perpetuating a paradigm of training that stimulates the creative mind and promotes a love of learning transcending traditional domestic borders and intellectual rigidity (Astley 1962; Morris 1992; Kernberg 2000). Shedding long-standing academic discourse and disagreements on what constitutes analysis and psychotherapy or the right kind of analytic patient, rigid psychoanalytic frameworks have now been modified to include the analyst's creative soul and independent thinking. Such transformations in the clinical and theoretical realms continue to intrigue us, and force us to examine the nature of transformation itself.

In contrast to this rather tarnished domestic image of psychoanalysis, one encounters a growing demand for psychodynamic and psychoanalytic training in other parts of the world, providing creative analysts an avenue to expand their psychoanalytic practices, broaden and deepen their reach (socially and culturally), and take psychoanalysis beyond its conventional European borders. Locally, this has translated into distance-learning psychoanalytic psychotherapy programs for some institutes, while others find themselves drawing analytic patients from a larger global pool. These and other changes provide compelling evidence of the cultural socialization that occurs as senior analysts now find themselves in positions of having to supervise and/or understand analytic patients who come from diverse and culturally nuanced backgrounds. The expansion of these programs to include psychoanalytic candidates is on the horizon (if not already prevalent), further forcing the entrepreneurially inclined analysts to shed their conservative hats and conventional methods in order to embrace contemporary and creative methods of engaging with the other. Perhaps the confluence of such external realities and internal personal dynamics propelled my own personal/professional journey upon graduation. This journey in the development of an analytic identity (as controversial as this may sound to some!) that shed conventional wisdom (and training) regarding clinical practice, while incorporating cultural and socialization practice prevalent in the communities I worked in (as I sought avenues to a "widening scope engagement" to broaden my theoretical and technical reach) proved to be the catalyst for my transformation. In doing so, it deepened my understanding of psychoanalysis and its ubiquitous relationship to the community in which it grows. This paper is an attempt to shed some light on this creative trajectory that has now spanned several decades of both professional and personal development. But before I embark on this project let me set the foundation to understand some basic premises of my work.

Community Outreach

The burgeoning of clinical outreach programs in the community, though mostly attributed to more recent times, is not new in the psychoanalytic world. I would be amiss if I did not describe and attribute the first call for community-based practice to Freud himself, who advocated for the use of psychoanalytic principles with disadvantaged populations. The establishment of free clinics for such a population shed light on Freud's vision of psychoanalysis as a cure for the masses, and serves now as the foundation for many programs that provide psychoanalysis to poor and socially disadvantaged populations in the United States (Altman 1993). However, despite such an early endorsement, the role of culture and creativity in analytic practice did not appear till much later in the literature. That is not to say that many did not grapple with such issues, from understanding the nuanced meaning of silence in the analytic dyad, to the use of humor, to self-disclosure, to the possibility of expanding the analyst's engagement with traumatized populations and incorporating cultural diversity into the analytical lexicon. As major theoretical and technical shifts began to appear in the literature it ushered in a new wave of thinking and working with individuals. The creative process inherent in psychoanalysis was now well underway and became further evident in the arena of applied psychoanalysis.

The mushrooming of psychoanalytically informed community outreach programs reflects the work of many analysts who work with the poor and disenfranchised (Leupniz, personal communication, 2015; Altman 1993), troubled and marginalized populations (Twemlow 2010), communities impacted by natural disasters (Krohn 2015) and societies devastated by the ravaging effects of manmade conflicts (First 2015). These analysts are just a few in the cadre of creative and culturally informed psychoanalysts who have broadened their vision and deepened their work by reaching into communities to help ameliorate human anxieties and suffering. However, while these analysts have concerned themselves with working with emotionally fractured communities, there are some who have adopted another creative avenue to go beyond their conventional borders. The China American Psychoanalytic Alliance (CAPA), founded by Elise Snyder, comes to mind as an example of a systematic, massive, and long-standing effort to reach out to another country (Fishkin et al. 2011). Established in 2001 during a fortuitous visit by its founder, Elise Snyder, to China, this outreach program has grown to encompass over 300 members who provide low-fee supervision, psychodynamic treatment and training, and now psychoanalysis using internet-based technologies. CAPA's phenomenal success is widely documented and it continues to grow exponentially. While CAPA is not the only outreach program in China (Scharff 2011) it has probably captured national and international interest by virtue of its substantial cyber presence and organizational outreach.

While the CAPA program undoubtedly grabs the national spotlight by its sheer size and reach, there are several other community-based programs that capture the spirit of creative psychoanalytic practice with cultural overtones. A 2015 special issue of *Psychoanalytic Inquiry* (Nayar-Akhtar 2015) presents the work of several psychoanalysts who work quietly and diligently to bring psychoanalytic understanding to the communities in which they operate. Their psychoanalytically informed explorations highlight the creative use of their clinical minds, their willingness to work in diverse and culturally complex settings, and a passion to take psychoanalytic practice beyond their domestic borders to reach people who would otherwise remain uninformed and in dire need of such clinical services. The cultural implications of the work of these analysts is implicit and compelling and provides the emotional and professional scaffolding for my work. Let me explore this briefly.

Cultural Trends

Contemporary literature in psychoanalysis has seen several movements to incorporate culture and its resulting impact on psychoanalytic practice. Concerning myself only with the American psychoanalytic community, one can trace the trajectory of incorporating cultural concerns to early descriptions of "culture shock" (Garza-Guerrero 1974), a term commonly used to describe changes in ego functioning following sudden and drastic changes in one's natural environment and the subsequent impact on the process of acculturation and assimilation encountered by an individual as they migrate from one country to another. While the earliest bastions of psychoanalytic thought in this country could undoubtedly be attributed to the migration of several European Jews who left during the time of the Holocaust to survive the oppressive Nazi regime, it is perhaps in more recent decades that the immigration process has been understood from a variety of different perspectives. A seminal paper by Salman Akhtar (1995) highlighted the complex relationship between the immigrant and his/her host country and country of origin. Paralleling the "second individuation" process of adolescence, Akhtar argues that the immigrant undergoes a significant transformation during the assimilation and acculturation process which is compounded by their ability to negotiate complex feelings of separation from both their country as well as their families of origin. This paper highlighted complex internal processes that accompany the journey of an immigrant, setting in motion a trajectory of cultural and clinical exploration that occurs with geographical dislocation.

Creativity in Practice

Psychoanalytically informed community outreach programs reflect the mind of the creative analyst at work. Some have documented their experience to demonstrate the complex and multiple ways they interact with the community to forge relationships and establish methodologies that effectively engage the population that they work with (Twemlow 2010). These cultural encounters appear to be transformative. There are several aspects of this process that are striking and would need consideration before one embarks on any venture to export psychoanalytic tenets across cultural borders, both symbolically and literally. Broadly speaking, one could identify several tracks that emerge in an analysis of such projects:

- The culture of the community itself;
- The psychoanalytic tenets being exported;
- The impact of the culture on the identity of the analyst; and
- And finally, the impact of the analyst on the culture they engage with.

In this chapter I present the expanding role of my work with my country of origin, India. In an effort to export psychoanalytic ideas to the larger Indian community, I developed several programs that emerged from various aspects of my psychoanalytic identity and training. The connection between India and psychoanalysis is not new, having originally been forged by Dr. Girish ChandreShekar Bose, who in the early 1900s corresponded with Freud to spark an ongoing communication in areas of mutual interest and discourse. While this did not exactly play out as anticipated, at least for Dr. Bose, it did lead to the creation of the Indian Psychoanalytic Society. Based in Calcutta, it grew to about sixty members who remained largely loyal to their founding father, Dr. Bose. However, the group remained local and did not spread to other parts of India. Psychoanalytic inroads were made in other metropolitan cities (Mumbai and New Delhi), but they remain regionally confined and somewhat isolated from each other. For example, an analyst practicing in Kolkata, Dr. Bose's original home, remarked to me one day that no national conference exists to bring these various groups together. In New Delhi, a group of psychoanalytically oriented individuals continue to hold lectures on psychoanalytic ideas and their application to the community at large, but their efforts for the most part appear to be restricted, with little impact on psychoanalytically informed training, and do not reach the larger community of which they are a part. Reasons for this are complicated and outside the scope of this chapter. But keeping all this in mind, I was guided by a singular motive, to broaden the reach of psychoanalytic thinking and create an atmosphere where a hunger for psychodynamic concepts in theory and practice could arise. The quintessential guiding posts for my ventures into this new world of professional development and analytic creativity included promoting community-based programs to reach a larger audience, sensitizing the regional (and beyond) mental health community to think dynamically, and reaching out to therapists who might not otherwise have any exposure to such ideas and technical considerations.

Having said this, any outreach model would need to be culturally sensitive, incorporating prevalent methods of viewing mental illness and resistances to treatment as well (Kakar 1985). Consistent with my counterparts who have established such programs in other communities, this model would have to be organic in nature, addressing the needs of the community and finding points or moments of intervention that would lend itself to future growth and exploration. Finally, I was aware that deviating from more traditional applications of psychoanalytic principles would challenge my internalized representations of analytic identity. This would force me to reassess and regroup some aspects of my internal analytic structures, especially those pertinent to the ongoing development and maintenance of my analytic identity. Let me elaborate on this further.

General Considerations

The application of psychoanalytic clinical skills to diverse cultural contexts is not new. In the history of the psychoanalytic movement, many analysts returned to provide instruction and help in the development of institutes worldwide, especially in areas where the knowledge of such skills was not readily available. In more recent decades, the influence of foreign-born psychiatrists/psychoanalysts in the United States has furthered the exploration of issues pertinent to the training of such doctors, using psychoanalytic psychotherapy with diverse cultural populations and with the increased sensitivity that is required when bridging cultural divides and schisms (Kakar 1995).

Leah Davidson (1987) identifies a critical difference between the East and the West. She states that in the West, a more formal logical process exists in any argument or discussion that prevails. In the East however, many different facts are set out "laterally for an authority to choose the correct combination of factors" (Davidson 1987, p. 230). According to Davidson, social mores and obligations determine how individuals in any particular society choose an option.

Davidson also identifies what she calls an emphasis in the East on an egoless state. People are more collective in their orientation, defined by their affiliation to a community, family, and by their actions towards each other. *Character and personality* (ibid., p. 231) are not necessarily stressed as concepts.

Challenges

I identified three main challenges that I would encounter as I embarked on this work.

a) My first concern was my clear and strong identification with my institute of training. Having trained at an institute that identifies with the structural model of training, I was guided primarily by a work ethic or work ego that adhered to a clear and definite paradigm for engagement. This included parameters for conducting psychodynamic psychotherapy and psychoanalysis, such as boundaries, both with the patient and within oneself, adherence to a particular psychoanalytic hour, and maintaining a certain analytic attitude. I was aware that my branching out to more community-based projects would challenge my "analytic identity" and that I would have to grapple with the

issues that arose from such encounters. I understood that the analyst's "work ego" (Olinick, Poland, Grigg, & Granatir 1973) in my case would have to undergo a transformation as I moved between countries and reestablished myself with a particular frame of reference that reflected my willingness to adapt and be "socialized" by the community that I engaged with. The analyst's work ego refers to mental functions that develop over several years of analytic training and beyond, and range from a variety of intrapsychic constructs that facilitate the analyst's ability to connect with the patient and conduct a proper analysis. These functions include but are not restricted to the capacity for empathy, self-reflection, reverie, and trial identification.

Contemporary perspectives on "work-ego" related mental functions have broadened this definition to include humor, judicious self-disclosure, and the capacity to learn from enactments; these are more relationally based and interpersonally anchored concepts. They are also more dependent upon the holding function of a familiar culture and susceptible to changes in the cultural setting.

b) This naturally led to my developing and adopting a more flexible approach in thinking and practice. Though originally from India, I could not assume that cultural norms once second nature to me would reemerge and give me an immediate and comfortable sense of belonging. I would therefore have to become more attuned to the cultural nuances that accompanied my journey, including my reentry to the United States where a different set of cultural values would reappear.

For example, one of the important distinctions that can be made between the Eastern and Western worlds is their concept of time. In the Western world the notion of time has become connected with productivity, as in "time is money, time matters," overtime, and so on. In the Indian subcontinent, the notion of time is not so strictly defined. Asian notions of time are more fluid, less punctuated by structure, and not equated necessarily with money-making and economic gain.

c) And finally, any community-based project that requires the creative use of one's time and energy forces us to make time for it in a more thoughtful and judicious manner. Making the best use of our time means condensing and using various community-based means to impart what we believe is quintessential in understanding how the mind works, how behavior is manifested, and what guides us unconsciously in the things we do.

Three Tracks

With this as a backdrop, I developed the following tracks of community outreach:

- Institutional Work

- Community Workshops
- Individual Supervision

Orphanage Work

My work with an orphanage in New Delhi, India, began in December 2011, when upon the request of a friend I contacted the Managing Trustee of an orphanage to offer my services as a psychologist/psychoanalyst. She had several concerns regarding the care and management of the orphaned children. By government policy, no child could be placed in an orphanage under the age of five and they were required to leave the institution by age eighteen. While the Managing Trustee was familiar with psychoanalytic ideas, she had found no systematic way to train a small cadre of social workers in understanding and working with her young charges. Sensing her dire need to get help, I set up a series of in-depth workshops on attachment and trauma for her group of social workers. Their overwhelmingly positive response led to monthly consultation meetings during which we discussed cases and I provided additional training to her social workers.

Community Workshops

My initial work informed me of the lack of any meaningful psychodynamic training in the area. Recognizing an imperative need to train the larger community, I developed a series of workshops that could be offered to mental health workers in the New Delhi Metropolitan area. To do this I needed to find an advocate on the ground. For me this appeared in the form of two individuals: Dr. G, a practicing child psychiatrist, and Dr. M, the managing trustee of the orphanage that sponsored my initial work and established ongoing parameters and contact for my involvement with orphans and the orphanage. Dr. G is one of three child psychiatrists in the Delhi Metropolitan area, and over his several years of practice he has established clinics with offices spread around the city. While clinically astute, Dr. G is committed to advancing his clinical expertise. His initial encounter with me convinced him that I could provide ongoing training programs that would enhance clinical knowledge in working with specific populations. Having attended my clinical workshops at the orphanage, Dr. G was quite enthusiastic about my establishing a teaching program in Delhi and collaborating with me to provide workshops in specific areas of concerns. The Indian Institute of Psychotherapy Training and Research was established by me in 2012 with the specific purpose of providing in-depth workshops, and it provided three-day workshop topics that were of significant concern. For example, the institute has offered psychodynamically informed programs in trauma, working with traumatized children and families, understanding attachment and adolescent

development, childhood sexual abuse, and more recently, in 2016, a three-day intensive workshop on psychodynamic psychotherapy. These programs have been well received, and in addition to furthering the understanding of psychoanalytic theory and technique have clearly established the overwhelming need for ongoing workshops in related areas. This is a personal and professional commitment that I honor every year. These workshops arise out of my ongoing work with the orphanage and in understanding the overwhelming societal problems that exist in the area. The following gives an example of how my workshop on childhood sexual abuse emerged.

Sexual abuse in orphaned children is ubiquitous. In perusing the regional literature on this subject, I learned of the overwhelming numbers of children who have been sexually abused in the country. In 2012, the Government of India launched a large-scale study to capture this data. Their findings were published in a report that documented unprecedented numbers of children, both boys and girls, who had been abused by family members as well as while they were placed in institutional care. The study attempted to provide guidelines for interviewing and working with such children of all ages. My workshop arose out of the recognition that a dearth of literature surrounded this profoundly disturbing issue, especially with respect to clinical understanding, to technical intervention, and to the establishment of age- and gender-sensitive protocols in working with young children and adolescents. My three-day workshop, attended by psychiatrists, psychologists, and social workers, addressed these issues in-depth and provided a psychodynamically informed understanding of the long-term impact of childhood sexual abuse.

Another example arose from a concern that Dr. G expressed during one of the informal meetings with me regarding clinical interests and concerns. Dr. G, committed to the community programs, worked with local school counselors to address the needs of their student population. Both behavioral and emotional concerns regarding their students were growing. The school counselors felt ill equipped to manage and deal with the problems of lying, fighting, and sexuality, in addition to several cases of severe anxiety and depression that kept cropping up in their case load. Of specific concern were their difficulties in helping students regulate their emotions and not resort to acting out in some form. A brief three-hour session on understanding and working with emotional dysregulation came out of this meeting in response to this specific need, and received the support of the local sponsoring organization and clinical community.

These aforementioned community-based programs, from their inception to their execution, offer a brief insight into the complexities of working with different communities. From developing local relationships, to maintaining ongoing consultation liaisons, to remaining sensitive to clinical needs, to incorporating culturally sensitive ideas, these workshops reflect the transfor-

mations that have occurred in me during the course of my journey in community outreach and involvement.

Supervision: Some Caveats

One of the greatest pleasures of analytic practice is the ability to train and provide supervision for those who wish to deepen their clinical thinking and work with their patients in a psychoanalytically informed way. As a result of my outreach efforts in my country of origin, I have been fortunate to come across therapists who, while having some introduction to psychoanalytic principles, felt woefully inadequate in their technique. However, prior to engaging in the provision of supervision with these therapists, I felt it was important for me the keep the following caveats in mind.

a) The role of boundaries:

In moving from the institution and community to the individual, the therapist is likely to encounter situations that call for a sort of engagement that in Western circles might cause discomfort and raise eyebrows. For example, sociocultural norms of how therapists begin and end sessions, whether by shaking hands, smiling, or engaging in some light verbal exchange, may vary from culture to culture. During the course of my work in New Delhi, I was often struck by the ease with which the therapists and counselors talked about physical contact with their patients and how much it became part of the treatment. For example, it was not unusual for me to hear of therapists who put their arm lightly around a patient's shoulder, or touched them on their forearm at the beginning or end of a session. To conclude that this constitutes a boundary violation is a misunderstanding if not an injustice, as it undermines some widely accepted and ego syntonic healing and holding aspects of one culture (India) and ignores the litigious qualities of another (America).

b) The role of affects and their expression:

Understanding affects and their expression is an integral aspect of psychoanalytic work. Having been part of the Indian culture (and still imbued in it), I can say with a certain degree of authority that Indians, especially in reference to professionals, are extremely hospitable and warm. Interpersonal relationships are governed by respect and deference to others (some Westerners might even refer to it as being subservient). There is a reluctance to confront adults older than oneself and a pattern of assuming a reverential stance when in the company of respected professionals. The personal and professional attention that I receive from my supervisees and colleagues assuages any feelings of physical and emotional burden (from having traveled such a long distance) that I might otherwise have, and quickly reminds me of the culture's inherently warm disposition. This translates into simple acts of human kindness, such as sensitivity to one's diet, to temperature, travel plans, and even a wish for narcissistic feeding. Putting all this

aside, it is the clinical realm that I wish to now comment upon. In this area, the following example illustrates some differences in how the therapist working in the Asian culture might view certain affects and their expression.

Tired after a long journey, I commented to an Indian colleague about an American patient's overwhelming demands on me to be available at all time. I added that I found this to be sadistic and was contemplating how I could draw attention to it in a therapeutic way. My colleague responded by a certain degree of awe, stating that he could never think of confronting a patient on their sadistic and aggressive maneuvers. This just did not happen in the clinical realm.

Family Involvement

It is not unusual in India for the family to be an integral part of the therapy regime. While this poses challenges in maintaining boundaries between the therapist and the identified patient, this is not an aspect of the therapeutic encounter that can be ignored by the supervisor. Familiarizing oneself with how the family serves to function as a containing and holding system for the patient, as well as their ubiquitous presence in the clinical setting, is an essential in this endeavor.

Individual and Group Supervision:

During the course of my repeated visits to New Delhi I have had the opportunity to meet young as well as mid-career therapists, practicing in public and private settings, who express a strong desire to deepen their understanding of their cases and incorporate more psychodynamic thinking in their case conceptualization and clinical technique. It was during one of my workshops that I encountered Ms. L. She attended several of my workshops before one day approaching me and asking me to provide weekly supervision via Skype. Ms. L was familiar with psychodynamic ideas, having received some training in counseling when she lived in London, England, a few decades ago. However, she felt insecure about her training, had clients who were from culturally diverse backgrounds, and felt challenged in trying to understand and work with them.

Supervision is a complex and nuanced exchange between two people, where a multitude of individual anxieties and fears are masked as the supervisee initiates a process of learning from another. This process is even more complex when there is a homoethnic identification (as was the case between myself and Ms. L) as well as a geographical rupture and subsequent displacement (my immigration). These subtle strands of complexity percolate in any supervision and are possibly less apparent when the supervisor and supervisee are face to face in the same structural space. The inevitable use of Skype in long distant supervision forces another "space," i.e., cyberspace, to enter the dialogue, forcing both the supervisor and the supervisee to contend with the inevitable and well-documented psychologically informed impact of such space on dialogue and exchange.

My work with Ms. L. certainly captured many aspects of these voiced concerns. I will elaborate on a few to highlight the creative process at work in a culturally informed setting, providing a model that incorporates many aspects of the supervisory/supervisee models that have been documented by others in the analytic literature.

As she brought her cases for discussion, I felt bombarded by Ms. L's desperate need to get clinical supervision. While I recognized this hunger for clinical insights, I needed to regulate the influx of information from my end (as I felt overwhelmed, running out of time, experiencing an impasse). While these were reflective of parallel processes in addition to the supervisory set-up, creating suitable parameters so that our supervisory sessions would be productive was essential to our work. These included a set time for our meetings and helping her to develop a system of keeping process notes. It also seemed imperative to ask her to limit our ongoing discussions to a few cases. This allowed us to embark on a journey that allowed for a creative exchange of ideas, rather than an influx of ideas guided by more Western notions of child development and adult functioning. For example, Ms. L was astonished when I asked her if the children in her practice had a transitional object. Though she knew what that represented, she had never seen that in her practice. She wondered if this was because the mother was always around for the child. While we could use this discourse to correct misconceptions of the functionality of a transitional object, it nevertheless remained a baffling omission, one that I continue to ponder upon from time to time.

One of my greatest pleasures in supervising Ms. L has been the abundance of child and adolescent cases that she has brought in for supervision. From children of divorced parents, to adopted children and adolescents, to children of parents who have moved from the United States or Europe, there was no dearth of cases. I will present one such case to illustrate the richness of the cases and the work that could be done via Skype supervision.

Four-year-old Jose was the son of an immigrant mother of Hispanic origin. She had recently moved to New Delhi following a work-related promotion. Jose's parents had never married, though his father had also relocated to a neighboring country, which afforded him periodic contact with his son. Jose had a series of nannies from different countries, often on a rotating basis as they moved from one job to another. Jose was referred to Ms. L when he began to experience difficulties in his new school. Usually an outgoing young child, he was now withdrawn, spending his time alone during recess, and he did not seem to want to socialize with his new playmates. At home, he clung to his nanny and had difficulties sleeping at night. He had nightmares and often woke up crying and crawling into his mother's bed to fall asleep again. His mother had a demanding workload and would spend hours at work having little time with her son. With Ms. L, however, Jose was an articulate young child who loved to play in the sandbox. He would make up elaborate stories using animals, which in displacement allowed for many feelings of anger, fear, and distress to emerge. Upon his return from his visits to his father, Jose had additional difficulty readjusting. I drew Ms. L's attention to the nannies that had been part of his life and asked her to obtain additional information from the mother. We learned that these nannies would leave abruptly with little time for preparing Jose to adjust to these departures. While there had been several such nannies, there was one he had been particularly fond of, and she had left to go back to her country of origin. Supervising Ms. L on the parent work, I asked her to educate the mother on the role of this person in Jose's life and the distress it caused him when he was no longer in contact, and suggested using Skype or FaceTime to stay in contact for a period of time so as to ameliorate his pain and confusion. Over time, Ms. L began to note changes in his behavior as he became quite attached to her and appeared more cheerful and less anxious even in school.

Broadening the Scope of Clinical Supervision

In more recent years, my scope of clinical supervision has extended to a larger group of therapists who practice as counselors in school settings, or as hospital-based psychologists or in private practice. Learning about my individual supervision, they approached me to conduct larger group-based supervision when I was in New Delhi. This has led to several meetings with them. Following are some examples of the training programs implemented and their outcome.

One of the serious deficits noted by me during the course of my interactions with these therapists is the absence of a comprehensive way of understanding a patient and diagnosing various aspects of their personality functioning that would be pertinent for the clinical work. Keeping this in mind, I introduced a two-day intensive training program to teach the therapists a theory of the mind as well as the theory of the developmental process. Drawing upon their cases as well as using clinical vignettes from my own practice, I introduced essential concepts of how a mind (the therapist) understands another mind. More specifically, I worked with ideas introduced and elaborated upon by Peter Fonagy and his colleagues (Fonagy & Target 2007), as well as concepts of the developmental process that would enhance their understanding of the case.

Broadening the Scope of Cultural Thinking

My regular visits to New Delhi have resocialized me with my country of origin. It has also drawn attention to significant gaps in cultural thinking that permeate society and impact children, adolescents, and adults. For example, while one could explore the rampant presence of child sexual abuse in society, one could not have a dialogue on sexuality and gender issues. Yet my supervisees were discussing cases where issues of sexuality, body image, and gender dynamics were prominent. Keeping in mind that sometimes "memes" (Dawkins 1976) can introduce sensitive topics for discussion, I proposed that I offer a workshop on contemporary psychoanalytic understanding of sexuality and gender. This workshop, offered in August 2017, was attended by therapists, pastors, and private school counselors, as well as my core group of supervisees, and was received with a great deal of enthusiasm. The eight-hour workshop was filled with clinical vignettes and discussions on child and adolescent sexuality. Contrary to what one might have thought, the group was quite vocal and willing to talk about various aspects of sexual development from masturbation to sexual fantasies and their role in adolescent identity consolidation. They brought in clinical material that illustrated their work with adult patients as well, providing us an opportunity to explore the dynamics underlying the complex nature of clinical cases and facilitating the process of talking about sexual and emotional intimacy. The following brief vignette presented by one of the attendees illustrates this aspect of the work.

Case #1

The therapist, a young woman in the later 20s, began working with a 40-year-old man who was disturbed by a revelation from his 7-year-old son that the biological mother had sexually abused him. The patient while seeking psychological counseling for his son soon realized that he too had been sexually assaulted by his mother when he was a young boy. The resulting emotions led to his referral to the therapist. While exploring these feelings the patient regressed, lying on the floor in a fetal position, crying uncontrollably. Distraught and confused, the therapist did not know what to do. We explored the imperative need to contain and hold the patient in the space while permitting the expression of his distress and deep emotions. The therapist then expressed concern for her safety (as her patient was a large man with a formidable presence), as she had recently moved to a new office and did not feel that if the patient were to attack her she would be able to draw attention to this, in contrast to her previous office where a guard posted at the entrance provided a modicum of safety. That the therapist was scared was quite evident, as was the fact that the patient was regressing as he retrieved memories that had hitherto remained unavailable to him. Stressing the importance of the therapist's safety, yet providing room for the work of therapy to proceed, we began to explore how the patient's life was paralleling that of his son's. My immediate reaction along with my supervisees was to be overly concerned for the therapist. I noted the alarm that I felt and wondered if the patient was on the brink of a psychotic break. However, as the therapist began to talk about the patient, I along with other members of the group noted her hesitation as well as her inclination to be overly critical of herself. When I asked her to present some process notes, it became clear that her actual work with the patient was far more containing, and the patient appeared healthier, than we had initially thought. When we began to explore this discrepancy, other aspects of the therapist's countertransference, as well as her rage toward him for some characterological aspects of his behavior, emerged. These characterological aspects included the patient using the bathroom and leaving it a mess every time. In fact, the supervisee was unaware of how angry she really was with the patient till she revealed that she had not informed the patient of the new bathroom in her new office! The exploration of her countertransference, the work that she was actually doing, and exploring the role of containment and holding when working with traumatized patients, strengthened her therapeutic resolve and eased the constraints that her superego was placing on her.

Case # 2

Ms. A, a therapist in her early 30s, began working with a young man who had recently graduated with a law degree but was unable to find any work. Unable to find a qualified therapist in his hometown, he traveled several hours by train to meet with her once a week. Ms. A reported that high school boys had sexually abused the patient when he was in middle school but he did not appear conflicted about these interactions. He reported an extensive history of ruptures, being moved from one home to another, his father a local gangster who was jailed when the patient was five years old and his mother an aspiring actress who would periodically have psychotic episodes. The biological father died when the patient was seven years old. The patient, despite a solid academic education, found himself unable to move forward, stuck with a family who he described as being exceedingly narcissistic and unaware of his internal struggles. The patient had recently broken up with his girlfriend of a few years, and was worried that he would not be able to sustain a relationship of any kind. He also reported that he was constantly bombarded with sexual thoughts and images, watched porn excessively, and was for all practical purposes hypersexualized. I asked the therapist to elaborate on his attire and presentation. She stated that he was a good-looking young man who dressed very well and was quite articulate and erudite. He was almost someone, she said, and paused: "that I could be friends with if we met outside." I remarked that I thought she was almost going to say she could have dated him had they met outside. She confirmed my suspicion and we explored what this might mean about the patient and how he presented himself. I remarked that he was probably seductive and she laughed and said "Yes," he was, with puppy dog eyes when he looked at her. From this we proceeded to explore the various types of countertransference reactions one could have and how she could find a way to expand her work with her patient.

CONCLUSION

Creativity in psychoanalytic practice incorporating culture and socialization is hardly a new phenomenon. Professional narratives that highlight the transformative nature of one's work provide only a glimpse of the complexity of internal and external processes that shape such encounters and trajectories in life. This chapter provides a glimpse in the complex trajectory of my professional development that furthered the exportation of psychoanalytic ideas, both theoretical and technical, to the New Delhi Metropolitan area. Traversing the great divide of cultural norms and societal taboos, this work involved the gradual shaping and molding of a community that is hungry for help in this realm. The work is far from over and continues with ever-expanding and far-reaching implications. That psychoanalysis is alive and well in this part of the world is amply evident from my ongoing visits and the persistent need for involvement. The pursuit of psychoanalysis in the twenty-first century is a creative enterprise and one that I hope will take us well into the twenty-second century.

REFERENCES

Akhtar, S. (1995). A third individuation: Immigration, identity, and the psychoanalytic process. *Journal of the American Psychoanalytic Association*, 43, 1051–1084.

Altman, N. (1993). Psychoanalysis and the urban poor. *Psychoanalytic Dialogues*, 3(1), 29–49.

Astley, R. (1962). Group 1 for Study of Curriculum, and Didactic Teaching—A sketch of their meeting and their work. *Journal of the American Psychoanalytic Assocation,* 10, 145–152.

Davidson, L. (1987). Supervision of psychotherapy East and West. *American Journal of Psychoanalysis*, 47, 230–236.

Dawkins, R. (1976). *The Selfish Gene*. Oxford University Press.

First, E. (2015) Siege: Marwan and Sahar, four years after the 2009 Gaza War. *Psychoanalytic Inquiry*, 35(7), 733–743.

Fishkin, R., Fishkin, L., Leli, U., Katz, B., and Snyder, K. (2011). Psychodynamic treatment, training and supervision using internet-based technologies. *Journal of the American Academy of Psychoanalysis and Dynamic Psychiatry*, 39, 155–168.

Fonagy, P. and Target, M. (2007). The rooting of the mind in the body: New links between attachment theory and psychoanalytic thought. *Journal of the American Psychoanalytic Association*, 55(2), 411–456.

Freud, S. (1919). Lines of advances in psychoanalytic therapy. In Strachey, J. (Ed.). *The Standard Edition of the Complete Psychological Works of S. Freud, Vol. XVII (1917–1919): An Infantile Neurosis and Other Works* (pp. 157–168). London: Hogarth and the Institute for Psycho-Analysis.

Garza-Guerrero, C. (1974). Culture shock: Its mourning and the vicissitudes of identity. *Journal of the American Psychoanalytic Association*, 22, 408–429.

Kakar, S. (1985). Psychoanalysis and non-Western cultures. *International Review of Psychoanalysis*, 12, 441–448.

———. (1995). Clinical work and cultural imagination. *Psychoanalytic Quarterly*, 64, 265–281.

Kernberg, O. (2000). A concerned critique of psychoanalytic education. *International Journal of Psychoanalysis*. 81(1), 97–120.

———. (2006). The continuing changes in psychoanalytic education: Part I. *International Journal of Psychoanalysis*, 87(6), 1649–1673.

———. (2007). The continuing changes in psychoanalytic education: Part II. *International Journal of Psychoanalysis*, 88(1), 183–202.

Krohn, A. (2015). Psychological struggles of children in alternative care settings. *Psychoanalytic Inquiry*, 35(7), 668–681.

Morris, J. (1992). Psychoanalytic training today. *Journal of the American Psychoanalytic Association*, 40, 1185–1210.

Nayar-Akhtar, M. (2015). On the seashore of Sunshine Homes: Psychoanalytic perspectives on working with institutionalized children in India. *Psychoanalytic Inquiry*, 35(7), 744–757.

Roland, A. (1993). *In Search of Self in India and Japan. Toward a Cross Cultural Psychology*. Princeton, NJ. Princeton University Press. 1988. 380 pp. *Psychoanalytic Quarterly* 62, 305–309.

Olinick, S. L., Poland, W. S., Grigg, K. A., and Granatir, W. L. (1973). The psychoanalytic work ego: Process and interpretation. *International Journal of Psychoanalysis*, 54(2), 143–151.

Scharff, D. E. (2011). Issue introduction: Psychoanalysis in China. *International Journal of Applied Psychoanalytic Studies*, 8(3), 191–195.

Twemlow, S. W. (2010). A community of schools: Psychoanalytic influences on peaceful and academically strong schools in USA, Australia, New Zealand and Jamaica. *International Journal of Psychoanalysis*, 91(5), 1258–1260.

Zhong, J. (2011). Working with Chinese patients: Are there conflicts between Chinese culture and psychoanalysis? *International Journal of Applied Psychoanalytic Studies*, 8, 218–226.

Chapter Thirteen

Psychological Testing for Psychoanalysis

Michael S. Garfinkle and Sara Lynn Richardson

The history of psychological testing has evolved to address myriad needs of individuals and institutions dating back four millennia, ranging from selection for employment and religious purposes to assessment of character and beyond. For much of the middle of the twentieth century, psychological assessment was considered a valuable source of information for psychoanalytic treatment, among other uses. In this chapter, we briefly review the history of psychological testing before considering why the disciplines of psychology and psychoanalysis became interrelated in the mid-twentieth century, and then follow with a description of the major components of psychological assessment, concluding with a consideration of the ongoing value of this practice to psychoanalysis.

A BRIEF SURVEY OF THE ORIGINS OF PSYCHOLOGICAL TESTING

The history of psychological testing has roots in Imperial China where measures were applied to predict the suitability of a candidate for civil service, which included, for example, assessment of penmanship as a means by which to determine the ability to communicate clearly (Gregory 2003, p. 4). In the West, historical antecedents of modern psychological testing can be traced to the work of Sir Francis Galton, who invented a series of psychosensory and psychophysiological tests in nineteenth-century Britain (Gregory 2003, p. 2). Galton's interest also included human evolution and heredity, especially in families of so-called geniuses. In a classic article published in *Macmillan's Magazine*, Galton wondered if humans could be bred "purely for intellectual power, and disregarding shape, size, and every other quality" (Galton 1865). He identified 605 individuals who met his criteria for genius and lived between 1453–1853, and he found "102 relationships" between those individuals, supporting his claim that genius runs in families. The luster of this work was lost over time, not only because the legacy of Galton's research produced enthusiasm for eugenics, but because Galton himself prepared the way for this appropriation, writing: "We are living in a sort of intellectual anarchy, for want of master minds. The general intellectual capacity of our leaders requires to be raised, and also to be differentiated" (Galton 1865, p. 165).

While the history of this appropriation led into the storminess of the experiments of the Third Reich, the legacy of intelligence research was also continued more generatively by researchers like Charles Spearman, who sought to define "general intelligence" (Spearman 1904). Spearman integrated the psychophysics work of Galton, Wilhelm Wundt, Camille Delezenne, and others, in an effort to produce a general intelligence quotient, defined as "Spearman's 'r,'" which bears relation to the modern term, "IQ." A contemporary of Spearman's, Alfred Binet, was committed to defining the intelligence of "subnormals," including "the insane type," a former, and rather unfortunate, description of individuals who showed signs of intellectual decay over time, and who today would be thought of as suffering from dementia or the cognitive effects of psychosis (Binet 1905/1916). Of significance to the present purpose was Binet's method, which integrated the "medical," "pedagogical," and "psychological" in his measurements of intelligence. As psychological science in the early twentieth century narrowly defined the psychological as "intelligence," Binet added to this conceptualization by considering "judgment" and "memory" as relevant elements of intellectual functioning, a novel contribution to the field. While the former was difficult to test, it stands that Binet made this intentionally so, as he sought to shift the focus of assessments of individuals from psychophysical features to emotional characteristics, now properly within the domain of the psychological.

Galton mentored the American psychologist James McKeen Cattell, who published the first significant articulation of the value of testing in measuring "mental processes, their interdependence, and their variation under different circumstances" (Cattell 1890, p. 1). Cattell proposed the use of ten tests that would measure sensory processes in terms of reaction and differential judgment, pain threshold, and memory. These, Cattell suggested, could be used to evaluate performance using psychophysiological terms which he advanced, such as "just noticeable sensation," and "least noticeable difference," which he judged as the most significant means to measure "mental intensity." Conversely, Cattell committed his research project to determining the minimum condition at which the human mind begins to react to novelty or difference. Notably, Cattell's tests of physical and psychological "character" were at some point made compulsory for freshmen entering Columbia University, where Cattell was on faculty (Gregory 2003). In the publication which outlined the findings from the Columbia data, Cattell remarked on his notion of the importance of psychological testing: "we must use our measurements to study the development of the individual and of the race, to disentangle the complex factors of heredity and environment" (Cattell and Ferrand 1896). Although Cattell's work in psychophysiology helped to legitimize psychology as an experimental science in its own right, his valuation of inheritable characteristics, like Galton, also supported the eugenics movement.

Also relevant is the history of neuropsychological testing, which ought to begin with the work of Pierre Paul Broca, the French physician and anatomist. Broca's interest in the brain was spurred by treating a fifty-one-year-old Louis Victor Leborgne, who presented to the Bicêtre Hospital in suburban Paris, having not been able to speak for thirty years (Broca 1861). This middle-aged man could only respond to questions with a single syllable, "tan," and it was only on postmortem evaluation that Broca was able to determine that a brain lesion in a section of the frontal region of the dominant lobe was responsible for the loss of speech. This region is now referred to as "Broca's area." Broca's early research on aphasia, or the inability to comprehend or formulate language, reflected a pivotal moment in psychological science that inspired generations of correlational research, often linking dysfunctional behavior with brain damage or underdevelopment. More specifically, Broca's work inspired a field of research that as early as 1930 was determined to account for human behavior in brain mechanisms, as seen in the work of Karl Lashley. Lashley led a paradigm shift in neuropsychology, from simply looking for single regions of the brain that could each be assigned a correlative function, to a more dynamic model of the brain built upon his theory of the "mutual influence of cerebral activities" (Lashley 1930). While Broca was indeed correct that the small sections of the frontal lobe he identified were implicated in the aphasia of Leborgne, Lashley's approach potentiated new theories that would, for example, connect language centers with affective areas of the brain.

The history of personality assessment has a considerably longer prehistory, with some sources citing the biblical account of Gideon using observations of how his men drank water from a stream as a selection criterion for who should join his army (Sundberg 1977). Examples from ancient Greece and Rome through to the Middle Ages reveal both formal and informal means to assess personality, including those designed to identify witches and heretics (Butcher 2010). The modern history of personality assessment can be traced to the nineteenth century as seen in the work of Franz Joseph Gall and Johan Spurzheim on phrenology, the study of contours of the head and their hypothesized connection to character and talent (ibid.). This pseudoscientific approach gained popularity in the United States in the 1820s, popularized by Charles Caldwell, and later the brothers Orson Squire Fowler and Lorenzo Fowler, who created a phrenology museum and a mail-order business. Galton, twice described above, who was a contemporary of, and influence on, Charles Darwin, expanded his research beyond psychophysiology to the study of "abnormal states" by the turn of the twentieth century (J. M. Cattell 1890). The use of survey methods to broadly assess personality was originated in The Netherlands by Heymans and Wiersma, who had "3,000 physicians rate people with whom they were well acquainted" (Heymans and Wiersma 1906, quoted in Butcher 2010). Contemporaneously, Carl Jung began studying personality using word association tasks, in part inspired by Sigmund Freud's preeminent work on free association (C. G. Jung 1907). A decade later, the U.S. Army hired Robert Woodworth to develop a psychodiagnostic self-report, the "Personal Data Sheet," or PDS, which produced a sum score hypothesized to correlate with the extent of psychiatric problems (Woodworth 1919). Woodworth's PDS became a model for a century of research and scale development, as well as raising the question of whether people could answer questions about themselves honestly and without being overly self-censorious.

As Lashley (1930) was developing more complex theories about the relationship between brain functioning and observable behavior, Herman Rorschach, who was influenced by Jung's work, was developing the field of psychodiagnostics through advancement of the inkblot test bearing his name, heralding the start of personality research not dependent on the deliberate self-report of patients (Rorschach 1921). The history of the Rorschach test, depicted in further detail below, is well-described in many works, including in the textbook that heralded a more objective interpretation system by the American psychologist John Exner (1974). Several years after the development of the Rorschach Inkblot Test, Henry Murray and Christiana Morgan, both Harvard psychologists, developed the Thematic Apperception Test (TAT) (Murray 1938), which was manualized five years later (Murray 1943). These tests moved away from the self-reports of Heymans and Wiersma (1906), and Woolworth (1919), in favor of deliberately vague tests that allowed the evaluator to gain insight into the unconscious processes at work in the mind, which were believed to be warded off from consciousness, especially when evoked with direct questioning.

This brief overview of several origin points in the history of psychological testing has been presented to describe the early efforts to determine and assess human behavior, as each produced a legacy of further research and the development of new tests of relevance to psychoanalytic work. In the next section, we will build upon this foundation as we describe the early stages of the relationship between psychological testing and psychoanalysis, as well as the status and potential uses of testing in psychoanalysis today.

The Origin of the Connection between Psychological Testing and Psychoanalysis

No person is better identified with the entrée of psychological testing into psychoanalytic treatment than David Rapaport, who, along with Merton Gill and Roy Schafer, published the first major textbook on the use of testing in psychoanalysis (Rapaport, Gill, and Schafer 1946). Rapaport and Schafer, who were teacher and student, are credited with developing the concept of administering a battery of tests, which formed part of the foundational identity of the field of clinical psychology that they helped to originate (Fritsch 2013). In turn, psychological testing became the specialty of clinical psychologists. Rapaport initiated a tradition of psychological testing at the Menninger Clinic in Topeka, Kansas, and then at the Austen Riggs Center in Stockbridge, Massachusetts, where this testing was, and is, used for diagnosis and treatment planning (Bram and Yalof 2015). The battery designed by Rapaport and his students drew from testing in the areas described above, and included cognitive, neuropsychological, and emotional tests. Another early articulator of the usefulness of "psychodiagnostics" to psychoanalysis was Saul Rosenzweig, who published on the subject in the mid-twentieth century (Rosenzweig 1949). Rosenzweig argued that every test could be interpreted psychodynamically, even cognitive and perceptual tests. He described any process of interpreting test data as both "art and science," emphasizing the relationship between the psychoanalytic approach and experimental science, which dovetails in the psychological testing situation.

That this work of integration was undertaken in the United States owes to at least two factors: first, that the Second World War displaced much of the European scientific community to American universities and clinical institutions; and, second, that the prevalent school of psychoanalysis, Ego Psychology, was already concerned with behavioral functioning as a criterion for the suitability of a patient for psychoanalysis, making an assessment of such functioning invaluable for determining "analyzability." Ego psychology derived primarily from the writings of Sigmund Freud's daughter, the psychoanalyst Anna Freud, who codified her theory in *The Ego and the Mechanisms of Defense* (1936/1992). This theory focused the consideration of psychoanalysts on how the ego allows the mind to accurately perceive and adapt to reality through a variety of "ego functions." This concept conceived of the mind as struggling to balance instinctual demands with other internal needs. The mind's role as protector-from-itself was accomplished through "defense mechanisms" which, in moderation, allowed for constructive, productive action, but when operating out of proportion produced pathological symptoms. Anna Freud's theory of defense mechanisms included: "regression, repression, reaction-formation, isolation, undoing, projection, introjection, turning against the self, and reversal" (ibid., p. 47). A contemporary of Anna Freud's who was influenced by her work, Heinz Hartmann shifted the line of thinking in ego psychology from imagining how the mind keeps itself in line, to considering how the mind allows for adaptation to the environment (Hartmann 1939/1958). Hartmann discriminated between "primary autonomous ego functions" like memory, perception, intelligence, language, and learning, and "secondary autonomous ego functions," which kept the unconscious mind in check, following Anna Freud. This complex theory postulated that the secondary layer of the ego could interfere with the former, meaning that, for example, excessive libidinal energy could interfere with memory. Hartmann's work, largely translated by Rapaport, became an essential framework for considering how to use psychological testing to discriminate between problems in the "primary functioning" system and the "secondary" system, or, conversely, how to determine if a patient's symptoms could be ascribed to problems of innate brain functioning on their own, or if the problems were caused or mediated by unconscious problems. Later in this chapter, a more contemporarily relevant description of how testing can address this concern is presented. Arguably, other theories of psychoanalysis have not produced systems as directly relevant to the nature of psychological testing as ego psychology, but this fact does not obviate the applicability of testing to those schools.

Psychological Testing Today: Major Areas of Evaluation and Examples of Tests

Since the origins of psychological testing outlined above, the field of assessment has expanded greatly. At present, there are over 25,000 tests used for myriad purposes (Educational Testing Service 2017). Within clinical psychology, testing is used for assessment of intelligence, academic achievement, functional behavior, biopsychosocial testing, vocational purposes, assessment of learning disabilities, school readiness, and a variety of neuropsychological purposes including attention, memory, and language, among others. Psychological testing has expanded because of developments in psychological science, new means to study the brain, and a trend over the past seventy years toward empiricism and behaviorism. Likewise, especially in the United States, testing has become part of the culture for children and adolescents, with the advent of college entry tests like the Scholastic Aptitude Test (SAT) and the use of testing to determine academic progress in children, as well as to evaluate the effectiveness of education systems. In this section, intelligence, neuropsychological, and emotional/personality tests are described to provide acquaintance with areas of testing and major tests that have the greatest potential value to psychoanalysis.

Intelligence Testing

Intelligence testing has evolved tremendously since the early days of Galton. Alfred Binet's work on intelligence produced the first formal test of intelligence, eventually called the Stanford-Binet Test. The original form of this test, developed by Binet and Theodore Simon and called the Binet-Simon Intelligence Test was published in 1905 (Binet and Simon 1905). This work was adapted and translated by Lewis Terman, a psychologist at Stanford University, who along with his colleague, Maud Merrill, developed the Stanford-Binet Test (Terman and Merrill 1937). This test, now in its fifth revision, assesses general intelligence, fund of knowledge, fluid reasoning, quantitative reasoning, visual-spatial processing, and working memory, and combines to produce IQ scores for verbal and nonverbal intelligence (Becker 2003). General intelligence follows from Spearman's pioneering work and describes the average expectable performance of an individual on a cognitive task, often thought of as hereditary or biological intelligence (Spearman 1904). Fund of knowledge refers to rote information that the test's designers believe people should know, and is highly culturally loaded. Fluid reasoning describes an individual's ability to reason in novel situations, as in recognizing and predicting patterns and other abilities implicated in inductive and deductive reasoning. Quantitative reasoning describes the ability to solve number problems, most directly applicable to mathematics achievement. Visual-spatial processing describes the integration of visual perception and ability to conceive of spatial relationships. Working memory describes a store of memory most often used in solving multistep problems when the first step's result needs to be stored long enough in memory to be applied to the next step, which is implicated in decision-making as well (Diamond 2013). The Verbal and Nonverbal IQ scores are derived from a statistical process that makes use of the standardized results of subtests in the aforementioned areas. Notably, the Stanford-Binet Test is primarily used today to assess degree of high intelligence, as it is much more sensitive at the higher end of that spectrum than it is at the lower end, and it is thus used for entry to schools for the gifted.

The other major tradition in contemporary intelligence testing derives from the work of David Wechsler, who published the Wechsler-Bellevue Intelligence Scale in 1939 while serving as chief psychologist at Bellevue Psychiatric Hospital in New York City (Wechsler 1939). Heavily influenced by American army tests of intelligence used for recruitment (cf. Fancher 1987, for a detailed history of the army Alpha and Beta intelligence tests), Wechsler selected subtests designed to measure verbal ability and "performance," the latter included because of Wechsler's contention that "an individual manifests intelligence by his ability to do things, as well as by the way he can talk about them" (Wechsler 1939, p. 138). Wechsler constructed his test using subtests that had already been statistically validated by other researchers and scientists; this made his test a more appealing choice than the work of Binet and Simon, who had developed their test based on their own samples of French schoolchildren (Boake 2002). Wechsler's work in intelligence testing also challenged Binet's concept of "mental age," and instead proposed a mean score for all people within an age range, which standardized the use of intelligence test scores across the life span (Sutton, Koller, and Christian 1982). Included in those impressed by the validity and reliability of Wechsler's test were Rapaport and his colleagues at the Menninger Clinic, who used it for the intelligence component of their testing battery. Many other tests of intelligence now exist, including those that exclude verbal intelligence to make the test less constricted by linguistic limitations, and others that are also comprehensive, most notably the Woodcock-Johnson Tests of Cognitive Abilities, originally developed by Richard Woodcock and Mary Bonner Johnson, which also include an assessment of long-term memory (Woodcock and Johnson 1977). Each of the major intelligence tests have undergone revisions to match advances in the theory and science of intelligence, as well as through ongoing assessment of the validity and utility of the measures included.[1]

Neuropsychological Testing

Neuropsychology is the study of the relationship between brain and behavior, and neuropsychological testing studies observable behavior to learn about brain functioning (Stebbins 2007). Neuropsychological testing is primarily employed for two purposes: diagnostic and descriptive uses. Diagnostic neuropsychological testing is used to determine the presence of attentional and other executive functioning disorders, dementia, learning disorders, etc. Descriptive neuropsychological testing is used to describe the strengths and weaknesses of a given individual. Neuropsychological testing is frequently in use in neurology clinics, which use extensive batteries like the Halstead-Reitan or Luria-Nebraska Batteries (Reitan and Wolfson 1985; Golden, Purisch, and Hammeke 1985). Both batteries are primarily used to discriminate brain-damaged individuals from healthy individuals and the former is more widely used than the latter, though both tests have been criticized for being insensitive to mild impairment. Aside from their use in neurology clinics and in research, neither test is widely used in psychological testing owing to the time each takes to administer—six hours for the more commonly used Halstead-Reitan battery—and because both produce more information than is commonly required for psychodiagnostic purposes.

More relevant to most requests for psychological testing and for purposes of considering appropriate treatment are tests that assess frontal lobe functioning. A good example of an assessment measure for frontal lobe functioning is the Delis-Kaplan Executive Function System, or D-KEFS, developed by Dean Delis, Edith Kaplan, and Joel Kramer and used for people ages 8–89 (Delis, Kaplan, and Kramer 2001). The D-KEFS is comprised of nine standalone tests that assess a range of different abilities including fluency, problem-solving, inhibition, planning, and multitasking, among others. Although there is no summary measure that describes functioning across the nine subtests, the results of the D-KEFS can be used for a variety of purposes, including in determining the presence of a mood disorder (Simonsen et al. 2008). Another test in wide use is the NEPSY, originally developed by Marit Korkman, Ursula Kirk, and Sally Kemp (Korkman, Kirk, and Kemp 1998, 2007). The NEPSY, an acronym for "a developmental NEuroPSYchological assessment," is a test for children ages 3–16, and in its current version includes tests of "Attention and Executive Functions," "Language," "Sensorimotor" functioning, "Visuospatial" functioning, "Learning and Memory," and "Social Perception."

Executive functions have become increasingly prominent in research and evaluation as brain imaging has become more sophisticated and as more emphasis has been placed on attentional disorders in children and adults (Friedman et al. 2007). These functions represent top-down brain functions, those implicated in mostly all brain activities, hence "executive." The "core" functions are thought to include inhibition, or self-control; working memory, described above; and cognitive flexibility (Diamond 2013). Executive functions can be improved with training and positively impact better personal, interpersonal, and societal functioning (Moffitt et al. 2011).[2]

Emotional/Personality Assessment

The field of personality assessment has greatly evolved from Woodworth's Personal Data Sheet. There now exists a wide range of measures used for broad and specific purposes, and these tests can be arranged on a continuum from most structured to least structured.

In the field of structured self-report, the most significant and perhaps best-researched test is the Minnesota Multiphasic Personality Inventory, or MMPI (Hathaway and McKinley 1940). Hathaway and McKinley recognized the problem of the extant self-report inventories as being too obvious in their phrasing and designed an inventory with "a large reservoir of items" designed to distract the respondent from the purpose of each and to generate data for future research (ibid., p. 249). The MMPI was designed from the outset to be atheoretical, seeking to produce as much description as possible, which could then be subjected to consideration along theoretical lines. This test has been continuously revised and now includes over 400 yes/no items and has parallel forms for adults and adolescents. The MMPI is interpreted via computer scoring and generates nine clinical scales, as well as a variety of supplemental scores concerning validity, as well as common contents, like anxiety and obsessiveness. Another important and equally well-researched self-report inventory is in the Millon Clinical Multiaxial Inventory, or MCMI, developed based on the "evolutionary theory" of its author, Theodore Millon (1969). Drawing from the work of Darwin and subsequent psychological theories of evolution, Millon advanced a view of human functioning that considers psychopathology a result of disruptions in the forces that promote survival and adaptation (Millon Personality Group n.d.). Millon rejected theories that deemed cognitive or unconscious processes as solely responsible for dysfunction, and instead based his assessment on how the individual views himself, how he regulates himself internally, how he conducts himself interpersonally, how he processes information, and how his emotions find expression in his behavior. In its current form, respondents administered the MCMI answer true or false to 195 items, which in turn produce fifteen personality scales, ten clinical syndrome scales, as well as five validity scales (Millon, Grossman, and Millon 2015).[3]

Projective testing describes tests whose purpose is deliberately obscured from the respondent to a partial or complete extent. The underlying theory of these tests is that when individuals are asked direct questions, they are more inclined to self-censorship owing to any number of factors including privacy, embarrassment, lack of insight, etc. This theory is basically unchanged from Heinz Hartmann's original conceptualization (1939/1958), explained above in the section on ego psychology. There are many projective tests, though several are used with far greater frequency than others.

Sentence completion tests are considered "semi-structured" because they offer the respondent a list of sentence fragments to complete, thus structuring the beginning of each effort. Hermann Ebbinghaus (1897) produced the first such task, designed to assess intelligence in children, and there exists many forms developed since then that are deliberately phrased to evoke thoughts about one's self, family, occupation or school, and friendships. Parallel forms also exist with phrasings intended for children or adults. The most common form for adults was designed by Julian Rotter, the "Rotter Incomplete Sentences Blank" (Rotter and Rafferty 1950). Related to but less structured than sentence completion tasks are word association tasks. First introduced by Carl Jung at his lecture at Clark University, the evaluator instructs the examinee by saying: "answer as quickly as possible the first word that occurs to your mind" (Jung 1931, p. 221). Jung's word-prompt list was described by him as selected to "strike easily almost all complexes of practical occurrence," (ibid., p. 220) and similar rationales have informed subsequent lists produced by others. Both tasks were influenced by Sigmund Freud's technique originally published in his treatment of Ilona Weiss, the first significant instance of instructing a patient to freely associate (S. Freud 1893/1955).

Born from the trend in projective testing made popular by Jung's Word Association Test, which highlighted the associative activity of the unconscious through tests using verbal material, several "form association" tests emerged as relevant to the field of psychological testing. The Rorschach Inkblot Test is arguably the psychological test best known to nonpractitioners, having been popularized in art and film. Hermann Rorschach, the Swiss psychiatrist whose interest in the technique of creating inkblots (klecksography) led him to explore the diagnostic applicability of association to form, published his results on his tests using his inkblot method in *Psychodiagnostik* in 1921 (Blum 1934). Notably, Rorschach produced the inkblots used in the current version of the test himself, by hand (Tibon-Czopp and Weiner 2016). He was inspired to apply the test for both diagnostic and therapeutic purposes after observing emotional relief in schoolchildren who associated to similar images in the Victorian game "Gobolinks" (Richardson 2011, p. 136). While Rorschach's original inkblots have remained the most common image-set used for this test, the instructions for administering it and for interpreting the patient's responses have undergone several modifications, most significantly by John Exner, who introduced a standardized, empirically researched model, known as the Comprehensive System (Exner, Jr. 2002). Common to the majority of approaches to administering the Rorschach Inkblot Test is an exposure phase where one inkblot is shown at a time, the patient is asked to tell what each might look like, and then, following this phase, each response is reviewed by the examiner for more information about the patient's approach. This test has been used to produce valuable data about an individual's ability to test reality, his ability to cope with stimuli, and his mood. Subsequent research has also evolved to determine potential suicidality in the respondent, among other clinically relevant data (cf. Fowler et al. 2001).

The TAT, mentioned above, is another common image-driven unstructured projective test developed at Harvard in the 1930s (Murray 1938). This test includes 31 pictures, though most practitioners use one-third of the images in a given administration (Cramer 2004). The images typically depict one or several people with facial expressions that tend to evoke wide-ranging interpretations, though some images have gained nicknames based on common responses to them. While attempts have been made to standardize the interpretation of images (cf. Rotter 1946), most practitioners rely on their own interpretive ability, lending the test to criticisms by those who decry excessive subjectivity on the part of examiners interpreting its results. The generally practiced administration of the test asks the patient to look at an image and to tell a story about it, with instructions recommended for children and those who would benefit from help knowing how to tell a story (Murray 1943).

Another commonly used projective test has the patient draw a series of pictures and then answer questions about each. Originally produced as an intelligence test and developed by Florence Goodenough (1926), in its original form a child was asked to "Make a picture of a man. Make the very best picture you can. Take your time and work very carefully" (quoted in Young 1926, p. 497). Since its original formulation, the instructions have been expanded and the patient is now instructed to produce several drawings, including drawing a person, a person of the opposite sex, a house, a tree, and a family drawing. The addition of a house and a tree integrate the work of John Buck, an early expander on Goodenough's original work, who also produced sample questions to interrogate the patient on his drawings (Buck 1948). The family drawing is likewise a product of integrating the work of another team influenced by Goodenough and involves asking the respondent to draw a picture of his family doing something together (Burns and Kaufman 1987). Like the TAT, these drawing tests have garnered criticism because of the subjective interpretation of their products, and also like the TAT, attempts to standardize these interpretations have not gained wide acceptance.

Despite a trend toward empirically validated measures, the projective tests that are subjectively interpreted have maintained popularity because they evoke creative, wide-ranging responses that are similar to the way that patients speak in psychotherapy and in social conversation.

Applying Psychological Testing to Psychoanalysis Today

The clinical data of concern to psychoanalysts vary considerably based on the theoretical grounding and preferences of the psychoanalyst. While one psychoanalyst might be concerned with whether his patient is employed or in a committed relationship, another may refrain from asking such questions of his patient and may also be relatively unconcerned with the details of his patient's practical reality. Because of the wide-ranging preferences and needs of psychoanalysts, also informed by the situations of their patients, the usefulness of psychological testing likewise varies.[4] In this section, consideration will be offered to the potential utility of psychological testing at different phases of a psychoanalytic treatment; and then two case examples are presented to illustrate this utility.

The question of suitability for psychoanalysis has a long tradition in the field, beginning with Sigmund Freud, who stated that his new treatment was ill-matched to individuals with psychosis or severe depression (S. Freud 1905/1953). Freud recommended a prolonged "examination period" for patients to determine their suitability for psychoanalysis, but offered little advice that has proven useful to practitioners (S. Freud 1913/1958). Despite the absence of consensus on what constitutes useful initial information to make a determination about treatment, the practice of interviewing remains common.

Moreover, efforts to research the practice of determining analyzability have not produced practically nor theoretically useful conclusions (Bachrach and Leaff 1978). One commonly held belief is that a patient's ability to free associate is a useful prognosticator for success in psychoanalysis (Varvin 2003). Further, there exists no meaningful consensus on what factors might explain premature termination of treatment by will of the patient, nor is there consensus on what factors ought to be in play to justify termination of treatment (cf. Gabbard 2009 for a review of some of the relevant literature in these two areas). Therefore, what follows are potentially useful sources of data from testing that will be more- or less-applicable given the predilections of a given psychoanalyst.

The patient seeking psychoanalysis may or may not have a concept of the treatment in mind, leaving the determination of suitability to the psychoanalyst. The psychoanalyst will likely determine the appropriateness of recommending psychoanalysis based on his experience conducting psychoanalyses with other patients, or may seek to consult with others to aid in this decision, especially if the treater is in training. Certain facets of a patient will emerge in any initial conversation, including some sense of his receptive and expressive language abilities, his ability to synthesize his thinking in a linear, cogent manner, and his affective range. Psychoanalysts differ in their practice of conducting initial meetings, with some seeking to develop a detailed sense of their patients' early histories, some emphasizing present functioning in their questioning, and others preferring to allow their patients to speak freely as useful preparation for the form of the treatment that might follow.

Independent of the technique or strategy that a given psychoanalyst selects as a regular practice, or that seems to address some aspect of a new referral's initial question or their presentation in person, it is common to learn later in a treatment of important clinical facts that were not mentioned initially, either for defensive reasons, or because they were inconsistent with what inspired the patient to seek treatment, and was thus less salient. In some instances, knowledge of certain facts would have modified the psychoanalyst's original recommendation for treatment. These facts could include a patient's addiction to a substance, their financial circumstances, or a history of significant psychiatric crises. Thus, psychological testing can serve many potential purposes in helping to determine the appropriateness of psychoanalysis for children and adults alike. First, psychological testing begins with extensive interviewing that typically includes a detailed developmental history, as well as a review of a patient's medical and psychiatric history. Even adult patients are often asked by their evaluator to produce grade reports from school and other information that may reveal useful facts of history that might not be evident from initial discussion. Other important factors like the ability to understand spoken language and to express oneself clearly are also readily testable, as is the ability to sustain attention, and to retrieve information from memory. Reality testing, quality of thinking, and absence or presence of severe character pathology are all discernible from structured and unstructured personality assessment tests.

While any of the aforementioned factors could bear usefully on a determination for psychoanalysis, nothing is more potentially useful to the psychoanalyst than the integration of test data on a psychological testing report. The skilled evaluator does not simply report high or low values; rather he can and should hypothesize the causal relations between test data. If a patient shows uneven ability to sustain attention or to express himself in language, comprehensive testing can place those phenomena alongside frustration tolerance, for example, and might find an interaction effect between the two. Thus, the psychological tester is in a unique position not only to report on relative strengths and weaknesses between skills, but to develop a complex model of individual functioning that can bear on indications for psychoanalysis and help the psychoanalyst decode complex phenomena that present during treatment. For example, a patient who on assessment shows poor stress tolerance that interacts with variable expressive language functioning might develop signs of decreased functional communication and interpersonal functioning during regressed states within the psychoanalytic situation. Psychological test data might discourage a psychoanalyst from misinterpreting this phenomenon as a negative treatment response, which could lead to a consideration of changing to a less-intensive, and potentially less-helpful modality, and instead might enable the psychoanalyst to offer himself and his patient a context for understanding why this is happening. Several case illustrations will describe this further.

Miss A was referred for psychological testing by her high school. She presented with symptoms of depression, inattention, and learning difficulties despite apparent high intelligence, mostly seen through her sophisticated written expression.[5] On assessment, her high intelligence was confirmed, but her facility with language decreased considerably on projective testing, where the vagueness of the test-frame caused her significant distress. In a distressed state, her thought process became more tangential and its content more depressed. Tests of attention confirmed her above-average ability to sustain attention, including while multitasking on monotonous tasks. The report produced from the evaluation emphasized her high ability but also noted that her loss of focus was marshaled for a defensive purpose, specifically to allow her to disengage from tasks that were emotionally evocative. With that disengagement and loss of focus, she also was less able to communicate, instead seeking refuge in tangential thoughts that protected her from "getting into" topics of concern to her. A recommendation for intensive treatment was made with the advice that her analyst anticipate that she would manifest resistance in the form of decreased expression, and that when that occurred, a move into nonverbal activity might allow her to continue to make productive use of the treatment. Miss A began a three-times weekly treatment with a child/adolescent psychoanalyst who felt that she was an excellent candidate for treatment, a judgment based mostly on the depth and high quality of her verbal productions in the initial sessions. Predictably, several months into treatment, Miss A suddenly became frustrated that she had "nothing to say" to her analyst and complained that the treatment was no longer useful to her. Miss A's analyst, heeding the advice of the report, suggested that they draw together, a technique that would not have been apparent in treating a seventeen-year-old, but the maneuver proved effective. Miss A's analyst was nevertheless surprised by the extensive drawings her analysand produced, which included family drawings depicting interpersonal conflict not previously described in months of treatment. As Miss A developed comfort expressing otherwise warded-off contents through her drawings, her language functioning was gradually restored, the drawing activity stopped, and the treatment returned to conversation that persisted for several more years with a positive outcome.

Referrals for psychological testing before beginning treatment are prompted by many possible features of clinical presentation. Bram and Yalof describe the case of "Betsy," a "young adolescent whose symptoms included chronic depression, self-harm, oppositionality, declining academic functioning, and multiple somatic complaints resulting in frequent absences from school" (Bram & Yalof 2015, p. 86). Betsy was referred to a psychoanalyst-psychiatrist for medication and the psychiatrist was struck "not only by the patient's refusal to engage in give-and-take in the consultation but by her parents' description of a series of previous unsuccessful psychotherapeutic and pharmacological efforts" (ibid.). A consultant psychoanalyst-clinical psychologist was sought for an assessment that would determine what impeded Betsy's ability to form a therapeutic alliance in the past and "what is the underlying developmental disruption driving her symptoms and that can guide treatment focus" (ibid., p. 87). In this example, the evaluator relied on TAT and Rorschach data exclusively to describe Betsy's internal object representations and relational expectations, and from that identified a treatment approach that would be more supportive at first, "engaging around conflict-free topics," before "pushing for reflectiveness" (ibid.).

Examples of phenomena during a treatment where psychological testing can be helpful include treatment impasses, diagnostic confusion based on the emergence of new symptoms, and concerns about decline due to aging or medical illness. Referrals for medical concerns, like dementia, are often best effected by referrals to specialty clinics or to clinical psychologists with relevant experience. While many psychoanalysts are wary of continuing an intensive treatment with patients who have dementia, some have published on the utility of ongoing treatment, for example, with people who have Alzheimer's disease (Sadavoy 1991). Diagnostic confusion in the middle of treatment can present for many reasons. Had the analyst treating Miss A not been able to anticipate the decline in her language secondary to feeling emotionally overwhelmed, she might have worried that her analysand was suddenly experiencing a neurocognitive deficit. Had she been less concerned about a somatic decline, Miss A's analyst might have correctly deemed this decline as a defensive reaction, or a resistance to treatment, but might have not found a useful strategy to progress past this impasse. A referral for testing might have, at that moment, provided similar help to the evaluation done before the treatment began.

Mr. B had been in a four-times-weekly psychoanalysis for three years with a senior psychiatrist-psychoanalyst, Dr. C, who despite her dedication and skill had not produced meaningful change in her sixty-year-old patient. Mr. B had a history of depressive symptoms that had him in treatment with many different clinicians for most of his life since childhood. When Mr. B began consulting with Dr. C, he presented his ongoing concern with his experience of limited recall, but this symptom was seen as secondary to his depression. After years of unsuccessfully trying to address Mr. B's depression in psychoanalysis, Dr. C became herself despondent and started worrying that she had underemphasized the role of possible memory dysfunction in Mr. B's presentation. By the time Mr. B was referred for a psychological evaluation, Dr. C felt she had slipped into providing a series of "ineffectual, supportive interventions." Mr. B responded very positively to the idea of an evaluation as he was very eager to find out if his memory was impaired; he seemed to the evaluator to be overexcited by this possibility. Mr. B's intelligence, neuropsychological, and emotional functioning were assessed and he was found to be a very intelligent person with high occupational potential if not for the presence of moderate-to-severe depression with connections to significant childhood, adolescent, and early adulthood traumata. Given the extent of his depression, it was unsurprising to the evaluator that tests that required more effort were more challenging for Mr. B than his intelligence alone would have suggested, though it was surprising that his ability to apply effort improved when a deeper rapport with the evaluator formed. Tests of Mr. B's memory found intact memory functioning for short- and long-term recall and for both verbal and nonverbal, or perceptual, stimuli. Based on the test findings, including the role that closer rapport had in increasing Mr. B's effort, the evaluator emphasized to Dr. C that her patient was indeed depressed and that his concern with memory was a symptomatic distortion. The evaluator moreover recommended to Dr. C that she work both supportively and interpretively to address Mr. B's low effort in participating in his treatment. Perhaps most important from the consultation was the encouragement to Dr. C to analyze as she might another patient and not become overly identified with Mr. B's depressive symptoms, including his fear of impaired memory.

After having worked one-on-one over multiple hours across multiple tests, the evaluator and his patient will have developed a comfortable rapport that may feel less threatening than the patient-psychoanalyst relationship. By the time patients in evaluation reach the projective emotional tests, usefully saved for last, they are less guarded, and are more inclined to freely associate to the stimuli. The rapport that emerges makes the final phase of testing, the feedback session, especially useful in reaching the patient. Here, the evaluator can carefully integrate findings and suggest to patients, like in the example of Mr. B, that long-held somatic worries indeed seem affective in origin, and with the weight of empirical data from the evaluation, this hypothesis will seem less doubtful than when the patient imagines his psychoanalyst saying the same thing. Because of the special rapport of the evaluation scenario, many psychoanalysts who treat children and adolescents frequently report the catalytic effect of an evaluation on their treatments (cf. Meersand [2011] for examples). If the evaluation scenario produces less threat and less resistance, it is because it can seem that the evaluator does not seek to work as "deeply" as the psychoanalyst, conveyed by the use of cognitive tests and structured self-reports. The psychological evaluator is also able to preserve a properly neutral position by allowing his impressions to emerge by observing his patient and from the test data. The evaluator ought not have any agenda or a priori assumptions and this position is facilitated by the deductive process of the evaluation.

CONCLUSION

While the history of psychological testing predates psychoanalysis, the disciplines of psychoanalysis and clinical psychology were significantly intertwined in the latter half of the twentieth century (Lerner 2007). Psychoanalytic training today tends not to include education about psychological testing, with the possible exception of child and adolescent psychoanalytic training. Psychological testing has potential use in determining the suitability of psychoanalysis when the psychoanalyst has testable criteria that can be evaluated, and in any case, can help predict what is likely to happen in psychoanalytic treatment and so prepare the potential analyst-analysand dyad. This then minimizes the likelihood of treatment ruptures. Testing can also help diagnose the cause for patient difficulties in engaging treatment and for impasses. Although psychoanalysts tend to wish to preserve the sanctity of their dyadic relationship with an analysand, soliciting this kind of consultation can provide for deeper psychoanalytic process and more long-lasting effects.

NOTES

1. Other current intelligence tests in common use include: the Cognitive Assessment System (Naglieri and Das 1997), the Differential Ability Scales (Elliott 1990), the Kaufman Assessment Battery for Children (Kaufman and Kaufman 2004), Raven's Progressive Matrices (Raven, Raven, and Court 2004), and the Test of Nonverbal Intelligence (Brown, Sherbenou, and Johnson 2010). These and the tests listed in the text have been translated into many languages.

2. Many neuropsychological tests exist and many of them have been included in battery-style tests like D-KEFS and NEPSY. Among those most commonly used as stand-alone tests, the Boston Naming Test (Kaplan, Goodglass, and Weintraub 1983), the California Verbal Learning Test (Delis, Kramer et al. 2000), the Rey-Osterrieth Complex Figure test (Osterrieth 1944), and the Stroop Test (cf. Stroop [1938] for a description of the foundation of this test) are noteworthy.

3. Noteworthy for their wide use are also the Personality Assessment Inventory (Morey 2007) and the NEO Personality Inventory-3 (McCrae, Costa, Jr., and Martin 2005), both theory-driven assessments of personality.

4. Because of the complex relationship between psychoanalysts and their theories, no effort is undertaken in this chapter to link specific theories of psychoanalysis with relevant elements of psychological testing. Instead, psychoanalysis is considered as a broad, varied practice, and the examples offered were selected for their broad applicability.

5. Details of this and subsequent case examples of been deliberately obscured to protect the confidentiality of those patients. The consent of Miss A's parents and Mr B was sought and received prior to describing elements of their presentation, even in its present, obscured form.

REFERENCES

Bachrach, H. M. and Leaff, L. (1978). "Analyzability": A systematic review of the clinical and quantitative literature. *Journal of the American Psychoanalytic Association*, 26, 881–920.

Becker, K. A. (2003). *History of the Stanford-Binet Intelligence Scales: Content and Psychometrics.* Service Bulletin, Itasca, IL: Riverside Publishing.

Binet, A. (1905/1916). New methods for the diagnosis of the intellectual level of subnormals. In Kite, E. S. (Ed.). *The Development of Intelligence in Children.* Vineyard, NJ: Publications of the Training School at Vineland.

Binet, A. and Simon, T. (1905). *Méthodes nouvelles pour le diagnostic du niveau intellectual des anormaux. L'Année psychologique*, 11, 191–336.

Blum, E. (1934). "Psychodiagnostik: By Hermann Rorschach (edited by W. Morgenthaler. Hans Huber, Bern and Berlin, 1932, Vol. I." *International Journal of Psycho-Analysis*, 15, 475–477.

Boake, C. (2002). From the Binet-Simon to the Wechsler-Bellevue: Tracing the history of intelligence testing. *Journal of Clinical and Experimental Neuropsychology*, 24(3), 383–405.

Bram, A. D. and Yalof, J. (2015). Quantifying complexity: Personality assessment and its relationship with psychoanalysis. *Psychoanalytic Inquiry*, 35, 74–97.

Broca, P. P. (1861). *Perte de la parole, ramollissement chronique et destruction partielle du lobe antérieur gauche du cerveau. Bulletin de la Société Anthropologique*, 2, 235–238.

Brown, L., Sherbenou, R. J., and Johnson, S. K. (2010). *Test of Nonverbal Intelligence: TONI-4.* Austin, TX: Pro-Ed.

Buck, J. (1948). The H-T-P technique, a qualitative and quantitative scoring method. *Journal of Clinical Psychology Monograph Supplement*, 5, 1–120.

Burns, R. C. and Kaufman, S. H. (1987). *Kinetic Family Drawings (K-F-D): An Introduction to Understanding Children Through Kinetic Drawings.* New York: Brunner/Mazel.

Butcher, J. N. (2010). Personality assessment from the nineteenth to the early twenty-first century: Past achievements and contemporary challenges. *Annual Review of Clinical Psychology*, 6(1), 1–20.

Cattell, J. M.(1890). "Cattell (1890)." *Classics in the History of Psychology*. Accessed Sept. 15, 2017. http://psychclassics.yorku.ca/Cattell/mental.htm.

Cattell, J. M. and Ferrand, L. (1896). Physical and mental measurements of the students of Columbia University." *Psychological Review*, 3(6), 618–648.

Cramer, P. (2004). *Storytelling, Narrative, and the Thematic Apperception Test*. New York: Guilford Press.

Delis, D. C., Kaplan, E., and Kramer, J. H. (2001). *The Delis-Kaplan Executive Function System: Technical Manual*. San Antonio, TX: The Psychological Corporation.

Delis, D. C., Kramer, J. H., Kaplan, E., and Ober, B. A. (2000). *Manual for the California Verbal Learning Test (CVLT-II)*. San Antonio, TX: The Psychological Corporation.

Diamond, A. (2013). Executive functions. *Annual Review of Psychology*, 64, 135–168.

Ebbinghaus, H. (1897). *Über eine neue Methode im Prüfung geistiger Fahigkeiten und ihre Awendung bei Schulkindern. Zeitschrift sur Psychologie und Physiologie der Sinnesorgane*, 13, 401–457.

Educational Testing Service. 2017. *Test Collection at ETS*. Accessed Aug. 10, 2016. http://www.ets.org/test_link/about.

Elliott, C. D. (1990). The nature and structure of children's abilities: Evidence from the Differential Ability Scales. *Journal of Psychoeducational Assessment*, 8(3), 376–390.

Exner, J. E. (1974). *The Rorschach: A Comprehensive System*. New York: Wiley.

Exner, Jr., J. E. (2002). *The Rorschach: A Comprehensive System*. 4th edition. New York: Wiley.

Fancher, R. E. (1987). *The Intelligence Men: Makers of the I.Q. Controversy*. New York: W. W. Norton & Company.

Fowler, J. C., Piers, C., Hilsenroth, Jr., M. J., Holdwick, D. J., and Paawer, J. R. (2001). The Rorschach Suicide Constellation: Assessing various degrees of lethality. *Journal of Personality Assessment*, 76(2), 333–351.

Freud, A. (1936/1992). *The Ego and the Mechanisms of Defense*. London: Karnac Press.

Freud, S. (1893/1955). Frälein Elisabeth von R., Case Histories from Studies on Hysteria. In Strachey, J. (Ed.). *The Standard Edition of the Complete Psychological Works of Sigmund Freud, Vol. II (1893–1895): Studies on Hysteria*, (pp. 135–181). London: Hogarth Press.

———. (1913/1958). On beginning the treatment. In Strachey, J. (Ed). *The Standard Edition of the Complete Psychological Works of Sigmund Freud, Vol. XII (1911–1913): The Case of Schreber, Papers on Technique and Other Works* (pp. 121–144). London: Hogarth Press.

———. (1905/1953). On psychotherapy. In J. Strachey (Ed.). *The Standard Edition of the Complete Psychological Works of Sigmund Freud, Vol. VII (1901–1905): A Case of Hysteria, Three Essays on Sexuality and Other Works* (pp. 257–268). London: Hogarth Press.

Friedman, N. P., Haberstick, B. C., Willcutt, E. G., Miyake, A., Young, S. E., Corley, R. P., and Hewitt, J. K. (2007). Greater attention problems during childhood predict poorer executive functioning in late adolescence. *Psychological Science*, 18(10), 893–900.

Fritsch, R. C. (2013). Roy Schafer's contributions to psychological testing: From clinical sensibility to the analytic attitude. *Psychoanalytic Quarterly*, 82(1), 9–21.

Gabbard, G. O. (2009). What is a "good enough" termination? *Journal of the American Psychoanalytic Association*, 57(3), 575–594.

Galton, F. (1865). Hereditary talent and character. *Macmillan's Magazine*, 12 157–166, 318–327.

Golden, C. J., Purisch, A. T., and Hammeke, T. A. (1985). *Luria-Nebraska Neuropsychological Battery: Form I and II*. Los Angeles: Western Psychological Services.

Goodenough, F. L. (1926). *Measurement of Intelligence by Drawings*. Yonkers-on-Hudson, NY: World Book Company.

Gregory, R. J. (2003). *Psychological Testing: History, Principles, and Applications*. Old Tappan, NJ: Pearson.

Hartmann, H. (1939/1958). *Ego Psychology and the Problem of Adaptation*. New York: International Universities Press.

Hathaway, S. R. and McKinley, J. C. (1940). A multiphasic personality schedule (Minnesota): Construction of the schedule. *Journal of Psychology*, 10, 249–254.
Heymans, G. and Wiersma, E. D. (1906). *Beitrage zur spezillen psychologie auf grund einer massenunterschung. Zeitschrift fur Psychologie*, 43, 81–127.
Jung, C. G. (1907). On psychological relations of the association experiment. *Journal of Abnormal Psychology*, 31, 249–257.
———. (1931). The association method. *American Journal of Psychology* 31, 219–269.
Kaplan, E., Goodglass, H., and Weintraub, S. (1983). *Boston Naming Test.* Philadelphia: Lea & Febiger.
Kaufman, A. S. and Kaufman, N. L. (2004). *Kaufman Assessment Battery for Children* 2nd edition. Circle Pines, MN: American Guidance Service.
Korkman, M., Kirk, U., and Kemp, S. L. (1998). *NEPSY: A Developmental Neuropsychological Assessment.* San Antonio, TX: The Psychological Corporation.
———. (2007). *NEPSY II: Clinical and Interpretive Manual.* San Antonio, TX: The Psychological Corporation.
Lashley, K. S. (1930). Basic neural mechanisms in behavior. *Psychology Review*, 37, 1–24.
Lerner, P. M. (2007). On preserving a legacy: Psychoanalysis and psychological testing. *Psychoanalytic Psychology*, 24(2), 208–230.
McCrae, R. R., Costa, Jr., P. T., and Martin, T. A. (2005). The NEO–PI–3: A more readable revised NEO Personality Inventory. *Journal of Personality Assessment*, 84(3), 261–270.
Meersand, P. (2011). Psychological testing and the analytically trained child psychologist. *Psychoanalytic Psychology*, 28(1), 117–131.
Millon Personality Group. (n.d). The Millon Personality Group. *Evolutionary Theory.* Accessed Oct. 3, 2017. http://www.millonpersonality.com/theory/core-components/EvolutionaryTheory.pdf.
Millon, T. (1969). *Modern Psychopathology: A Biosocial Approach to Maladaptive Learning and Functioning.* Philadelphia: Saunders.
Millon, T., Grossman, S., and Millon, C. (2015). *Millon Clinical Multiaxial-Inventory-IV.* Bloomington, MN: NCS Pearson.
Moffitt, T. E., Arseneault, L., Belsky, D., Dickson, N., Hancox, R. J., Harrington, H. L., Houts, R. et al. (2011). A gradient of childhood self-control predicts health, wealth, and public safety. *Proceedings of the National Academy of Sciences of the United States of America*, 108(7), 2693–2698.
Morey, L. C. (2007). *The Personality Assessment Inventory: Professional Manual.* Lutz, FL: Psychological Assessment Resources.
Murray, H. A. (1938). *Explorations in Personality.* New York: Oxford University Press.
———. (1943). *Manual for the Thematic Apperception Test.* Cambridge, MA: Harvard University Press.
Naglieri, J. A. and Das, J. P. (1997). *Cognitive Assessment System.* Itasca, IL: Riverside Publishing Company.
Osterrieth, P. A. (1944). *Filetest de copie d'une figure complex: Contribution a l'étude de la perception et de la memoire. Archives de Psychologie*, 30, 286–356.
Rapaport, D., Gill, M., and Schafer, R. (1946). *Diagnostic Psychological Testing.* Chicago, IL: World Book.
Raven, J., Raven, J. C., and Court, J. H. (2004). *Manual for Raven's Progressive Matrices and Vocabulary Scales.* San Antonio, TX: Harcourt Assessment.
Reitan, R. M., and Wolfson, D. (1985). *The Halstead-Reitan Neuropsychological Test Battery: Theory and Clinical Interpretation.* Tucson, AZ: Neuropsychology Press.
Richardson, J. (2011). *Howard Andrew Knox: Pioneer of Intelligence Testing at Ellis Island.* New York: Columbia University Press.
Rorschach, H. (1921). *Psychodiagnostik.* Bern, German: Hans Huber.
Rosenzweig, S. (1949). *Psychodiagnosis.* New York: Grune and Stratton.
Rotter, J. B. (1946). Thematic Apperception Tests: Suggestions for administration and interpretation." *Journal of Personality*, 15(1), 70–92.
Rotter, J. B. and Rafferty, J. E. (1950). *The Rotter Incomplete Sentences Blank: Manual.* New York: The Psychological Corporation.

Sadavoy, J. (1991). Psychodynamic perspectives on Alzheimer's disease and related dementias. *American Journal of Alzheimer's Disease & Other Dementias*, 6(3), 12–20.
Simonsen, C., Sundet, K., Vaskinn, A., and Andeassen, O. A. (2008). Neurocognitive profiles in bipolar I and bipolar II disorder: Differences in pattern and magnitude of dysfunction. *Bipolar Disorder*, 10(2), 245–255.
Spearman, C. (1904). "General Intelligence," objectively determined and measured. *American Journal of Psychology*, 15, 201–293.
Stebbins, G. (2007). Neuropsychological testing. In C. G. Goetz (Ed.). *Textbook of Clinical Neurology* (pp. 539–557). Philadelphia: Saunders.
Stroop, J. R. (1938). Studies of interference in serial verbal reactions. *Journal of Experimental Psychology*, 18, 643–662.
Sundberg, N. D. (1977). *Assessment of Persons.* Englewood Cliffs, NJ: Prentice-Hall.
Sutton, G. W., Koller, J. R., and Christian, B. T. (1982). The Stanford-Binet Mental Age and WISC-R Test Age: A comparison study. *Psychology in the School*, 19(3), 287–289.
Terman, L. A. and Merrill, M. A. (1937). *Measuring Intelligence.* Boston: Houghton Mifflin.
Terman, L. M. (1916). *The Measurement of Intelligence: An Explanation of and a Complete Guide for the Use of the Stanford Revision and Extension of the Binet-Simon Intelligence Scale.* Boston: Houghton Mifflin.
Tibon-Czopp, S. and Weiner, I. B. (2016). *Rorschach Assessment of Adolescents: Theory, Research and Practice.* New York: Springer.
Varvin, S. (2003). Which patients should avoid psychoanalysis, and which professionals should avoid psychoanalytic training? A critical evaluation. *Scandinavian Psychoanalytic Review*, 26, 109–122.
Wechsler, D. (1939). *The Measurement of Adult Intelligence.* Baltimore: Williams & Wilkins.
Woodcock, R. W. and Johnson, M. B. (1977). *Woodcock-Johnson Psycho-Educational Battery.* Allen, TX: DLM.
Woodworth, R. S. (1919). Examination of emotional fitness for war. *Psychological Bulletin*, 15, 59–60.
Young, K. (1926). "Measurement of Intelligence by Drawings. Florence L. Goodenough, Lewis M. Terman." *American Journal of Sociology*, 32(3), 497–498.

Index

actual neuroses, 204
Adult Attachment Interview (AAI), 58, 59, 60
affects, 9, 123; in adolescents, 19; body language and, 17; bonds with caregiver, 11, 13, 15; character and, 20; classification of, 8; contagious, 8; culture and, 8, 17, 19, 21; development of, 10; Freud on, 9, 10, 11; in infancy, 11; innate expression, 8; mental representation, 12, 20; negative, 9, 14, 15, 17, 19; preverbal, 10, 20; psychoanalytic concepts of, 9, 17; regulation of behavior, 11; self-regulation, 14, 16, 19; social regulation, 11, 16; somatization and, 7, 9, 10, 11, 17; verbalization of, 9, 14, 15, 16, 19, 20. *See* somatization
affect theory, 8
aggression, 48, 55–56, 59–60, 63, 94, 95
Ainsworth, Mary, 13, 44
alexithymia, 17, 202; autism and, 204; empathic failure and, 205; functional somatic disorders, result of, 206; trauma and, 204, 206
analytic third, 213
annihilation anxiety, 97
anxiety, 9, 10, 11, 13, 17, 96; signal, 9, 13, 14. *See also* somatization
Asperger's syndrome, 83, 88
attachment, attachment theory, 7, 13, 43, 44, 46, 53, 55, 63, 64, 66; Adult Attachment Interview (AAI), 14; attachment organizations, 54, 58, 60, 65, 66; attachment theory and psychosomatics, 201, 205–206, 208, 220; caregiving and, 65; clinical examples, 58–63; internal working models (IWMs), 65, 67, 91; and neurobiology, 130–131
autism, 83, 88, 89

babies: agency of, 50, 53, 56, 59, 66; "love affair with the world," 50; mental life of, 44, 46, 47–49, 66; mental representations in, 49, 50, 51, 52, 53, 55, 56, 60; observations of, 44, 45, 48; psychological birth of, 47
Beebe, Beatrice, 44, 53, 64, 66
Bergman, Anni, 45, 46, 53, 54, 55, 59, 67
betrayal, 132
biology: in early development, 46, 48, 58, 65. *See also* babies
bodily states, 57, 93
body: boundaries in infancy, 49, 50, 56–57, 58; in clinical work, 57; of mother, 65, 66
Bowlby, John, 13, 44, 45, 46, 53
brain, 227; and mind, relationship of, 227, 228, 229–230, 230, 234; scaffolding, 234

brain injury, 219–220
breakdown (mental), 96
Broca, Paul, 271

cancer, 202
caregiver, 11, 13, 16, 19. *See also* motherhood
caregiving or caregiving system, 65, 66
cathexis, 229
chaos, 86, 96, 97
child abuse, 91
childbirth, 65
childhood psychosis, 83, 89
childhood schizophrenia, 83, 87–88, 89
chronic fatigue, 206, 216, 219
cognition, 232
conflict (intrapsychic), 94
countertransference: Driver and, 219; Katz and, 215; McDougall and, 209–210; Ogden and, 212–213; with psychosomatic patients, 207
customs inspection, 49

dead mother, 212, 213, 219
delay of gratification, 234
depersonalization, 180
depression: anaclitic, 154; introjective, 154
depressive position, 152
derealization, 180
developmental challenges, 96
developmental deficit, 86
developmental delay, 85, 93, 94
developmental lines, 47
developmental moment, 95–98
disaffected, 203
dissociation, 132
dissociative amnesia, 180, 185
dissociative identity disorder (DID), 179; and alters, 185, 186, 187; biology of, 182–183; cultural context of, 180–181; etiology, 183–184; experience of analyst in treating, 188; phenomenology of, 181–182, 185; splitting in, 186; treatment of, 189–190, 190–192
dyadic expansion of consciousness model (DECM), 25–26, 27, 40

eating disorder, 206

emotion, 7, 9, 17, 19; the arts and, 19; James-Lange Theory of, 8. *See also* alexithymia
emotional growth, 91, 92, 93, 98
emotional refueling, 50, 53, 66
emotional/personality assessment, 277–280; Minnesota Multiphasic Personality Inventory (MMPI), 277; projective testing, 278–280
environment in early development, 46
externalization, 247

failure to thrive, 156
fathers, 54
Freud and neuroscience,. *See also* caregiving system; parents 227, 228–229
Freud, Anna, 44
Freud, Sigmund, 9, 10, 11, 13, 44, 149, 150, 151, 179–180, 227, 228–229

gender identity, 71, 72; development of, 72

hatching, 49
hate, 15, 17
hypothalamus-pituitary-adrenal (HPA) axis, 201, 220

impingement, 127
implicit knowing, 231
incest, 132
infants, 10, 11, 12, 13, 14, 15, 19. *See* babies
intelligence testing: early attempts at, 270–271; Stanford-Binet, 270, 275; Wechsler-Bellevue Intelligence Scale, 275
intentionality, 232
internalization, 232, 232–233, 247
insufficient, 238

Kohut, Heinz, 156

language, 9; and development, 16, 117–119. *See also* alexithymia; motherhood; narcissistic development
la pensee operatoire, 202

Mahler, Margaret, 44–46, 47, 48, 53–54, 55, 56, 58; contemporary relevance of, 48, 57, 67; critique of, 48, 57, 67
Masters Children's Center (MCC), 44, 45, 58, 59, 67
match, mismatch, and repair, 25, 26, 39
melancholia, 150, 151
mentalization, 14, 46, 54, 56, 63, 66, 130, 201, 205–206, 230; eating disorders and, 206; history of concept, 228–230; impairment in functional somatic disorders, 206; and internalization, 232–234, 247; and mothers, 235–236; treatment using, 208, 209
mental representations, 12, 228
mindfulness, 131
misattunement, 128, 130
models of reality, 96
motherhood, 10, 11, 12, 14–15, 21; and language, 16
mothers: aggression in, 55–58, 59–60, 61; anxiety of, 47, 53, 58, 235; clinical work with, 58, 61, 62, 63, 64–65; interviews with, 48, 54, 58; mental health or illness of, 46, 50, 54, 55, 58, 61, 62, 63, 64; and neurodevelopment, 235; role in development of narcissism, 109–110
mourning, 151
multiple simultaneous meaning-making, 25–26, 27, 40

narcissism: definition, 103, 104; description of normal, 105–106, 114, 116, 121, 124; disruption of, 115, 121; pathological, 104–105, 121, 125; primary, 124; secondary, 107, 116, 124
narcissistic development: 0-2 months, 111–112; 2-9 months, 112–116; 9-18 months, 115–116; 18-24 months, 119–122; 24-36 months, 123; 36 months and beyond, 124–125; in adolescence, 125; and language, 117–119
neglect, 91
neurobiology, 8, 14, 17, 227; neurobiological deficit, 94; oral sensitivity, 85
neurocircuitry, 234, 247
neurodevelopment, 228, 230–232, 233; and mental representation, 230–231, 235
neuronal pathways, 227, 229
neuroplasticity, 96
neuropsychological testing, 276–277; and assessment of frontal lobe functioning, 276; and executive function, 277
neuroscience, 227, 228
nonneurotypical children, 236, 237, 247; therapy with, 237
nonverbal learning deficit, 90, 91, 93, 94

object constancy, 47, 48, 52, 59, 60, 63, 66, 123, 229
object permanence, 49, 119
object relations, 46, 47, 50, 51, 52
observational research, 45
oedipal, 94
operatory thinking. *See* la pensee operatoire

parenthood, 45, 46, 60, 62, 66
parents, 45, 58, 63, 64, 67; role in development of narcissism, 110; *See also* parenthood; caregiver
pattern-making, 234
peek-a-boo, 12
personality assessment, history of, 271–272
personality disorder, 17
pervasive developmental disorder, 83, 89
pleasure-unpleasure principle, 10
posttraumatic stress disorder, 204, 206, 214
preferential smiling, 49
pregnancy, 45, 57, 64, 65
psychic trauma, 204, 206, 214
psychoanalysis, 160, 227, 251; and community outreach, 252–253, 257–258; consultation and outreach in India, 258–259; creativity in, 254–255; cultural issues, 254, 256, 264; expansion of practice, 252; in India, 255, 257; supervision and cultural issues, 260–262
psychoanalytic work ego, 256–257
psychological testing: historical antecedents, 269–270; and

psychoanalysis, 273, 280–282, 283, 285
psychoneuroimmune effects, 201
psychosomatic illnesses, 204
psychotherapy, psychodynamic, 161
psychotherapy, short term psychodynamic, 162
puberty, 98–100

reflective function. *See* mentalization
regression, 88, 171
relatedness: dyadic, 106, 116; triadic, 107, 116
representational world development of, 230
resilience, 52. *See also* babies, mental representations in; object constancy; self-constancy
Rorschach, Herman, 272

schizophrenia, 83
self-constancy, 47, 52, 63, 66, 123
self-object, 125
self-reflection, 129
self-regulation, 234, 247
self-representations, 120; *See also* self-constancy
self states, alien, 202, 206, 216, 217, 219
sensory integration deficit, 83, 88, 90, 91, 92, 93, 94
separation, 13. *See also* anxiety; separation anxiety; separation-individuation.
separation-individuation (theory), 7, 10, 11, 15, 44, 45–46, 47–57, 67, 123, 133; aggression in, 55–56; body in, 48, 49, 57; clinical examples, 58–63, 67; contemporary relevance of, 54–57, 64, 66, 67; differentiation, 49–50, 53, 57; practicing subphase, 50–51, 123; rapprochement subphase, 14, 15, 51, 59, 107, 119, 120–121, 123; refueling, 119, 122. *See also* object constancy
separations, 45, 50, 53
severe emotional disorder, 83–100
sexual abuse, 132
somatization, 203–204; alexithymia and, 203–204
soul murder, 133
speech delay, 85
symbolic function, 230, 234, 247

therapeutic process, 27–28, 39–41; data used to study, 29; study of, 28–29; videotape analysis of, 29
thought disorder, 83
torticollis, 218
Tourette's syndrome, 216, 217
transgender people, 71; analysis and therapy with, 71–73, 81; parents of, 80; sense of self, 80; treatment of, 72
transitional objects, 122
transitional phenomena, 122
trauma, 9, 10, 13, 17, 19, 83, 91, 127; cumulative/strain trauma, 128
trust development of, 112–113
type A personality, 202

vulnerable child, 83, 90

Winnicott, D. J., 44, 48, 53

About the Editors

M. Hossein Etezady, MD, is a board-certified adult, as well as child/adolescent, psychiatrist, and is certified in psychoanalysis by the American Psychoanalytic Association. He trained in child and adolescent psychoanalysis at the Philadelphia Psychoanalytic Institute (currently called the Psychoanalytic Center of Philadelphia). He is a faculty member at the Psychoanalytic Center of Philadelphia and is head of faculty at the Tehran Psychoanalytic Institute. Currently Dr. Etezady is in the private practice of child and adult psychiatry and psychoanalysis in Malvern, Pennsylvania.

Inga Blom, MD, is senior psychologist at Lenox Hill Hospital/Northwell Health in New York City, where she initiated a comprehensive treatment and intervention program for women in the perinatal period. She is also assistant professor, Department of Psychiatry, Zucker/Hofstra Northwell School of Medicine, Hofstra University, and is in private practice in New York City. Her training includes several years of psychoanalytic training at New York Psychoanalytic Institute (NYPSI), a postdoctoral fellowship in Neuropsychology at Bellevue Hospital Center/NYU Langone Medical Center, a PhD in Clinical Psychology from the New School for Social Research, and a BA (hons) in Psychoanalytic Thought from Trinity College, University of Toronto.

Mary Davis, MD, is a child and adolescent psychiatrist and psychoanalyst in private practice in Lancaster, PA. She has been in practice since 1980, working in inpatient, outpatient, residential, and partial hospital settings and is on the faculty of the China American Psychoanalytic Alliance. Currently she is co-chair of the Vulnerable Child Discussion Group that meets yearly at the American Psychoanalytic Association annual meetings, and is co-editor of the Vulnerable Child Series by Rowman & Littlefield. She has one published book, *Language and Connection in Psychotherapy: Words Matter.*

About the Contributors

Harold P. Blum, MD, is Executive Director Emeritus of the Sigmund Freud Archives and a Distinguished Fellow of the American Psychiatric Association. He is Clinical Professor of Psychiatry, Emeritus and supervising and training analyst at the New York University School of Medicine, and has been the editor-in-chief for the *Journal of the American Psychoanalytic Association.* He is also a past vice president of the Internal Psychoanalytical Association, and has more than 170 psychoanalytic papers and multiple books to his credit.

Alexandra M. Harrison, MD, is training and supervising analyst at the Boston Psychoanalytic Society and Institute, and a clinical professor of psychiatry at Harvard Medical School. She is consulting psychiatrist to the Cambridge-Ellis School, where she directs the application of Reflective Network Therapy. She has authored, with Susan Sherkow, the book *Autistic Spectrum Disorder: Reflections from Psychoanalysis and Neuroscience*, as well as numerous papers published in professional journals and presented at professional conferences around the world.

Gabriel Ruiz, MA, is on the faculty of the Chicago Institute for Psychoanalysis, the Institute for Clinical Social Work, and visiting lecturer at the Saint Louis Psychoanalytic Institute. He maintains a private practice in psychoanalysis and psychotherapy with children, adolescents, and adults in Chicago. His areas of interest include technique, development, culture, and dreams.

Theodore Fallon Jr., MD, has twenty-five years' experience as a child and adult psychiatrist and psychoanalyst, and has prior training as an internist and epidemiologist. He is the director of the Child and Adolescent Psychoanalytic Training Program at the Psychoanalytic Center of Philadelphia, and is clinical associate professor at Drexel University College of Medicine. His publications include *Disordered Thought and Development: Chaos to Organization in the Moment*, as well as multiple articles in professional journals and in edited collections of professional articles.

Ann G. Smolen, PhD, is a supervising and training analyst in child, adolescent, and adult psychoanalysis at the Psychoanalytic Center of Philadelphia. She is in private practice in Ardmore, Pennsylvania. She is the author of *Mothering without a Home: Attachment Representations and Behaviors of Homeless Mothers and Children*, and *Six Children: The Spectrum of Child Psychopathology and Its Treatment*.

Corinne Masur, PhD, is a licensed clinical psychologist, a child and adult psychoanalyst and an adult supervising psychoanalyst at the Psychoanalytic Center of Philadelphia (PCOP). She has been in private practice for over thirty years. She is the co-director of the Parent Child Center in Philadelphia, a founder of the Philadelphia Center for Psychoanalytic Education (PCPE) and the Philadelphia Declaration of Play, an organization which advocates for the right of all children to have access to free, imaginative play. She has written, lectured, and taught on a variety of subjects including early childhood bereavement, mourning, mortality, and the denial of death in psychoanalysts and psychotherapists, child development, the development of trust in childhood, and the effect of divorce on children. She is a member of the faculty at PCOP and has been awarded the J. Alexis Burland Award for Teaching on three occasions.

Richard P. Kluft, MD, PhD, is clinical professor of Psychiatry at Temple University School of Medicine and on the faculty of the Psychoanalytic Center of Philadelphia and the China America Psychoanalytic Alliance. The author of over 250 scientific papers and book chapters, he has written extensively about trauma, the dissociative disorders, boundary violations in psychotherapy, and hypnosis. He is also the author of three novels.

Richard Cruz, MD, has a private practice in psychoanalysis, adult and child/adolescent psychiatry in Wilmington, Delaware and Chadds Ford, Pennsylvania. He is on the faculty of the Department of Psychiatry, Thomas Jefferson University, Philadelphia, and the Philadelphia Psychoanalytic Center.

Susan P. Sherkow, MD, is in private practice in adult, child, and adolescent psychiatry and psychoanalysis in New York City, and is the founding director of the Sherkow Center for Child Development and Autism Spectrum

Disorder, a not-for-profit center for research and treatment of ASD and developmental differences (2012). She is also a supervising analyst at the New York Psychoanalytic Institute (Child and Adolescent Division); a training and supervising analyst and founding member of the Berkshire Psychoanalytic Institute; and Assistant Clinical Professor in Psychiatry at both Albert Einstein College of Medicine and Mount Sinai College of Medicine. In 2011 she received the Samuel Ritvo Prize in child psychoanalysis, and she has multiple publications in professional journals and delivered many presentations at professional conferences.

Kate Lieberman, PhD, is a clinical psychologist obtaining postdoctoral training with Susan Sherkow, MD, and at Columbia University Center for Psychoanalytic Training and Research.

Monisha Nayar-Akhtar, PhD, is a licensed child, adolescent, and adult psychologist/psychoanalyst located in the Greater Philadelphia Area. She is the founder of the Indian Institute of Psychotherapy in India and has been a pioneer in research related to orphaned and vulnerable children in the South Asian region. Dr. Nayar-Akhtar holds several positions in the American Psychoanalytic Association related to multicultural and child issues, and is a member of the International Psychoanalytical Association. She recently received the Ticho Foundation Award, which includes a presentation at the American Psychoanalytic Association annual meeting. She has published extensively, with several books as well as articles appearing in journals such as *Psychoanalytic Inquiry* and the *Journal of the American Psychoanalytic Association.*

Michael S. Garfinkle, PhD, is a licensed clinical psychologist and psychoanalyst in private practice in New York, New York. He is on the psychiatry faculty of the Icahn School of Medicine at Mount Sinai and on the voluntary faculty in the psychology departments of Adelphi University, the New School, and Teachers College at Columbia University. He is an associate member of the Institute for Psychoanalytic Training and Research (IPTAR) and is on the editorial boards of *Frontiers in Psychoanalysis* and *Neuropsychoanalysis*, as well as the *Journal of the American Psychoanalytic Association.*

Sara Lynn Richardson, MA, is a doctoral candidate in clinical psychology at Adelphi University's Derner Institute. She is currently working on completing her clinical training, as well as her dissertation, which explores the theoretical and practical uses of temporality in psychoanalytic theory